Behavioral Treatment for Substance Abuse in People with Serious and Persistent Mental Illness

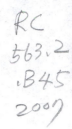

Behavioral Treatment for Substance Abuse in People with Serious and Persistent Mental Illness

A Handbook for Mental Health Professionals

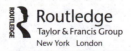

Alan S. Bellack ◆ Melanie E. Bennett ◆ Jean S. Gearon

Routledge
Taylor & Francis Group
New York   London

Routledge is an imprint of the
Taylor & Francis Group, an informa business

Routledge
Taylor & Francis Group
270 Madison Avenue
New York, NY 10016

Routledge
Taylor & Francis Group
2 Park Square
Milton Park, Abingdon
Oxon OX14 4RN

International Standard Book Number-10: 0-415-95283-2 (Softcover)
International Standard Book Number-13: 978-0-415-95283-5 (Softcover)

Library of Congress Cataloging-in-Publication Data

Bellack, Alan S.
    Behavioral treatment for substance abuse in people with serious and persistent mental illness : a handbook for mental health professionals / Alan S. Bellack, Melanie E. Bennett, Jean S. Gearon.
        p. ; cm.
    Includes bibliographical references.
    ISBN 0-415-95283-2 (pb : alk. paper)
    1. Drug abuse--Treatment. 2. Behavior modification. 3. Mental illness--Patients--Medical care. I. Bennett, Melanie E. II. Gearon, Jean S. III. Title.
    [DNLM: 1. Substance-Related Disorders--therapy. 2. Behavior Therapy--methods. 3. Mental Disorders--complications. 4. Schizophrenia--complications. 5. Substance-Related Disorders--complications. WM 270 B4356b 2007]

RC563.2.B45 2007
616.86'06--dc22   2006014121

Visit the Taylor & Francis Web site at
http://www.taylorandfrancis.com

and the Routledge Web site at
http://www.routledgementalhealth.com

ASB: To Sonia McQuarters, who blossomed professionally with this project and who kept the machine running through thick and thin. It would not have been possible without her.

MEB: To Stephen and Sondra Bennett for their help and support.

JSG: To Matthew, Vicky, and my brother Don for all their strength and courage.

CONTENTS

PREFACE

The seeds of this book were planted in Philadelphia in the early 1990s. ASB and colleagues had been conducting clinical trials and psychopathology studies at Medical College of Pennsylvania (MCP) with people who had schizophrenia. As was standard practice at the time, we excluded people from our studies who had comorbid drug abuse. It was assumed that they were behaviorally difficult to engage, and that they had a different, more severe disease course with greater cognitive impairment. MCP was located in central Philadelphia and, during the late 1980s and early 1990s, drug abuse, especially abuse of crack cocaine, was an epidemic in the area. This tragic circumstance increasingly affected people with schizophrenia, and over time more and more patients were being excluded from our studies due to drug abuse. Kim Mueser, PhD, a colleague at MCP, recognized the significance of this problem and was lead author on an early, seminal paper that identified the magnitude and possible causes of this problem (Mueser, Yarnold, & Bellack, 1992), and a subsequent paper that discussed the implications for treatment (Mueser, Bellack, & Blanchard, 1992). In examining the literature it quickly became apparent that there was no empirically sound treatment available for people with dual disorders and we began conceptualizing what an effective treatment might entail. A fortuitous circumstance about the same time was that the National Institute of Drug Abuse (NIDA) issued an innovative program announcement for *treatment development* grants. Most NIH funding mechanisms at the time required extensive pilot data, which required the availability of local resources. In contrast, this mechanism was designed to provide pilot costs for investigators interested in developing new treatments: essentially venture capital. ASB and MB submitted an application and were funded to develop an innovative program that we called Behavioral Treatment for Substance Abuse in Schizophrenia (BTSAS). Shortly after the grant was funded, MEB moved to New Mexico, and ASB moved to Baltimore, where he hired JSG to help run the project. Preliminary data were sufficiently promising that we received funding for a competitive renewal in 1998. To our great good fortune MEB moved to Maryland at about the same time, and she rejoined our team.

This book is the culmination of 10 years of work. It evolved gradually as we learned more about how to conduct the treatment. We dropped some elements that did not work as planned or were not relevant to our subjects. Similarly, we refined many elements and added others. In many respects the consumers who volunteered for our studies were our tutors. However, the changes have primarily been evolutionary rather than revolutionary. The content of the current program is very similar to what we initially proposed, although it is much more clinically sophisticated. In the course of conducting our studies we also expanded the treatment beyond schizophrenia to include other consumers with serious mental illness; hence, the current title: *Behavioral Treatment for Substance Abuse by People with Serious and Persistent Mental Illness: A Handbook for Mental Health Professionals.*

As indicated by the second part of the title (*A Handbook for Mental Health Professionals*), the book is designed to be a practical guide, not a didactic overview of dual disorders and their treatment. It contains *skill sheets* that provide detailed lesson plans, and extensive examples of the specific language to be used by clinicians. It also discusses problems that frequently arise and issues involved in implementing treatments in public mental health clinics. It is our intent that a clinician who has some experience working with dual disordered clients can read the text and actually *do* the treatment, not simply understand how it is done by experts. There is a significant lag in our field between research on evidence-based practices and application of these practices on the front lines. *Behavior Treatment for Substance Abuse* has an evidence base, and we hope this book will provide enough clinical guidance that the evidence can be effectively disseminated.

The text is divided into three sections. Part I contains five chapters that provide a background for the approach and describes some general clinical parameters of the intervention: chapter 1 provides an introduction to the treatment of people with dual disorders; chapter 2 gives an overview of the scientific background; chapter 3 describes training philosophy and general strategies; chapter 4 discusses social skills training, and chapter 5 discusses assessment strategies.

Part II contains six detailed chapters that cover each component of BTSAS: chapter 6 discusses motivational interviewing; chapter 7 looks at urinalysis and goal setting; chapter 8 discusses social skills and drug refusal skills training; chapter 9 considers education and coping skills training; chapter 10 discusses relapse prevention and problem solving; and chapter 11 covers graduation and termination.

Part III includes two chapters that deal with a number of ancillary topics that are important for some clients and some settings; chapter 12 discusses dealing with problem situations, and chapter 13 discusses implementing BTSAS for substance abuse in clinic settings, along with strategies and potential modifications.

There is also an Appendix that contains handouts for participants. The handouts duplicate materials presented by group leaders during group sessions. They are given to participants when new material is introduced so they can follow along during group, as well as take the material home to serve as reminders.

We are indebted to the large group of clinicians who worked on the project over the years, without whom the background research and manual development would have been impossible. We are also indebted to the consumers who graciously volunteered to be research subjects in our studies.

Alan S. Bellack
Annapolis, MD
Melanie E. Bennett
Clarksville, MD
Jean S. Gearon
Washington, DC

Part I

Chapter 1

INTRODUCTION TO TREATING PEOPLE WITH DUAL DISORDERS

Drug and alcohol abuse by people with severe and persistent mental illness (SPMI) is one of the most significant problems facing the public mental health system. Referred to variously as people with dual disorders or dual diagnosis, mentally ill chemical abusers, and individuals with co-occurring psychiatric and substance disorders, these patients pose major problems for themselves, their families, clinicians, and the mental health system. Lifetime prevalence of substance abuse was assessed at 48% for schizophrenia and 56% for bipolar disorder in the Epidemiological Catchment Area study (Regier et al., 1990), and estimates of current abuse for the SPMI population range as high as 65% (Mueser, Bennett, & Kushner, 1995). Rates of abuse are likely to be even higher among impoverished patients living in inner city areas where drug use is widespread. Substance use disorders (SUDs) in people with SPMI begins early in the course of illness, and has a profound impact on almost every area of the person's functioning and clinical care. People with SPMI and SUDs show more severe symptoms of mental illness, more frequent hospitalizations, more frequent relapses, and a poorer course of illness than do those with a single diagnosis. They also have higher rates of violence, suicide, and homelessness. They manifest higher rates of incarceration, greater rates of service utilization and cost of health care, poorer treatment adherence, and treatment outcome. People with schizophrenia are now one of the highest risk groups for HIV, and there are ample data to indicate that substance use substantially increases the likelihood of unsafe sex practices (Carey, Carey, & Kalichman, 1997), the primary source of infection in this population. Women with schizophrenia and comorbid substance use disorders are at substantial risk of being raped and physically abused (Gearon, Kaltman, Brown, & Bellack, 2003). Substance use also impairs information processing, which is particularly problematic for people with schizophrenia, given the range of cognitive deficits characterizing the disorder (Tracy, Josiassen, & Bellack, 1995).

The toxic effects of psychoactive substances in individuals with schizophrenia and bipolar disorder may be present even at levels of use that may not be problematic in the general population. Although people with SPMI may abuse lower quantities of drugs, they are more likely to experience negative effects as a result of even moderate use. There is evidence to suggest that they are more sensitive to lower doses of drugs (supersensitivity model). For example, in challenge studies, patients with schizophrenia have been shown to be highly sensitive to low doses of amphetamine that produce minimal response in controls (Lieberman, Kane, & Alvir, 1987). Other studies have shown that people with SPMI can experience negative clinical effects, such as relapse, following self-administered use of small quantities of alcohol or drugs (Mueser, Drake, & Wallach, 1998).

Why do people with SPMI use street drugs if the consequences are so severe? It is widely assumed that they use substances as a form of self-medication: to reduce symptoms of mental illness and to alleviate side effects of medications, especially the sedating effects of many neuroleptics. However, the data suggest that substance abuse by many people with SPMI is motivated by the same factors that drive excessive use of harmful substances in less impaired populations: negative affective states, interpersonal conflict, and social pressures. Empirical data do not document a consistent relationship between substance use and specific forms of symptomatology. Alcohol is the most commonly abused substance by people with SPMI, as well as in the general population. Preference for street drugs varies over time and as a function of the demographic characteristics of the sample. For example, Mueser, Yarnold, and Bellack (1992) reported that between 1983 and 1986 cannabis was the most commonly abused illicit drug among people with schizophrenia, whereas between 1986 and 1990 cocaine became the most popular drug, a change in pattern similar to that in the general population. For many people with SPMI, availability of substances appears to be more relevant than the specific neurological effects. Poly-drug abuse is also common, with availability determining which drugs are used when.

In addition, the pattern of use appears to be somewhat intermittent or adventitious, rather than a persistent daily activity. For example, in our research, carefully diagnosed subjects meeting DSM-IV criteria for drug dependence reported using drugs on about nine days each month, primarily on weekends and when they received their benefit checks (American Psychiatric Association, 1994). Many dual disordered people also seem to be able to go for periods of time (weeks or months) with little or no drug use, and then resume regular use. Relatively few of these individuals fit the profile of the daily (or almost daily) cocaine or heroin abuser, whose daily activity is focused on how to get money and access drugs. Given this pattern of intermittent drug use, people with dual disorders generally do not report extreme cravings or withdrawal symptoms. Rather, they seem to be very much affected by social and environmental cues, especially including people with whom they often use drugs, and time (e.g., the week before benefit checks arrive). It is also worth noting that many people with SPMI do not have enough money to maintain an expensive drug habit. They often access drugs from friends and family. Some dually disordered women exchange sex for drugs, but it appears as if they are more likely to be taken advantage of than to be active sex workers.

TREATMENT OF SUBSTANCE ABUSE IN PEOPLE WITH SPMI

There is extensive literature on the treatment of dual disordered SPMI patients (Bellack & Gearon, 1998; Drake, Mueser, Brunette, & McHugo, 2004), and there is a broad consensus on a number of elements required for effective treatment, including: There should be integration of both psychiatric and substance abuse treatment (Mueser, Noordsy, Drake, & Fox, 2003). The traditional service models in which substance abuse and psychiatric (mental health) treatment are implemented by distinct clinical teams with different funding streams does not work for these very impaired individuals. They are unable to coordinate services between two distinct clinical systems, and they need a consistent message from all relevant clinicians: drug use is harmful. We will discuss some models of integrated care in chapter 13). Treatment should be conceptualized as an ongoing process in which motivation to reduce substance use waxes and wanes (Bellack & DiClemente, 1999). BTSAS is designed to be a six-month program because the literature suggests that this is a reasonable minimum time frame. However, that duration was partly determined by the exigencies of our NIH grants; a longer duration will often be desirable or necessary. An extended treatment period is required for two reasons. First, it is necessary for the participants to experience both successes and failures in reducing drug use. Failures, in particular, provide an opportunity for the therapists to teach the person how to cope with lapses, and how to prevent lapses (an occasional bad day or weekend) from turning into relapses (i.e., full return to pretreatment rates of use). Second, motivation to reduce drug use waxes and wanes over time. It is important to have the person engaged in group when motivation is waning, so the group can provide a motivational boost, and so the person can learn how to cope with periods of low motivation and strong urges to use drugs. Third, a *harm reduction* model is more appropriate than an abstinence model, especially during the early stages of treatment when the patient has uncertain motivation to change (Carey, Carey, Maisto, & Purnine 2002). The term *harm reduction* refers to an approach that values anything that reduces risk or *harm* associated with drug use. As indicated above, people with dual disorders are at risk for a host of adverse consequences, ranging from psychiatric relapse to sexual abuse to HIV infection. Any day that they avoid drugs decreases the risk of those adverse consequences. Of course, abstinence is the most appropriate long term goal for everyone. But, the evidence suggests that if abstinence (or a commitment to become abstinent immediately) is a precondition to entering treatment most dual disordered persons will not enroll. Further, if the clinician persistently and aggressively promotes abstinence and is critical of efforts to cut down use, the attrition rate is very high. Thus, the program should promote reduced drug use in the short term, and keep abstinence in mind as a long term goal.

While there is widespread agreement that integrated treatment employing a psychoeducational approach that is sensitive to motivational level is the best treatment strategy (i.e., a general structure for delivering treatment), there is a dearth of empirical data on effective techniques for producing change (i.e., specific treatment procedures). This literature has been surveyed in three recent reviews, each of which used somewhat different criteria for identifying and evaluating clinical trials. Drake, Mueser et al. (2004) found 16 studies of outpatient treatment, 4 using quasi-experimental designs and 12 using experimental designs. Nine studies tested brief interventions (1 to several sessions) to increase engagement or motivation to change. Seven studies evaluated integrated treatment (primarily some form of assertive case management), of which only three tested the effects of a specific substance abuse intervention. Jerrell and Ridgely (1995) compared a 12-step program, behavioral skills training, and intensive case management. While each of the latter two interventions was more effective than the 12-step condition on a variety of outcome domains, the effects on substance use were quite modest. Barrowclough et al. (2001) compared a multimodal intervention that included cognitive behavioral therapy and family psychoeducation to routine care in a study conducted in the United Kingdom. They found a modest advantage for the experimental treatment initially and at an 18-month follow-up (Haddock et al., 2003). While Drake, Mueser et al. (2004) were generally positive about the effectiveness of available treatments, they concluded that, "As yet there is little evidence for any specific approach to treatment...."

Dumaine (2003) and Ley, Jeffery, McLaren, and Siegfried (2003), in an analysis done for the *Cochrane Review*, each found only six randomized trials of psychosocial treatments for dually disordered clients. While still advocating the use of integrated, psychoeducational interventions, Dumaine (2003) reported that the largest effect size, which was for intensive case management without a specific psychoeducational component, was only 0.35, and the largest effect size for a specific psychosocial treatment procedure was only 0.25. In the least optimistic view of the literature, Ley et al. (2003) concluded that: There is no clear evidence supporting an advantage of any type of substance misuse program for those with serious mental illness over the value of standard care, and no one program is clearly superior to another. These reviews were each written before the most recent outcome data for BTSAS became available. As indicated below and described more fully in a paper published in the *Archives of General Psychiatry* (Bellack, Bennett, Georon, Brown, & Yang, 2006), BTSAS may be the most promising approach developed to date.

WHY IS IT SO DIFFICULT TO REDUCE DRUG USE BY PEOPLE WITH SPMI?

An extensive body of research on substance abuse and addiction in the general population indicates that critical factors in abstinence and controlled use of addictive substances include high levels of motivation to quit, the ability to exert self-control in the face of temptation (urges), cognitive and behavioral coping skills, and social support or social pressure. Unfortunately, people with SPMI, especially those with schizophrenia, often have limitations in each of these areas. First, several factors can be expected to diminish motivation in people with schizophrenia. They frequently suffer from some degree of generalized avolition (lack of motivation or drive) and anergia (lack of energy or initiative) as a function of neurological dysfunction (hypoactivity of the dorsolateral prefrontal cortex), medication side effects, or other social, psychological, and biological factors that contribute to negative symptoms. Thus, they may lack the internal drive to initiate the complex behavioral routines required for abstinence. This hypothesis was supported in a survey of dually diagnosed persons, which found that depending on the substance abused, as many as 41% had little motivation to reduce their substance use and only 52% were participating in substance abuse treatment. Another negative symptom, anhedonia, may compromise the experience of positive emotions, thereby limiting the ability to experience pleasure and positive reinforcement in the absence of substance use and restricting the appraisal of the advantages of reduced substance use. While people with other diagnoses (e.g., bipolar disorder) have a different neurobiology, they may also suffer from secondary negative symptoms (e.g., negative symptoms driven by medication side effects, cumulative effect from failure experiences and frustration in life).

A second issue is the profound and pervasive cognitive impairment that characterizes schizophrenia and is often present in bipolar disorder. Research since the mid-1990s indicates that persons with schizophrenia have prominent cognitive impairments, including deficits in attention, memory, and higher level cognitive processes, such as abstract reasoning, maintenance of set, the ability to integrate situational context or previous experience into ongoing processing, and other "executive" functions. They have been shown to have profound deficits in problem solving ability on both neuropsychological tests (e.g., the Wisconsin Card Sorting Test), and on more applied measures of social judgment. There are several lines of evidence, which suggest that cognitive impairment is largely (but not completely) independent of symptoms, and that many of these higher level deficits may result from a subtle neurodevelopmental anomaly reflected in frontal-temporal lobe dysfunction. Moreover, cognitive performance deficits are not substantially ameliorated by treatment with typical antipsychotic medications.

These higher-level cognitive deficits would be expected to make it very difficult for people with schizophrenia to engage in the complex processes thought to be necessary for self-directed behavior change. They may have difficulty engaging in self-reflection or in evaluating previous experiences to formulate realistic self-efficacy appraisals. Deficits in the ability to draw connections between past experience and current stimuli may impede the ability to relate their substance use to negative consequences over time, and modify decisional balance accordingly. Deficits in problem solving capacity and abstract reasoning may impede the ability to evaluate the pros and cons of substance use or formulate realistic goals. Problems in memory and attention may also make it difficult for people with SPMI to sustain focus on goal-directed behavior over time.

Third, people with schizophrenia have marked social impairment. They are often unable to fulfill basic social roles, they have difficulty initiating and maintaining conversations, and they frequently are unable to achieve goals or have their needs met in situations requiring social interaction. These deficits are moderately correlated with symptomatology, especially during acute phases of illness, but the disruptive effects of acute symptoms do not account for the panoply of interpersonal deficits exhibited by most of these patients. The precursors of adult social disability can often be discerned in childhood, and may be associated with early problems in attention. This pattern of social impairment would leave people with schizophrenia who abuse drugs vulnerable in a number of ways: they would have difficulty developing social relationships with individuals who do not use drugs; would have difficulty resisting social pressure to use; and they would have difficulty developing the social support system needed to reduce use.

BEHAVIORAL TREATMENT FOR SUBSTANCE ABUSE BY PEOPLE WITH SPMI (BTSAS)

BTSAS is an innovative behavioral treatment to address illicit drug use among people with SPMI. We have developed BTSAS over a 10-year period with the support of a series of grants from the National Institute of Drug Abuse (NIDA). BTSAS was specifically designed to address the special needs of dual disordered persons, especially those with schizophrenia. It will be apparent to experienced clinicians that many of the elements of BTSAS are similar to techniques widely used in interventions with less impaired populations of substance abusers. However, we have systematically modified the techniques to accommodate to people with SPMI. Notably, a variety of strategies and tactics are employed to address cognitive impairment, and the typical pattern of low and variable motivation.

BTSAS contains six integrated components:(1) motivational interviewing to enhance motivation to reduce use; (2) structured goal setting to identify realistic, short-term goals for decreased substance use; (3) a urinalysis contingency designed to enhance motivation to change and increase the salience of goals; (4) social skills and drug refusal skills training to teach participants how to refuse social pressure to use substances, and to provide success experiences that can increase self-efficacy for change; (5) education about the reasons for substance use and the particular dangers of substance use for people with SPMI, in order to shift the decisional balance towards decreased use; and (6) relapse prevention training that focuses on behavioral skills for coping with urges and dealing with high risk situations and lapses. Each of these components will be described in more detail in later chapters of this book.

Several steps are taken in consideration of cognitive deficits. Sessions are highly structured, and there is a strong emphasis on behavioral rehearsal. The material taught is broken down into small units. Complex social repertoires required for making friends and refusing substances are divided into component elements such as maintaining eye contact and how to say, "No." Patients are first taught to perform the elements, and then gradually learn to smoothly combine them. The intervention emphasizes *overlearning* of a few specific and relatively narrow skills that can be used automatically, thereby minimizing the cognitive load for decision making during stressful interactions. Extensive use is made of learning aides, including handouts and flip charts, to reduce the requirements on memory and attention. Participants are prompted as many times as necessary and there is also extensive repetition within and across sessions. Participants repeatedly rehearse both behavioral skills (e.g., refusing unreasonable requests) and didactic information (e.g., the role of dopamine in schizophrenia and substance use), and receive social reinforcement for effort. Rather than teaching generic problem solving skills and coping strategies that can be adapted to a host of diverse situations, we focus on specific skills effective for handling a few key, high risk situations (e.g., what do you do when you are offered coke by your brother or by one specific friend, rather than what to do when *anyone* offers it to you). While this might be viewed as placing a limit on generalization, data clearly show that people with schizophrenia have great difficulty in abstraction and applying principles in novel situations. Hence, they are more likely to benefit from a narrow repertoire of skills to minimize demands on these higher-level processes.

Training is done in a small-group format (4 to 6 is preferred). The group format allows participants to benefit from modeling and role-playing with peers. The small size provides ample opportunity for all group members to get adequate practice, while minimizing demands for sustained attention (i.e., they can rest while peers are role-playing, etc.). This group size also allows therapists to control even highly symptomatic participants. The treatment can be adapted for either a closed membership or open-enrollment format. The open membership format is convenient in settings where enrollment is slow, so consumers do not have to wait long to begin treatment. Groups for people with SPMI generally do not develop the cohesiveness that is seen in groups for less impaired persons, so that new admissions are not disruptive to current members. Moreover, the modular nature of the teaching units and the highly tailored nature of the training make it easy to filter in new members. Units (e.g., conversational skills training) can be repeated in whole or in part as needed. Presenting previously covered units for new members has the added benefit of giving existing members additional practice, which is always advantageous in working with persons with schizophrenia.

Abstinence is generally viewed as the most appropriate goal for less impaired substance abusers, and it has been suggested that it is the most appropriate goal for people with SPMI as well. Nevertheless, abstinence is not a viable goal for all people who enter treatment. Many will "vote with their feet" and drop out if pressured to abstain. There also is increasing evidence with less impaired populations that outcomes are better when people select their own goals than goals being imposed by programs. Consequently, we employ a harm avoidance model and promote abstinence, but do not demand it as a precondition for participation. Moreover, our experience is that some people with SPMI profit from substance abuse training without ever formally admitting that they have a problem and want to reduce usage. As long as they actively participate in the education and training, they can acquire skills and information that may be of use at some time in the future. In addition, we also assume that they may become more amenable to making changes if they have first acquired some skills and developed an increased sense of efficacy for resisting social pressure and saying no to drugs. Hence, we increase social pressure on reducing drug use very gradually so as to avoid conflict or early termination. We begin goal setting for reduced substance use (via motivational interviewing) and the urinalysis contingency in the second week of treatment, but we are less proactive in setting goals for change in the early sessions than we are once subjects have acquired some substantive training in social skills and coping skills.

In contrast to traditional substance abuse programs, the atmosphere in BTSAS groups is supportive and positively reinforcing. Therapists actively search for ways to provide social reinforcement and encouragement. Even when members have used drugs or express waning motivation, the therapists support effort and encourage participation. Notably, they are *never* critical or punishing. Members are never admonished to do better or work harder, and they are never made to feel guilty or unwanted. Rather, therapists acknowledge how difficult it is to reduce drug use and work to support participants during difficult times. Group members are encouraged to provide social reinforcement and encourage one another as well. It is common for members to applaud for one another when they provide clean urine samples or work hard in a difficult role play rehearsal.

While the treatment is very supportive, it is also highly structured. As will be apparent in subsequent chapters, BTSAS has a very detailed curriculum. Each session has a structure, in which treatment procedures are carried out in a standardized order and in a prescribed manner. Many of the session worksheets presented in later chapters contain specific language for how material is to be presented. There is relatively little chitchat in sessions. The bulk of the time is devoted to urinalysis procedures, goal setting, role-play rehearsal, and didactic teaching. BTSAS is *not* a verbal psychotherapy. Participants will often raise questions and problems that warrant therapeutic discussion, but they are generally referred to other clinical staff for help with these issues. This style takes some getting used to for many experienced clinicians whose proclivity is to do conversational therapies; conversely, it works quite well for new therapists because it provides the structure they generally need in order to be effective.

EMPIRICAL SUPPORT FOR BTSAS

BTSAS was developed in a systematic, empirical manner. There was no established treatment for substance abuse in schizophrenia or other people with SPMI when our program was initiated in the mid-1990s. A number of promising strategies were employed in programs for less impaired populations, but most procedures could not be applied in their standard format given the cognitive and motivational impairments that characterize people with schizophrenia and other SPMIs. For example, a common strategy to enhance motivation for less impaired persons who abuse substances is to enlist the aid of supportive family members, friends, and employers. However, many people with SPMI do not have contact with family members or friends who are not also drug users, and they generally are unemployed. Less impaired persons often can identify meaningful life goals associated with reduced drug use, such as better employment opportunities, and reconciliation with spouses. In contrast, many people with SPMI are not married and do not have good employment options, even when clean and sober. Consequently, our first step was to identify strategies that were applicable for people with SPMI, and that could be adapted to their special needs and difficulties. We focused exclusively on strategies that had good empirical support. Our plan was to develop a new intervention de novo by sequentially administering preliminary treatment modules to small groups of SPMI volunteers, and adding and refining elements as needed, based on our observations. One of our primary goals was to develop a treatment manual that could be used in research to evaluate BTSAS and, if the results were positive, could be disseminated to the clinical community. The evolution of the treatment and development of the manual was very much a bootstrapping process in which we drafted manual sections, recruited and treated a cohort of subjects with it, revised as needed, and applied the new iteration to a subsequent cohort. When we were satisfied that the module was working effectively and could be administered in a consistent manner, the next draft module was added. By the conclusion of the initial five-year NIDA grant we had completed a draft manual and had collected sufficient pilot data to justify funding of a subsequent trial. We had also demonstrated that therapists could be trained and could deliver the intervention appropriately, that the intervention is safe, and that people with SPMI would attend.

The pilot development work was followed by a controlled trial that compared BTSAS with a contrasting group treatment that represented good clinical practice in the community (Bellack et al., 2006). Subjects were 110 patients at community clinics and a VA outpatient clinic in downtown Baltimore, MD. All subjects met DSM-IV criteria (American Psychiatric Association, 1994) for current dependence on cocaine, opiates, or cannabis, along with objective criteria for severe mental illness, including: (1) a diagnosis of schizophrenia or schizoaffective disorder or other severe mental disorder including bipolar disorder, major depression, or severe anxiety disorder; (2) has worked 25% or less of the past year; or (3) receives payment for mental disability (SSI, SSDI, VA disability benefits). The sample was representative of community samples of SPMI patients in the United States. Participants were 59.5% male, 88% ethnic minority (primarily African American), and 42.9% never married. Mean age was 42.2 years (sd = 7.17), with 11.6 years of education (sd = 2.24). Diagnostically, 48.4% had a current psychotic disorder, 54% had a current mood disorder, 35.7% had a current alcohol use disorder, and the large majority (80.2%) met criteria for a past alcohol use disorder. The mean number of past psychiatric hospitalizations for the sample was 5.62 (sd = 7.43) and the mean age of onset of psychiatric disorder was 26.2 years (sd = 10.8). The sample reported a mean of 5.43 years of heroin use (sd = 8.23), 10.22 years of cocaine use (sd = 8.53), 10.01 years of marijuana use (sd = 10.23), and 11.7 years of polydrug use (sd = 10.6).

After providing informed consent and participating in baseline assessments, subjects were randomly assigned to BTSAS or the contrast condition, Supportive Treatment for Addiction Recovery (STAR). STAR is a manualized intervention based on a sophisticated treatment model developed by Osher, Drake, Noordsy, and their colleagues at Dartmouth. Like BTSAS, STAR was administered in small groups twice per week for six months. STAR groups are interactive, supportive, flexible, and unstructured, and are intended to help participants understand how substance use complicates their lives. The therapist stance is nondirective, and there is an emphasis on having members share with one another, rather than having the therapists dictate the content of group sessions. The primary goals of the therapists are to engage participants in treatment and to generate discussion among them. The groups are designed to be supportive and encouraging, and to provide a safe and nonjudgmental place for members to talk about substance use and their ideas and feelings about it. Some didactic education is provided about the effects of drugs and factors involved in reducing drug use when it fits into the discussion, but there is no formal curriculum or session by session plan regarding these issues. The group sets its own pace and determines its own topic, and the therapists encourage, but do not require, participant interaction.

Therapists for both BTSAS and STAR were trained to administer the respective treatments before they were certified to conduct protocol groups. Most therapists were relatively inexperienced clinicians with a master's degree in psychology, counseling, social work, and related disciplines; none were drug counselors. Therapists were closely supervised throughout the project. All sessions were videotaped for supervision sessions and for subsequent (blinded) ratings of therapist performance. All therapists in both treatment conditions were shown to be very effective in administering the respective treatments appropriately.

Overall, the data provide strong support for the efficacy of BTSAS. Urine samples were collected from all subjects at every session beginning in session 3, providing an objective measure of drug use throughout the six months of the trial. Subjects in BTSAS had a significantly higher proportion of clean urines over the six months of treatment than subjects in STAR: M = 0.70 vs. 0.51 (p = 0.0434). Urine tests provided an indication of cocaine and heroin use over the preceding two to three days, and cannabis use over the previous 28 days. The twice per week urine samples thus provide a rough estimate of periods of continuous abstinence. These data also show a pronounced advantage for BTSAS. Subjects in BTSAS had significantly more four-week blocks of continuous abstinence (M = 44.12% vs. M = 8.82%, p = 0.001), and more multiple four-week blocks of abstinence (M = 29.41% vs. M = 2.94%, p = 0.003). There was also a trend for BTSAS subjects to have more eight-week blocks of continuous abstinence. BTSAS subjects also attended significantly more sessions (M = 27.2 [out of 50] vs. 17.5, p = 0.0042). That is noteworthy in this difficult-to-treat population, as patients who attend drug treatment generally do better than those who do not (Timko & Moos, 2002). In addition, 57.4% of subjects enrolled in BTSAS completed the six months of treatment vs. 34.7% for STAR, a highly significant difference. The relative risk of dropout (hazard ratio, HR) for BTSAS was about half that for STAR (HR [95% CI] = 0.51[0.30, 0.85]).

We assessed subjects on a variety of clinical measures. At Baseline and Posttreatment, inpatient admissions (psychiatric reasons or substance abuse) declined from 27.3% in the 90 days prior to Baseline to 8.0% in the 90 days prior to the Posttreatment assessment for subjects in BTSAS (X^2 = 4.36, p = 0.0368), compared to 26.5 and 20.7%, respectively for STAR (ns). Prior to treatment, 48.5% of BTSAS subjects reported having enough money for food, clothing, housing, and transportation compared with 69.2% at the end of treatment (X^2 = 6.61, p = 0.0102). This could reflect reduced expenditures on drugs. There was no change for subjects in STAR (48.5% prior to treatment and 50.0% afterwards). Subjects in BTSAS also reported a small, but significant increase in General Life Satisfaction from pre- to posttreatment (M = 4.12 [1.87] to M = 4.69 [1.85], t_{66} = 1.95, p = 0.0549), and there was a trend toward increased ability to independently perform activities of daily living on the SFS: M = 27.8 (6.65) to 30.2 (5.69), t_{66} = 1.76, p = 0.0838). Again, neither of these variables was significant for STAR. These data suggest that the treatment effects were clinically meaningful as well as being statistically significant.

BTSAS is not a panacea for people with dual disorders. Some 30 to 40% will not participate in treatment, and others will participate for a while and then drop out. Even among those who stick it out, only a small percentage become abstinent during the six months of the intervention. However, our data indicate that our ability to engage and retain participants is at least as good as in the best trials of drug treatment for less impaired people, and our rates of reduced drug use are comparable. Despite common wisdom to the contrary, our experience is that people with SPMI and drug abuse can be effectively engaged in treatment and can be helped to substantially reduce their drug use over time. Without trying to sound like Pollyannas, we can attest that a large percentage of people who have participated in BTSAS actually like it! They receive considerable positive reinforcement for attending and doing well, which takes the form of social approval from peers and therapists, as well as small financial incentives. Participants applaud for one another when they provide clean urine samples and report success experiences between sessions, and they get extensive praise and encouragement for their work during sessions. Conversely, as will be discussed further below, a cardinal rule of BTSAS is that problems and failures are *never* followed by criticism or censure. Thus, BTSAS provides a safe and supportive environment in which participants can work hard to deal with a very, very difficult problem. It may be the only such environment most participants have ever experienced. Based on watching hundreds of hours of videotaped sessions, as well as examining the data, we believe that the positive environment, with its emphasis on harm reduction and success, is among the critical elements of BTSAS.

ORIENTATION TO THE REMAINDER OF THIS VOLUME

The material presented above is intended to provide an overview of the issues surrounding drug use by people with SPMI, and introduce the reader to BTSAS. There is an extensive literature on drug use and its treatment in this population, and the interested reader is referred to papers and chapters contained in the reference list as a good starting point for more detailed information. The remainder of this book will focus on the clinical application of BTSAS. We will provide much greater detail about each element of the treatment and how they should be administered. We make ample use of visual support materials in sessions, and provide participants with many handouts to reduce the need for them to memorize material. Samples of these materials are reproduced throughout the chapters. BTSAS has been successfully administered by a large number of therapists during the 10 years of our development work and clinical trial. Most therapists have been relatively young, with recent master's degrees in psychology, counseling, and social work. They are representative of clinicians in the public mental health system in the United States, who are typically thrown into the clinical fray after graduation with little direct supervision or continued training. This book is designed with them in mind. In contrast to most books in the field, it provides little in the way of theory or conceptualization. Rather, it provides a step-by-step guide for what to do and how to do it. Some clinical experience with dual disordered clients is desirable, but we have often found that many experienced clinicians have developed bad habits along the way (e.g., they find it easier to be critical than to be positively reinforcing), and need to unlearn things, as well as learn how to do BTSAS. We have attempted to provide a manual that can be picked up de novo and used effectively by someone who has good clinical instincts and some technical knowledge about mental illness and substance abuse. We cannot guarantee that it has to be done exactly the way we recommend in order to be effective, but we can guarantee that most clinicians will not have good results if they simply borrow scattered ideas and techniques. Remember, in our controlled trial, STAR was a thoughtful, highly regarded *treatment as usual* administered by trained and motivated clinicians, yet it did not fare very well in comparison to BTSAS.

Chapter **2**

SCIENTIFIC BACKGROUND

INTRODUCTION

When we began to develop BTSAS, several things were clear. First, there is a great need to treat substance use disorders among people with SPMI. As we have reviewed in chapter 1, people with SPMI show alarmingly high rates of substance use disorders and a range of severe and persistent negative consequences of use (for reviews see Bennett & Barnett, 2003; Dixon, 1999). Moreover, the toxic effects of psychoactive substances in individuals with schizophrenia and bipolar disorder may be present even at use levels that may not be problematic in the general population (Bergman & Harris, 1985; Lehman, Myers, Dixon, & Johnson, 1994; Mueser et al., 1990). Clearly, substance abuse by people with SPMI is one of the most significant problems facing the public mental health system.

Second, there is general agreement that treatment needs to address both psychiatric and substance use disorders, and that these interventions are likely to be most effective if they are delivered in an integrated fashion. "Integrated treatment" refers to treatment that occurs within the same overall system, in which there are trained and knowledgeable staff members with experience of both types of disorders, and medication is perceived as an option for patients who require it (Drake et al., 1998). This means having substance abuse treatment services housed within mental illness treatment systems as well as mental health services available in substance abuse treatment facilities, along with staff within each system who are trained to recognize, diagnose, refer, and treat dual disorders. Evidence suggests that such an approach can make a difference in terms of treatment outcome. Moggi and colleagues (1999) examined the impact that the strength of dual diagnosis treatment orientation had on substance abuse treatment outcome among male inpatients with dual disorders. Patients in programs with a strong emphasis on dual diagnosis treatment had substantially better outcomes than those in programs lacking such emphasis, including fewer psychiatric symptoms, higher rates of employment, and longer time in the community after one year.

Third, despite the widespread belief that integrated treatment is the best treatment *strategy* (i.e., a general structure for delivering treatment), there is a lack of empirical data on effective *techniques* (i.e., specific treatment procedures) for producing change. This literature has been surveyed in three reviews, each of which used somewhat different criteria for identifying and evaluating trials. Drake et al. (1998) reviewed 36 reports on integrated substance abuse and mental health treatment, of which only two employed experimental designs and two others employed *quasi-experimental* designs. While the authors were optimistic about the potential benefits that could be achieved by integrated treatments, they were unable to specify which specific strategies were most effective in reducing drug use among SPMI clients. Dumaine (2003) and Ley, Jeffrey, McLaren, and Siegfried (2003) conducted wider searches of the literature on psychosocial treatment for dual disordered patients, and each found six randomized trials. While still advocating the use of integrated treatment, Dumaine (2003) reported that even the strategy that showed the largest effect size (general intensive case management without a specific psychoeducational component) appeared to be only minimally effective (effect size of 0.35). Ley et al. (2003) concluded that there was no clear evidence supporting any one or set of strategies in treating substance use disorders in dually diagnosed SPMI clients.

With this as background, we decided to develop BTSAS as a specific program (set of strategies) that would decrease substance use in SPMI clients as part of an integrated system of mental health and substance abuse care. To select a set of strategies that would have the greatest likelihood of being effective, we decided to turn to the substance abuse treatment literature more generally (i.e., in primary substance abusers) that finds several effective interventions for substance use disorders in primary substance abusing populations. Our goal in developing BTSAS was to take strategies that have been found to be effective in primary substance abusers, tailor them to meet the needs of the SPMI population, and integrate them with strategies that have been found to be helpful in managing patients with SPMI more generally. In this chapter, we review the different literatures that guided our development of BTSAS, as well as the strategies that have been incorporated into the BTSAS program. We present a brief review of the literature that supports the efficacy of each in treating substance abuse. In later chapters we will present more detail regarding how these strategies have been tailored to meet the unique needs of SPMI clients.

THE BTSAS PHILOSOPHY

There are several core characteristics of the BTSAS program: (1) The treatment environment must be positive, supportive, and reinforcing. (2) Attention must continually be paid to helping clients overcome obstacles to treatment participation. (3) The program must emphasize enhancing motivation to change and teaching and practicing skills for drug-free living. (4) Treatment must be broad based and integrated with mental health services. The strategies that are a part of the BTSAS program each play into one or more of these core features.

Creating a Positive, Supportive, and Reinforcing Treatment Environment For BTSAS

At the outset, the BTSAS program was designed to be positive (not negative), supportive (not harsh), and reinforcing (not punishing) in how it guided therapists to interact with clients. There is evidence that this is the sort of setting that tends to help clients make changes in their substance use. For example, Bien, Miller, and Tonigan (1993) reviewed the literature on brief interventions for alcohol problems in primary alcohol clients. First they reviewed studies of brief interventions for drinking in a range of treatment contexts (general health care settings, self-referred drinkers, specialist treatment settings), followed by an analysis of the methodological issues that were found among these studies. Overall, the authors found that brief interventions are more effective than no treatment, are often more effective than more extended treatments, and can be useful to improve the effectiveness of any further treatment for alcohol problems. Following this review, these authors identified some of the common elements found in effective brief interventions. In this way, the authors examined the underlying elements that make effective brief interventions just that, effective. In other words, effective brief interventions have certain characteristics. Bien and colleagues summarized these characteristics with the acronym FRAMES (Feedback, Responsibility, Advice, Menu, Empathy, Self-Efficacy). We wanted to incorporate these characteristics into BTSAS.

First, effective interventions were marked by therapist–client collaboration. Rather than telling clients what was best or what to do, these interventions all involved assisting clients in figuring out what they felt they could do and what they wanted to do in terms of their substance use (**R**esponsibility), and then allowed the client to pursue options from there. Therapists were direct and honest, providing explicit feedback (**F**eedback) to clients on the exact nature and extent of their drinking problems and offered clear advice (**A**dvice) to change. However, therapists and clients in these interventions worked together to develop goals, explore, and select treatment options (**M**enu), and pursue change. Importantly, effective brief interventions stressed that change was possible, and overall were optimistic and strived to instill in clients the belief that they could change (**S**elf-efficacy). The underlying message conveyed by such strategies is that change is possible, is ultimately in the hands of the client, and that the role of the therapist includes helping the client figure out the ways in which substance abuse is affecting his or her life, and collaborating with patients to identify appropriate goals and interventions.

Incorporating this sort of underlying philosophy required some tailoring to the unique needs of a dual-diagnosis population. The strategies that comprise BTSAS involve clear and direct feedback and advice for change. Importantly, feedback and advice are not conveyed via confrontation or communicated with a tone of disappointment. Rather, feedback is provided in a matter-of-fact way, one that gives information without judgment. For example, as described in more detail in Chapter 10, feedback is given in each session on urinalysis contingency results. Clients with positive urine tests are provided with this information, reinforced for attending in spite of a dirty urine sample, and directed toward problem solving with the goal of developing a plan so that the client can cope more effectively in a high risk situation in the upcoming week. BTSAS also incorporates the idea of a menu of treatment options and therapist–client collaboration. When describing the BTSAS program to new clients, therapists tell them that they will learn many skills and need to decide for themselves which skills and strategies will be the most useful for them. Clients are encouraged to attend sessions that might not, at first, seem relevant to them, in order to learn something new to try out and to discover if this new skill can be of use to them. Importantly, clients are not told to "do what we say" and their substance use problems will be gone. Rather, clients are urged to comment on the skills, to try them out and change them around if need be in order to see what will work best for them in different high risk situations.

Second, Bien and colleagues found that effective brief interventions were marked by high levels of therapist empathy: showing support and being understanding, patient, and importantly, nonjudgmental (**E**mpathy). Primary substance abusing clients have been found to show better outcomes when treated by empathic therapists (see Miller, Benefield, & Tonigan, 1993 for a review). That empathy is an important component of effective treatment for substance abuse may seem obvious, but substance abuse treatment is not typically characterized by the kinds of support and encouragement that is more often shown to treatment of other patient populations. It is not unusual in substance abuse treatment as it is practiced in this country to see a harsh or confrontational tone to therapist–client interactions and to programming more broadly. This is most aptly illustrated by the fact that in many substance abuse treatment programs, clients who use drugs—even once—are often immediately terminated from the program. Given that clients come to such programs for treatment of their drug use, and the fact that achieving complete abstinence can take some amount of time, having a requirement of stable abstinence for continued enrollment in treatment would seem to set clients up to fail. These harsh attitudes toward substance abusers, and the idea that these clients are weak or flawed and need only show strength, smarts, or willpower in order to stop their drug use, are longstanding biases that impact treatment to this day (see Miller & Hester, 1995 for a review).

In developing BTSAS, we wanted to make sure that such biases were not a part of the work we did with SPMI clients. These clients experience biases and stressors of their own, live lives that are difficult and oftentimes filled with hardship, and are likely to decompensate psychiatrically when under stress. It was important to us to develop BTSAS as unequivocally positive, reinforcing, and nonjudgmental, so that clients would feel comfortable, calm, and safe during their time in the BTSAS program. Therapists continually reinforce clients for any positive behaviors, including attendance at BTSAS sessions, other clinic appointments, reduced use, self-reported use of the skills learned in session, and clean urines.

Helping Clients Overcome Obstacles to Treatment Participation

SPMI clients generally have a long list of problems that stand in the way of them ever connecting with and engaging in substance abuse treatment, let alone completing treatment and benefiting from it. We wanted the BTSAS program to set clients up to succeed by building into the program a focus on enhancing motivation to change as well as practical strategies to overcome common obstacles to treatment participation. We had two important influences in this regard. The first was the Transtheorectical Model of Change (TTM), also referred to as the Stages of Change model, developed by Prochaska and Diclemente (1982). The idea guiding the model is that people come to treatment at different stages of motivation or readiness for change, and many clients are opposed to or ambivalent about change. In the precontemplation stage, clients are not considering change. In this stage, clients view the positive aspects of substance use as more important or salient than the negative consequences they incur. Precontemplators may be coerced into substance abuse treatment, or they may come for help with another issue that they believe is their central problem and they see as unrelated to their substance use. In the contemplation stage, clients are more aware of the costs of substance use and the benefits of change, but are not fully convinced that change is the best path for them. Here the client starts to understand the benefits of change, but he or she remains ambivalent about actually changing due to strongly held beliefs about the positive aspects of drug use. In the action stage, the client makes attempts to reduce or stop substance use. In the action stage, the client attempts to cut down or quit using, and in the maintenance stage the client is trying to stick with changes he or she has made. Finally, many clients will relapse, return to an earlier stage, and begin the process again.

The TTM illustrates that clients need different kinds of help depending on their readiness to change. While the assumption is that a client is ready for change when he shows up for treatment, a relatively large proportion of clients are undecided, don't think change is necessary, or have attempted change and failed. This is particularly true of clients with SPMI, who, as we reviewed in chapter 1, are generally not considering changing their substance use and face a number of practical and symptomatic barriers to change. That is, given the difficulties of working with a dually diagnosed SPMI population, it is critical to figure out how to help clients in any of these stages of change when they present for treatment. An SPMI client who is in the precontemplation stage of change may need a therapist to help her talk about her substance use in a nonjudgmental atmosphere, which might then allow for a more candid and realistic discussion of the negative consequences of her use. For the SPMI client who is in the contemplation stage, a therapist needs to help that client think more seriously about change, recognize how life would be better without drug use, and reinforce any small steps the client makes toward change. SPMI clients who are ready to make a change need help in developing skills and strategies to achieve their goals. This is a situation in which SPMI clients likely differ in important ways from less impaired populations. Many primary substance abusers are able to figure out ways to change their drug use once they have made a commitment to change: "The underlying view is that change is ultimately in the hands of the client, who has unique skills and resources to draw upon once a commitment to change is made" (Miller et al., 1998, p. 209). By contrast, SPMI clients often have few if any ideas as to how to practically achieve substance use reductions, they have few role models or sources of support, and they typically have cognitive deficits that make delaying gratification and thinking about the future consequences of some present-day action extremely difficult.

Our goal with BTSAS is to teach SPMI clients what to do and have them practice doing it so that when they are ready to change their use they have the skills and strategies to do so. Overall, the emphasis of the TTM on there being something that can be done for clients at any stage of change, and that a therapist must adjust how he or she works to the differing needs and motivational levels of clients, is a useful framework for substance abuse treatment for SPMI clients, and the one on which BTSAS is based.

In addition to using the TTM as a foundation for thinking about how to approach substance abuse treatment for dually diagnosed SPMI clients, we wanted to figure out how to assist clients in very practical ways so that substance abuse treatment was seen as "do-able." That is, what could we do to help clients be able to attend BTSAS sessions? This sort of active approach characterizes many types of interventions for SPMI clients in the mental health field, including case management, assertive community treatment, and other active outreach programs that help clients in practical ways to function in the community. We believe that the same sort of active, persistent quality was needed in order to get SPMI clients to engage in, participate in, and benefit from substance abuse treatment. Not surprisingly, this was being applied to primary substance abusers. For example, Miller (1995) reviewed ways to increase motivation for change in substance abuse treatment clients, including removing barriers to treatment, utilizing external contingencies where appropriate, and using what Miller termed "practical persistence" with clients. First, Miller stressed that seemingly simple problems can derail clients on the way to treatment, and removing practical barriers makes treatment more accessible. Applied to clients with SPMI, these practical barriers include but are not limited to paying for transportation to the clinic; scheduling conflicts (with other treatment appointments or work schedules); discomfort in group treatment sessions; poorly managed symptoms that leave clients too ill to negotiate meeting their basic needs; poorly organized lives that lead to forgotten appointments; general stress and chaos that make substance abuse treatment low on the list of a client's acute needs. Removing these sorts of practical barriers at the start of substance abuse treatment involves learning about a particular client and being creative in terms of problem solving potential solutions. For example, clients who do not have regular transportation need to be helped at the start of treatment to obtain a bus pass or other regular ride so that they know how they are getting to the clinic for treatment sessions. Schedules need to be coordinated from the beginning of treatment, with the substance abuse therapist interacting with mental health service providers to make sure that sessions do not conflict and that the client understands when and where he has to be each day. Other practical solutions include encouraging a client who oversleeps to get and use an alarm clock or have someone provide him with a wake-up call, enlisting the help of family members or other concerned people in a client's life in getting clients to and from appointments, and helping the client manage money so that he or she can pay for transportation to and from sessions if needed. Confronting and removing practical barriers to treatment attendance was an essential component of BTSAS.

Second, Miller defined use of external contingencies as using "leverage or pressure from the outside…to persuade or coerce a client to change or seek help" (Miller, 1995, p. 97). With primary substance abusers, the "outside" can include spouses, jobs, or legal authorities. Applied to a client with SPMI, this could take the form of working to coordinate all mental health and SA treatment so that all providers could reinforce treatment attendance and help one another find clients who were not attending their appointments. That is, the SPMI client needs to understand that all involved in his care (both substance abuse and mental health) are interested in his substance abuse treatment, and are working together to help this along. In addition, for those clients with legal problems, substance abuse treatment should utilize any possible legal consequences of nonattendance as a strong reason for keeping up with treatment appointments. Importantly, it is critical for this to be done within a reinforcing and positive framework, rather than have it take on a punitive tone. For example, a substance abuse treatment provider can remind an SPMI client on probation that attendance at SA treatment will help the client stick to the conditions of his probation, and any reductions in use would also help the client be seen as hard working and making progress by his probation officer. In this example, probation was not used as a potential punishment (if you don't come to substance abuse treatment groups, I'll tell your probation officer and you will go to jail). Rather the situation is being framed as one that could help the client with his probation, as well as signal to the client that the two systems (substance abuse treatment and legal troubles) are connected and impacted by one another. Another useful area of outside influence for SPMI clients can be housing, because many clients are in housing situations that require drug abstinence. This is another situation in which any collaboration needs to be implemented in a positive and supportive way that communicates that the two domains are working together to help the client. For example, a substance abuse treatment provider can link with a housing program that requires abstinence in order to create a program in which the client is rewarded for nonuse (perhaps with additional privileges within the housing program). The two systems work together in the event of a slip or relapse (i.e., the client can maintain housing if he or she is actively working in substance abuse treatment to limit the slip and to prevent a full-blown relapse). Often these concepts (slips vs. relapse, maintaining housing through a slip as a way to help a client get back on track) will be new to housing programs and so should be addressed at the start of substance abuse treatment.

Third, Miller stressed the benefits of what he termed "practical persistence"—therapists being active and assisting clients in concrete ways. Miller cited studies that found that contact (such as a note or call) after a missed visit can greatly increase the likelihood that a client will return to treatment, and that when making a referral, the probability that a client will actually get there is dramatically increased by placing the call and making the appointment from the office, rather than just giving the client the phone number to call him- or herself (see Miller, 1995 for a review). This sort of active assistance to help clients receive services or achieve goals is a standard part of many types of mental health care for SPMI clients, such as case management or assertive community treatment (ACT). Incorporating this sort of active assistance into substance abuse treatment for dually diagnosed SPMI clients is critical in that these are clients who often lack the skills to remember appointments, follow through on referrals or other treatment recommendations, or reengage with treatment after a period of absence. BTSAS therapists make frequent calls to clients to reinforce attendance, to check in with clients who have missed sessions, and to remind clients of important upcoming appointments (whether related to substance abuse treatment, medical treatment, or mental health treatment).

Emphasis On Enhancing Motivation and Teaching Skills for Drug-Free Living

BTSAS has as its focus to help clients learn ways to reduce or stop drug use and maintain a drug-free or drug-limited lifestyle in the future. To do this, we developed BTSAS with a behavioral approach that emphasized enhancing motivation to change and teaching and practicing skills for drug-free living. The primary substance abuse treatment literature provides support for this approach. Miller and colleagues, both in 1995 (Miller, Brown et al., 1995) and again in 1998 (Miller, Andrews, Wilbourne, & Bennett, 1998), did large-scale reviews of the alcohol treatment outcome literature. In the 1995 chapter, the authors reviewed 219 studies of alcohol use disorder treatment, and the 1998 chapter added an additional 85 studies. Studies had to meet several criteria: Studies examined at least one treatment for alcohol problems; there was some comparison between the study intervention and a control or alternative intervention; some procedure was used to equate treatment groups; and there were some measures of drinking outcome (quantity, frequency, level of drinking-related problems). Importantly, the authors made ratings of these studies that took into account the size of the treatment effect for the different interventions that were included in a study; the methodology (more rigorous studies were rated higher than less rigorous ones); and the features of treatment (inpatient or outpatient setting, group or individual format, harm reduction or abstinence focus). Based on these ratings, the treatment strategies that were used in these studies were assigned a score (cumulative evidence score) that took into account the number of studies in which the strategies were found to have some effect on drinking outcomes and the methodological quality of those studies. The findings of these reviews offer a complete look at the alcohol treatment literature and a rigorous rating system for different treatment strategies.

Several important findings emerged from these reviews. To begin with, brief interventions and motivational enhancement approaches received some of the highest ratings for treating alcohol problems in both reviews. These findings further illustrated the great importance of developing BTSAS as a program that included collaboration between clients and therapists, direct feedback and advice to change, and adjusting the intervention to different levels of motivation to change. Next, both reviews identified a range of behavioral treatment approaches that had high evidence scores. This list included social skills training (2nd highest rating in the 1995 review and 3rd highest rating in the 1998 review); behavioral contracting (ranked 5th and 7th in 1995 and 1998 respectively); community reinforcement approach (4th highest score in both reviews); relapse prevention (8th highest score in the 1995 review); behavioral self-control training (11th highest score in the 1998 review); and behavioral marital/family therapy (12th highest score in the 1995 review and 10th highest in the 1998 review). Cognitive therapy (restructuring dysfunctional thoughts that lead to drinking) also received top ratings (10th highest score in the 1995 review and 12th highest in the 1998 review). While these approaches differed in terms of their specific areas of focus and the extent to which they included cognitive techniques along with behavioral ones, taken together they illustrate the effectiveness of broad-based behavioral approaches that emphasize skills training and practice, goal setting, and positive reinforcement of both reduced drinking and other nondrinking related activities. Importantly, skills training also has been shown to be an effective intervention for improving functioning in SPMI clients, and behavioral approaches have been widely used in a range of contexts with this client population (see Bellack, Mueser, Gingerich, & Agresta, 1997 for a review). Finally, client-centered approaches earned high ratings (7th highest score in the 1995 review and 8th in the 1998 review), further illustrating the importance of an empathic approach with substance abusing clients.

Treatment Must Be Broad-Based and Integrated With Mental Health Services

Drake and colleagues (2001) summarized several important elements of integrated treatment for patients with dual diagnosis, including matching interventions to patients' stage of change, assertive outreach aimed at treatment engagement, addressing motivation to change as part of treatment, a long-term approach to treatment with ongoing support, skills building, relapse prevention, and comprehensive treatment that addresses functioning in all areas in addition to substance use and connects with other systems of care. Of particular importance to SPMI clients are issues related to symptoms, medications, housing, poverty, lack of social support, and overall coordination of these diverse aspects of treatment. Treatment for substance abuse in SPMI clients also needs to be tolerant of lapses, relapses, sporadic attendance, and low motivation for change. Efforts to develop substance abuse treatment for dually diagnosed SPMI clients have shown good results when they have been broad-based and included attention to a range of issues in addition to substance use.

Drake and colleagues (Drake, McHugo, & Noordsy, 1993) designed an integrated program for drinking that involved a long-term approach to treatment; extensive use of case managers to coordinate treatment, medication, and crisis intervention; housing, skills training, vocational rehabilitation, and family education. After four years, 61% of the participants remained abstinent from alcohol. Addington and el-Guebaly (1998) developed a group intervention for schizophrenia patients with substance abuse that combined attention to treatment engagement, psychoeducation, support, and social skills training, along with features aimed at behaviorally reducing substance use, including goal setting, identifying reasons for relapse, coping with high risk situations, and money management. After one year, 44% of participants were abstinent. Moggi and colleagues (Moggi, Ouimette, Finney, & Moos, 1999) evaluated a four-month inpatient program designed for patients with dual diagnosis that included stabilizing the psychiatric disorder, enhancing motivation for change, relapse prevention, and involvement of concerned significant others in treatment, as well as groups on money management, employment, and housing issues. While substance abuse did not change over time, most patients at follow-up were involved in mental health programs, and they reported improved compliance with medication and decreases in positive symptoms. Barrowclough and colleagues (2001) conducted a randomized controlled trial comparing routine care alone with routine care plus motivational interviewing, CBT, and family or caregiver intervention for substance abuse in SPMI patients. Patients in the integrated program showed greater improvements in functioning at the end of treatment and at the 12-month follow-up, including reduced positive symptoms and a greater percentage of abstinent days over the 12 months of the study. Overall, these studies show that interventions that combine components central to good care of clients with SPMI, such as an emphasis on long-term treatment, use of case managers and other support systems, and attention to engagement in treatment and issues of crisis and daily functioning, can be effective in treating substance abuse in SPMI clients.

COMPONENTS OF BTSAS

BTSAS contains six integrated components: (1) motivational interviewing to enhance motivation to reduce use; (2) a urinalysis contingency designed to enhance motivation to change and increase the salience of goals; (3) structured goal setting to identify realistic, short term goals for decreased substance use; (4) social skills and drug refusal skills to enable patients to refuse social pressure to use substances, and to provide success experiences that can increase self-efficacy for change; (5) education about the reasons for substance use and the particular dangers of substance use for people with SPMI, in order to shift the decisional balance towards decreased use; and (6) relapse prevention training that focuses on behavioral skills for coping with urges and dealing with high risk situations and lapses.

Motivational Interviewing (MI)

Motivational Interviewing (MI; Miller & Rollnick, 1991) is nonconfrontational and directive, and involves providing clear feedback and advice along with negotiating goals and problem solving to overcome barriers to treatment. MI combines the therapeutic elements that have been found to be successful components of brief interventions for substance abuse (Bien et al., 1993), including giving clear advice and feedback, utilizing an empathic counseling style, and addressing barriers to treatment. There have been numerous tests of MI as both a precursor to treatment and as an add-on to treatment-as-usual in both inpatient and outpatient settings, with a range of patient populations (see Miller & Heather, 1998 for a review). Overall, the literature supports MI as an effective strategy for raising client motivation, increasing treatment attendance, and reducing substance use (Miller, 2000). Importantly, MI was revised into a four-session intervention called Motivational Enhancement Therapy, which was one of the three treatments tested in Project MATCH, a large, multisite intervention study for individuals with alcohol dependence. The four-session MET intervention was compared to 12 sessions of either cognitive behavioral therapy or 12-step facilitation training (Project MATCH Research Group, 1997). The first two MET sessions consisted of assessment, feedback, and the development of an individualized change plan delivered in a motivational interviewing style. The third and fourth sessions reviewed client progress, reexamined reasons for change, and made adjustments to the change plan if necessary. Results showed that MET produced outcomes comparable to the other treatments involving up to three times as many sessions.

While MI began as an intervention for problem drinking, it has since been applied to a range of behavior change efforts. There have been a number of studies of MI with drug abusing populations that show promising results. Studies have included amphetamine users, patients on methadone maintenance, marijuana users, and patients with cocaine dependence, and have found that drug abusing patients who received MI showed greater attendance at and retention in treatment, lowered use, and lower rates of problems (Baker, Boggs, & Lewin, 2001; Saunders, Wilkinson, & Phillips, 1995; Stephens, Roffman, & Curtin, 2000). Importantly, MI seems especially useful with drug abusing clients who report low motivation to change (Stotts, Schmitz, Rhoades, & Grabowski, 2001).

Importantly, MI also has been used successfully in dually diagnosed clients to improve treatment engagement and outcome. Kemp and colleagues (1996, 1998) studied the impact of a brief motivational intervention on observer-rated compliance and attitudes toward treatment in patients with psychotic disorders. Patients who received the intervention showed greater compliance with treatment at 6- and 18-month follow-up intervals, as well as better improvements in social functioning and longer survival in the community prior to readmission as compared to those who did not. Daley and Zuckoff (1998) added a one-session motivational session prior to discharge for dual diagnosis patients and found their rates of attendance at aftercare increased from 35% prior to instituting the intervention to 67% for clients who received the one-session intervention. In a study of patients with depression and cocaine dependence, Daley and colleagues (Daley, Salloum, Zuckoff, Kirisci, & Thase, 1998) found that a brief motivational intervention was associated with greater treatment attendance and completion and lower one-year readmission rates. Swanson and colleagues (Swanson, Pantalon, & Cohen, 1999) examined the impact of MI on attendance at aftercare appointments for patients with dual diagnosis and found that the proportion of patients who attended their first outpatient appointment was higher for the MI group (42%) than for the standard treatment group (16%). Martino and colleagues (Martino, Carroll, O'Malley, & Rounsaville, 2000) compared the use of a one-session preadmission MI to a standard interview for dual diagnosis patients in a partial hospital program and found that those in the MI group had lower rates of treatment dropout and greater treatment attendance. Overall, the literature finds that MI does much to enhance behavior change generally, to reduce substance use specifically, and is an effective strategy for raising client motivation, and increasing treatment attendance in a range of clinical populations, including clients with SPMI (see chapter 6 for a discussion of the way in which we have tailored MI to fit into the BTSAS program).

Urinalysis Contingency Program (UCP)

Contingency management as part of substance abuse treatment typically involves providing immediate reinforcement of a positive behavior in order to increase the likelihood that the behavior will be repeated. In standard CM programs aimed at reducing drug use, clients are provided with some reward for providing a clean urine sample. The rewards vary, but usually involve money or vouchers that can be traded for desired goods, services, or activities. Contingency procedures and voucher-based incentives have been shown to be beneficial in reducing substance use in samples of primary substance abusers (see Higgins, Alessi, & Dantona, 2002 for a review; Petry, 2000).

Small-scale contingency management programs have also been used with SPMI clients with dual disorders. Both Shaner and colleagues (1997) and Roll, Chermack, and Chudzynski (2004) utilized CMPs with small samples of dually diagnosed schizophrenia patients. In the Shaner study, two clients with schizophrenia who were also homeless provided urine specimens twice per week, and the clients received $25 for drug-free urine samples. Compared to baseline, clients had a much lower rate of cocaine-positive samples during the intervention. Roll and colleagues found similar reductions in use of crack cocaine using a CMP with three clients with schizophrenia. In a larger sample, Peniston (1988) developed a contingency program that successfully reduced drinking among 15 clients with schizophrenia who were receiving inpatient mental health treatment. The program used rewards such as praise, day passes, and money to reward abstinence when patients were out of the hospital on day passes in the community. Sigmon and colleagues (Sigmon, Steingard, Badger, Anthony, & Higgins, 2000) used a CMP to reduce marijuana use in a small sample of outpatients with schizophrenia. These sorts of findings support the use of UCP in clients with SPMI. While UCP has not yet been used with large samples of SPMI clients, it is included in BTSAS as a way to concretely reinforce reductions in substance use in a way that likely has great applicability to this client population (see chapter 7 for a detailed description of how we have integrated the UCP into the BTSAS program).

Behaviorally Based Strategies

A number of behavioral treatment programs have been developed for treating addictive behaviors (Annis & Davis, 1989; Carroll, Rounsaville, & Gawin, 1991; Chiauzzi, 1991; Monti, Abrams, Kadden, & Cooney, 1989). The programs differ in specifics, but they each emphasize the use of social learning principles to teach a variety of cognitive and behavioral skills. As reviewed earlier, there is ample evidence to document that the generic behavioral approach is effective, but the data do not clearly favor one specific strategy over another (Miller, 1992). In BTSAS, we have adapted a number of these procedures that seem especially relevant to the problems faced by SPMI clients and that these clients are likely to be able to learn and implement effectively. These include: behavioral contracting (goal setting); resisting social pressure to use; identifying high risk situations; and identifying alternatives to substance use in a given situation. In teaching all of these skills, the same basic social learning strategies are used: instruction, modeling, role-play, and feedback. Each of these components was selected in order to make the process of reducing substance use less a task of willpower and more one of a series of learned steps that could be used in a range of situations.

Social Skills Training

BTSAS is based on social skills training (SST; Bellack et al., 1997), a structured intervention that uses instruction, modeling, role-playing, and social reinforcement. Complex social behaviors are broken down into component elements. Patients are first taught to perform the elements, and then gradually learn to combine them. There is a strong emphasis on behavioral rehearsal and overlearning of a few skills to minimize the cognitive load during stressful interactions. The social skills training component of BTSAS includes two sections: (1) General social skills training is included to teach clients how to make plans with and refuse requests of other people. There is clear evidence that social skills training is an effective way to teach clients with SPMI how to interact more successfully and less stressfully with other people (see Bellack et al., 1997 for a review). (2) Drug refusal skills training, in which clients learn and practice how to refuse offers of drugs from others, is viewed as a logical extension of social skills training that is needed for dually diagnosed clients. We view drug refusal skills training as a central component of BTSAS. Dually diagnosed SMI clients generally need to deal with other people—either to get drugs or to use drugs—in order to maintain their drugs use. That is, drug use is a social experience, and clients have social interactions in a range of situations that support and maintain their drug use. Friends and family members are typically among those who provide and offer drugs to clients, and often clients receive offers of drugs in settings that most of us would think should be safe, such as where they live. Clients are often enlisted to purchase drugs for others and are vulnerable and so open to easy manipulation by drug dealers. The goal of drug refusal skills training is to teach clients how to interact with other people in ways that support nonuse. By giving clients a language for refusing offers of drugs, drug refusal skills provide clients with a tool for successfully coping with social interactions without drug use.

Education

An important aspect of reducing substance abuse with any population is getting the individual to recognize that they have a problem and that they need to do something about it (Hall, Wasserman, & Havassy, 1991). Prochaska and DiClemente (1982) have hypothesized that this recognition and the decision to reduce consumption is a process rather than an event; the inclination to change evolves gradually over time, during which motivation to change behavior waxes and wanes. Characteristically, there are many false starts and failures before durable change occurs. The education component of BTSAS is designed to enhance motivation to change. Education about the negative consequences of excessive use is a standard component of most substance abuse treatment programs. It serves to increase the perceived value of behavior change, disabuse patients of myths that facilitate consumption, and provide information that makes change easier. The educational component of our intervention is administered in six group sessions, modeled after the educational training used in other substance abuse programs (Heather, 1989). Emphasis is placed on providing information that is personally relevant to group members, rather than presenting a general admonition about the dangers of drug use.

Coping Skills Training

The coping skills training component of BTSAS is based on several cognitive behavioral treatment programs (Monti et al., 1989) that emphasize building skills for coping with daily problems and stressors (listening skills, conversation skills), reducing social conflicts (i.e., improving general communication with others, addressing relationship problems), and managing intrapersonal factors (i.e., managing urges to use drugs, managing negative thinking) that contribute to substance use. In order to adapt these principles, we have streamlined the topics in the coping skills component of BTSAS to those that we feel are most relevant to SMI clients. Specifically, our emphasis in this section is on teaching clients how to identify triggers for substance use and the high risk situations in which these triggers present themselves, and then learn to escape or avoid these situations. We have intentionally reduced the number and complexity of topics in our coping skills component. As is evident in our approach to skills training more generally, we emphasize behavioral rehearsal and overlearning of a few specific and relatively narrow skills that can be used automatically, thereby minimizing the cognitive load during stressful interactions. For SMI clients, providing the level of detail needed to think through specific skills to cope with many different drug-related situations would require a level of cognitive functioning that most clients do not have. Instead, we focus on two general skills—avoidance and escape—that clients can easily understand and can be applied to a range of drug-related situations without much tailoring for different situations.

Relapse Prevention

The relapse prevention component of BTSAS is based on Marlatt and Gordon's (1985) work on relapse prevention with primary alcohol abusers. Marlatt and Gordon emphasized the importance of teaching patients to expect lapses, and proposed a number of strategies to prevent lapses from becoming relapses. A significant aspect of their strategy involved changing attributions, increasing self-efficacy, and employing self-control. Within this framework, alcohol abusers are encouraged to develop sources of social support that they can contact when they feel vulnerable, to develop appropriate health habits (e.g., exercise), to develop hobbies and other sources of entertainment and reinforcement, and to participate in marital or family therapy (McCrady, 1993). While this approach is useful with SPMI clients (expect lapses, develop a plan so that lapses do not become relapses), these specific techniques are generally not going to be useful for most SPMI clients due to their information processing deficits, lack of economic resources (most SPMI clients are unemployed), and their relative social isolation (they tend not to have a network of peers or relatives they can access). We have tailored relapse prevention to make it more relevant to SPMI clients (see chapter 10). Briefly, as we developed BTSAS, we listened to our clients in order to figure out what some of the most important high risk situations were that led to use or relapse in this client population. We then developed sessions that involved discussion about the difficulties clients have in coping with these situations without using, as well as problem solving to create an individual plan for each client to use when in this situation. Situations include coping with boredom, coping with medication side effects, coping with symptoms of mental illness, and having money.

SUMMARY

The components of BTSAS are all strategies that have been studied and used effectively in primary substance abusing populations. By basing BTSAS on concepts and strategies from the substance abuse treatment literature, we did not have to start from scratch, and we were able to utilize what has been shown to be important or effective in reducing substance use. The key to BTSAS is in the tailoring of these strategies to the needs and deficits of clients with SMI.

Chapter 3

TRAINING PHILOSOPHY AND GENERAL STRATEGIES

BTSAS includes a detailed procedural manual. The exact content of every session is not predetermined, and will be partly a function of the idiosyncratic characteristics of each group member. However, there is a specified structure or organization plan for each session, and there is a comprehensive curriculum that is presented in a standard order. This level of specification may be a bit off-putting to experienced clinicians who are used to *flying by the seat of their pants*. But, it actually makes the process easier for clinicians because they know pretty much what to do, and when and how to do it. The structure is also very effective at shaping members' behavior and keeping the sessions focused on the target: reducing drug use. In our experience, too much time is wasted in most therapy groups as the lack of structure fosters free-wheeling discussion on the topic of the moment. These wide ranging discussions may be helpful at times, but more often than not they are not productive for most group members, and they may be counterproductive by distracting the group from the primary focus of treatment.

In addition to the curriculum a key aspect of BTSAS is therapist style and behavior. BTSAS therapists are warm, but directive. They are therapists, but they function more as teachers than traditional verbal therapists; finally, they are positive and supportive. The structure of each session is outlined in Table 3.1.

OVERVIEW OF TREATMENT COMPONENTS

Treatment components include motivational interviewing, urinalysis, goal setting, social skills training, education, and coping skills.

Motivational Interviewing (MI)

MI is conducted in individual sessions, during the first week of treatment, after three months, and at the end of treatment (6 months). The purpose of the MI sessions is to identify a few key reasons to decrease drug use and to develop both short- and long-term goals for decreased use. The emphasis is on concrete goals that are relatively short term. Notably, goals should have a reasonable likelihood of

Table 3.1 Format for BTSAS Sessions

1. Members provide urine samples.
2. Group convenes while tests are being read.
3. Results of urinalysis are presented to each member in turn, and reinforcement is provided for those with a clean sample.
4. Therapist provides support to members with a dirty urine sample, and directs goal-setting discussion focused on the situation in which the person used drugs.
5. Goal setting takes place with each member in turn.
6. Review of material/skills covered in preceding session.
7. Therapists describe the content/focus of the day's session.
8. Skills training/didactic presentation is conducted.
9. Goals are briefly reviewed, homework is assigned if applicable, and members are reminded of time/date of next session.

being achieved so the person does not become frustrated and use the failure as a reason to drop out of treatment or resume drug use. Subsequent sessions are used to review progress, identify problems in achieving goals, and revise goals as needed.

Urinalysis Contingency

Participants are required to provide a urine sample prior to each session beginning in week 2. We do not require a sample during the first week because we do not want the person to begin treatment with a failure experience or feeling self-conscious about having a dirty sample. By the second week it is likely the person has seen one or more peers provide a dirty sample without being criticized or berated in public. Participants receive ample social reinforcement (congratulations and applause) from the therapists and other group members if the urine is clean for the substance targeted during the MI session (the primary substance of abuse). They also receive a small financial reinforcement. Our clinical trial provided $1.50 for the first clean sample, and that amount increases by $.50 up to a maximum of $3.50 for every third consecutive clean sample. Because dual disordered persons will sometimes skip a session when they have used drugs, the reinforcement amount is reset to $1.50 after each absence. In the case of a "dirty" sample, the therapists do brief problem solving training to key identify factors that contributed to drug use (e.g., running into an old friend with whom the person often used coke), and the member then receives guidance or practices skills to avoid using in the same situation in the future.

Goal Setting

A critical aspect of reducing substance use is establishing reasonable goals and objectives. Goal setting is a formal process in BTSAS that immediately follows the administration of the urinalysis contingency. Each member in turn reports on her or his success with the previous week's goal and establishes a goal for the intervening time until the next session. The therapists provide guidance and structure so goals are focused on reducing use of the goal drug and are likely to be accomplished. Examples might be not smoking crack over the weekend, or not going out socially with a friend who uses drugs. Problem solving strategies are introduced as needed if the person has had difficulty achieving the goal in the past, and simpler targets are selected to avoid continued frustration. The goals are written into a formal contract that the therapist and member each sign. The member keeps one copy of the contract and is requested to identify someone in his or her immediate environment to whom he or she can publicly announce this goal. Such public announcements have been shown to be helpful in changing a variety of behaviors.

Social Skills Training

The social skills training curriculum covers three topics: conversation skills, general refusal skills, and substance use refusal skills. It is intended to teach participants how to develop relationships with people who do not use drugs and how to effectively refuse drugs from peers, family members, and other people with whom they use or from whom they receive drugs. The emphasis is on *substance use refusal* skills. Conversation and general refusal skills provide an orientation to the skills training approach, and insure that all participants have a minimum competence in basic social skills before they begin the more difficult training in how to deal with stressful drug related situations.

Education and Coping Skills

The purpose of this component of treatment is: (1) to provide information that will increase motivation to abstain from drugs by helping participants understand why they use drugs and why they should not, and (2) teaching them how to cope with urges to use, and to identify and avoid or escape from high-risk situations. Training includes both didactic presentations and skills training with rehearsal. As with all components of BTSAS, we provide general information that is relevant to most participants, but we also focus in on specific issues that are germane to each member. We make ample use of visual aides (flip charts and whiteboards). Each member gets a loose-leaf binder at the beginning of treatment in which copies of all the written materials are stored. Depending on the member's living circumstance, he or she may take the binders home after each session or leave them in the clinic. Of course, the member takes home the completed binder when treatment concludes.

The topics covered in this unit include:

- Positive and negative consequences of using substances
- Biological factors in substance use which are especially relevant to people with SPMI
- Impact of substance abuse on symptoms of people with SPMI
- Habits, cravings, and triggers
- High-risk situations
- Avoidance-based coping strategies
- Escape and refusal-based coping strategies
- HIV prevention skills
- Hepatitis prevention

Problem Solving and Relapse Prevention

The purpose of this segment is: (1) to apply to life events and problems that arise over the course of time, the core skills and generic coping strategies that have previously been taught; (2) to shift the focus of goal setting and the urinalysis contingency to any secondary drugs that the person abuses after success is achieved with the primary substance; (3) relapse prevention, including dealing with lapses; and (4) review of material covered earlier, including repetition of units as needed for new members in the group or existing members who continue to have difficulty in a particular area. A key feature of this segment is helping members apply skills and coping strategies to new problems that develop in their lives, and to deal with decreases in motivation for abstinence.

Termination

Subjects in our research program participated for six months of biweekly sessions. As indicated previously, this time frame is widely considered to be a minimum for effective treatment of dual disordered persons. In a clinical setting the duration can easily be extended, especially with open-enrollment groups.

In fact, our groups continued for several years, but members *graduated* after six months. We do not have data on this issue, but we think it is important for members to have an ending or graduation date.

Otherwise, participation is apt to reach a point of diminishing returns in which the same issues are addressed over and over. There is also a natural time limit for the utility of the contingency, because either the person has maintained abstinence for an extended period , or he or she is clearly not going to become abstinent and has a predominance of dirty samples. In any case, we recommend making graduation a celebratory event, with a diploma and refreshments. Decreasing drug use and attending a drug abuse group is difficult, and participants deserve recognition and congratulations.

TRAINING PHILOSOPHY AND TECHNIQUES

This training program is based on social skills training (SST), a social learning approach for rehabilitation that has been successfully employed with a wide variety of people with SPMI since the early 1980s. SST is a highly structured educational procedure that employs instruction, modeling, role-playing, and social reinforcement. Complex social repertoires, such as making friends and refusing substances are broken down into component elements, such as maintaining eye contact and providing social reinforcers. Participants are first taught to perform the individual elements, and then gradually learn to smoothly combine them. There is a strong emphasis on shaping (learning new skills piece by piece), behavioral rehearsal (practice), and overlearning of a few specific and relatively narrow skills that can be used automatically, thereby minimizing the cognitive load for decision making during stressful interactions. This same basic teaching/rehearsal model is adapted for presentation of didactic material, goal setting, and problem solving. In each case, material is broken down into simple elements or components, members are required, behaviorally or verbally, to demonstrate learning, and expectations are gradually increased such that members have a maximal chance of being successful and being reinforced (see chapter 8 for skills training). The following are general guidelines for how the techniques can be successfully applied in BTSAS

Training Philosophy

Skills Training Is Teaching, Not Group Psychotherapy

Most people working in mental health became interested in the field because they wanted to help people, and it is generally assumed that the way to help is through some form of verbal psychotherapy. Regardless of the specific brand, these approaches all assume that conversation about emotionally important issues is a central ingredient for change. That is absolutely not the case with SST or other skills training units employed in BTSAS. These are educational, skill building procedures. Conversation is a vehicle to transmit information and make people feel comfortable with one another, not for teaching. A piano or tennis instructor does not bring a group of students together to talk about striking the piano keys or the tennis ball, and discussing how the students feel about it. The participants in BTSAS are often willing to discuss their problems; sometimes they prefer talking to working at learning. Nevertheless, talking and self-exploration are issues for other groups. The leader must make up her mind before beginning that she will be conducting a skills group, not doing a little skills training in the course of a more open-ended verbal psychotherapy. The former is the only way to really develop complex new behaviors and help people reduce drug use.

Learn to Do Skills Training

Doing skills training effectively is a skill. Consequently, the leader must learn how to do it in the same way that participants learn their new skills. That means starting slowly, practicing, and securing feedback. Where possible, it would be very helpful to observe skills groups conducted by experienced skills trainers, or to watch videotapes. Short of that, training can be bootstrapped by soliciting feedback from coleaders or supervisors who are familiar with the approach. As with all new skills, it is important to start slowly. Select easy skills to teach, work with a coleader, and set very minimal goals. Practice doing skills training and don't worry too much about the outcome. Get used to role-playing and to running a structured group. Become comfortable with the role of teacher and in keeping a group on task. Keep in mind that the structure (how you teach) is much more important than the content (what you teach). Most neophyte leaders function as if the opposite is true, and spend too much time talking.

The level of organization referred to above, is particularly important for learning. Prepare written materials (handouts and poster boards) in advance, come to session with a set of role-play scenarios already prepared, and stick as close as possible to the script. When we suggest doing two to three role-plays with each member we mean two to three brief role-plays with each member, not one or two, sprinkled with conversation, and differing wildly in content or length. Keep in mind that role-plays are not vehicles to stimulate discussion about social situations, or to rehearse a single, long-winded, idiosyncratic dialogue. Think of learning to serve in tennis by serving once, hitting a few volleys, talking about your grip, volleying a little, and then trying another serve, vs. hitting 10 serves in a row and getting corrective feedback after each shot. Finally, keep in mind that every group is a little different. Learning to be an effective leader requires that you practice implementing the structure with different groups, whose members present somewhat different challenges.

Never, Never Underestimate the Cognitive Deficits of Your Members

We have previously highlighted the problems people with schizophrenia and other SPMIs face in memory, attention, and higher-level problem solving. This is one of the most important and most difficult points for most clinicians to understand. People with schizophrenia who are asymptomatic can appear to maintain lucid conversations, seem to learn and understand well, and respond affirmatively to questions about whether or not they understand. We have regularly observed such apparently well-functioning group members nod appropriately in response to instructions, parrot the leader's role-played responses, and be totally unable to generate an appropriate response when the situation is slightly changed. Whether they don't remember, are easily distracted, or are so concrete that they can't transpose ideas from situation A to situation B, they often lack the capacity to learn from continuities across situations. The only solutions to this dilemma that we have found to be effective are: (1) impose as much structure as possible and minimize demands on abstraction (use prompts and handouts, identify simple commonalties across situations for the person to focus on, and keep instructions very simple and straightforward); (2) practice, practice, practice (the more automatic the response is in situation x, the less the demand on working memory and analysis). Finally, do not ask if your participants understand: have them demonstrate that they understand! Similarly, do not preach or lecture. Keep your instructions brief, and always use audiovisuals (handouts, posters) for anything you want them to remember. Finally, keep role-plays brief and narrowly relevant to what you are trying to teach. It is typical of new leaders to get caught up in role-playing, staying in role too long, and leading the interaction far from the few specific points the participant is supposed to practice. The longer the role-play lasts the greater the likelihood that the participants will forget what they are supposed to be focusing on.

Never, Never Underestimate How Difficult It Is For People With SPMI To Reduce Drug Use

This caveat will not be surprising to clinicians experienced in working with dual disordered persons, but it is worth repeating to them as well as to novice clinicians. Most of us have made New Year's resolutions or otherwise tried to change behaviors, such as going on a diet, stopping smoking, saving more money, and most of us have failed. It is extremely difficult to change addictive behaviors and ingrained habits.

People with dual disorders have all the same problems we face, but magnified by the problems and disabilities associated with SPMI, including cognitive impairment, vacillating motivation, lack of good social supports, psychiatric symptoms, behavioral disorganization, poverty, and associated stresses from the environment. The clinician must be prepared to be tolerant of these problems, and adapt the intervention and adjust tactics accordingly. This will certainly include tolerance for intermittent attendance, for failure to complete homework assignments, for lapses, for members seemingly not paying attention or agreeing to do things that it is obvious the person cannot or will not do, and for being difficult to manage in group. To be sure, there will be some persons in group who will have little or no desire to reduce drug use, and some people will be sufficiently disruptive as to jeopardize their peers' participation in group. As will be discussed below, there are clear rules that participants need to follow to make the environment safe and allow other members to achieve their goals, and some individuals need to be directed to leave group, for one session or permanently. But, that should be a rare event. For the most part, the onus is on the therapists to create a supportive environment and reinforce effort and baby steps in the general direction of reduced drug use and abstinence at some time in the future. Keep in mind that a person who is not really motivated to reduce drug use now may acquire information or learn skills that will increase motivation, or help the person be more successful at some time in the future.

Be Reinforcing

It is natural for most of us to tell others what they have not done or what they have done wrong when we are giving instructions. A key to making this intervention work well is to be consistently positive and reinforcing. Some new skills trainers interpret this caveat to mean that they must be bubbly and effusive and praise everything. To the contrary, a laid-back style will work fine as long as participants hear that they are doing OK and that the therapist and the other group members approve. Most people with SPMI have long histories of failure and frustration. SST is one place where they can be assured of success because: (1) the level of demand is geared to their capacity, not some abstract or unreachable standard; and (2) communications are always positive, emphasizing what the member has done well, not what he or she has done poorly. This caveat about being positive also does not mean that therapists should be dishonest and say something is good or correct when it is not. However, one can imply that an idea is bad or stupid, which will have an iatrogenic effect, or one can be supportive and still correct misinformation or faulty ideas. For example, in goal setting a therapist might say: "Susan, it's great that you plan on never using cocaine again, but that is a very difficult promise to keep. Let's figure out a short-term goal that will be easier for you. How about not using cocaine between now and our next group?"

Even difficult group members (and some are difficult) can be controlled without much negativity and censure if the leader can focus on rules and the situation, rather than the person's bad behavior (e.g., "It is important that we don't make fun of one another here. Fred, if you are having trouble not laughing when Jon tries to talk maybe you would like to take a brief break"; "Steve, Susan may find it distracting when you touch her during group; why don't you come over here and sit next to me. Then it will be easier for you to not touch her."). Remember, you can't lose your temper, be sarcastic, or speak in an angry tone of voice and be an effective teacher. Group members will turn off or, if they are really testing you, will be reinforced for their inappropriate behavior. Of course, everyone must feel safe, including the leaders. If a member is really posing a threat he or she should be asked to leave and the overall positive tone must be temporarily suspended.

Be Persistent

Conducting highly structured, skills-based interventions with dual disordered persons is not easy. The leaders must do more homework than in other treatments in order to be adequately prepared. The intervention is fun for both leaders and participants (it really is!), but everyone works hard. There is no sitting back and letting others do all the work. Many times it will seem easier to just talk about something or move on to a new topic, rather than repeat the same role-play for what seems like the umpteenth time. Nevertheless, remember our tennis and music analogies. It's like the old joke: "How do you get to Carnegie Hall?" "Practice, practice, practice."

Don't Work In Isolation

In all likelihood, the participants in your groups will be receiving psychotropic medications, have a caseworker, and (potentially) one or more other therapists. Keep in touch with your colleagues. Find out when the person has been put on a new medication, or has received a major change in dosage. Learn how she is doing in other settings (is this a particularly bad time for her? Is she showing prodromal signs of relapse?). Of special note is the issue of whether the member is giving the therapist a hard time that she is not giving others or vice versa. Similarly, what else is going on in the person's life outside of the treatment center? Are there conflicts at home? Do you need to be in touch with family members or residence managers to insure that the member's new skills are being reinforced, or to teach a specific skill needed to avoid conflict in the home (e.g., the member is fighting with a sibling or housemate and you can teach a skill to alleviate the conflict). As a general rule, generalization of the effects of training will be enhanced to the extent that the skills taught are: (1) relevant to the person's immediate environment, and (2) are reinforced by the environment (see chapter 13 for ways to implement BTSAS in a clinical center).

General Strategies

The role of therapists in group and the ways in which the treatment can be tailored, are two very important strategies.

The Role of the Therapists in Group

Each session is conducted by two group therapists. To differentiate their roles and responsibilities, one will be identified as the presenter, or group leader. The second therapist, identified as the coordinator, acts as an aide to the presenter and will assist in various ways throughout the different sessions. Therapists often vary their roles across sessions, and different teams will develop slightly different ways of interacting and helping one another. The therapists should clarify with each other their roles for that day before the beginning of each group session. Also, both co-facilitators should give individual, positive feedback to group members during each session. *The presenter* is responsible for leading the group members into the session topics, eliciting feedback, and providing positive and corrective feedback from members. During the role-play introductions, the presenter will model the skills with the assistance of the confederate coordinator and then direct group members in subsequent role-plays. He or she will review previous sessions and homework, assign new homework, and model role plays.

The coordinator also participates in eliciting feedback, and provides positive and corrective feedback to members. The coordinator serves as the confederate in initial social skill role-plays and in all drug and alcohol refusal role-plays with group members. As a participant in the role-play, the coordinator will still give positive feedback to group members when appropriate at the end of practice. In addition, the coordinator will manage group disruptions when necessary: For example, in the event that a group member arrives intoxicated, the coordinator will act appropriately in escorting that member out of group so as not to disrupt the flow of the session or call unnecessary attention to the situation. The coordinator will also be responsible for dissemination of group handouts, props for alcohol and drug refusal skills and visual aides to emphasize pertinent topics of discussion.

A dry erase easel or flip chart are important elements of group. Member feedback, role-play instructions, or definitions will all be highlighted in one or both ways during sessions by the group coordinator. The information generated in one session should also be recorded whenever possible to be used as reference material in later group sessions.

At the end of each session, a preprinted homework sheet is given to each group member. Any member-specific lists or ideas generated during that session that will be useful for homework and retention should be recorded on these homework sheets. As is possible, both the facilitator and the coordinator will fill these out and hand them out at the end of group.

Tailoring the Treatment to Group Members

People who suffer from chronic mental illness and substance abuse problems are diverse in their cultural backgrounds, socioeconomic status, and cognitive and behavioral abilities. Because of this, each individual substance abuse treatment group will need to be tailored to the needs of its members. Each member's ability to function in the group should be assessed during initial sessions. Group format can then be adjusted based on the average level of functioning for the entire group. This can be done by the facilitator(s) by first making judgments—both clinical and behavioral—about group member abilities. The following are some areas for facilitators to look at when making these judgments:

- How effective is the group member in performing the skill when first modeled?
- How quickly does the group member learn to perform a skill after it is first modeled?
- Can the group members stay focused on all steps of a multistep skill?
- When using the blackboard as a visual aid, do subjects need entire sentences or simple phrases/key words as prompts for role-plays?

For persons who are quick to learn, are more easily engaged, and have greater ability to deal with abstractions, group facilitators should use clinical judgment to increase the complexity of the material and difficulty level of role-play situations. For example, for a group member who is able to recognize his problems regarding communicating or staying sober/drug free and is willing to share feelings about this from the outset (this may be the case with persons who are actively involved in 12-step recovery), refusal role-plays should be developed that are highly personalized. More time can be spent on elaborating scenarios and asking group members for feedback. On the other hand, with group members who are difficult to engage due to symptomatology or other factors, or who have difficulty attending to the steps of a skill, the focus should remain on learning the basics of the skill. This should be done by performing simple role-plays and much effort on the part of facilitators to keep all engaged by asking members to repeat steps of skills and give positive feedback to one another.

Tailoring for New Members in Open Enrollment Groups
Tailoring is particularly important for new group members. They should be faded into group such that expectations and demands are only gradually increased. They should be included as participant observers during the first week as they learn about the group by observing existing members. It is helpful to have the new member sit next to one of the therapists, who can quietly explain or describe what is going on. They should be invited to provide feedback to role-plays and to engage in role-plays if they choose. In the latter case, the scenarios should be kept briefer than for experienced group members and performance criteria should be simpler. Expectations for participation in all aspects of treatment should be increased beginning in the second week of attendance. As is the case for all members when the group begins, they should begin to participate in the urinalysis contingency and goal setting in the second week as well. References to material from education sessions (e.g., role of dopamine, high-risk situations) should be briefly explained to new members as needed until units are formally repeated. It

is often helpful to have experienced members explain points to new members in their own words. This process reinforces the material for the "teacher," as well as teaching the new member. For example:

Therapist: (Talking to new member) Ramon, one of the most important steps in reducing drug use is knowing what situations to avoid: what we call "high-risk" situations. Carlo (experienced member), can you explain to Ramon what a "high-risk" situation is?

Carlo: A high-risk situation is when there are lots of triggers for drug use and you really want to use.

Therapist: Thanks Carlo, that's right. Susan (experienced member) can you give Ramon an example of one of your high-risk situations?

Susan: Well, I always used with my boyfriend Bob. So Bob would be a trigger and seeing him would make me really want to use. So seeing Bob would be a high-risk situation.

Therapist: That's a good example. Ramon, what is a high-risk situation for you?

In most cases, new members should be well acclimated to the group process within two weeks, and should be functioning as full members within three to four weeks. The one constraint on adding new members is when all existing members started together and are due to graduate in the following four to five weeks. In that case it is very difficult for the new member to catch up, and it is better to hold the patient until a new group can be formed.

Teaching Members to be Good Group Participants

Prior to participating in BTSAS, most dual disordered persons will have experienced other group therapy approaches that were less structured, more insight oriented, and where members were encouraged to "just let their feelings out." When first attending a BTSAS group, people might be surprised at its structure and at its teaching approach, and at first they may have difficulties adapting to the group format.

The leaders should provide a clear description and explanation for the format of BTSAS groups in their initial interviews with prospective members, and again when they start. Early sessions should include a brief orientation/lesson plan so members know what to expect that day. In general, members should be provided with a curriculum so they are attuned to what will be coming in the future, as well as what will happen in a particular session.

When members drift from the format, the leaders can gently but firmly redirect them to the task at hand ("Right now I'd like you to hold your comments while you watch Steve do a role-play"). Praising group members who make progress in following the format is also beneficial. For example, to a person who previously interrupted role-plays and has now begun to observe them quietly, the leaders could say, "Miguel, I liked the way you waited until Steve finished his role-play before you gave feedback."

Usually people are able to follow the group format after several sessions. The open enrollment format is especially conducive to orienting new members because we do not ask much of them during the first week. New participants can observe other group members and learn appropriate behavior by modeling from their peers.

Group participants also should be taught how to provide appropriate, supportive feedback to one another. When people are first involved in a BTSAS group, they sometimes give feedback to each other that is either critical or vague. This is not surprising because this is the kind of feedback most people have received in the past. Also, many people find it is easier to find fault than to praise, and learning how to give helpful feedback takes time. With practice, however, almost anyone can learn to give feedback that is both positive and specific. There are many ways that the leaders can facilitate this. As indicated above, members learn via social modeling: by observing the therapists and other group members. The leaders can also remind people to give positive feedback by saying something like this: "Isabel, what did you like about how Frank refused drugs in that role-play?" It is common for members to respond to such a question by speaking to the therapists, rather than the member who did the role-play. This is easily corrected by directing the person to, "Please, tell Frank what you thought."

If a person starts to criticize someone in the group, the leaders need to interrupt the criticism as soon as possible. It is important to nip criticism in the bud. The leaders can say something such as "Let's stop there, Susan. I'd like you to tell Maria what she did well. Later we can offer a suggestion for improvement." It is also important to praise people who begin to make positive comments after having been critical in their previous feedback. For example, the leaders might say, "Thanks, that was very helpful feedback. You really noticed what Maria did well."

After the group has met for several weeks, a sense of cohesion usually develops, and group members become more supportive of each other's efforts. They may begin to offer positive feedback spontaneously and might even applaud group members who accomplish something that was very difficult for them in the past. If appropriate feedback does not occur after several weeks, it might be helpful to review what is meant by constructive feedback and to provide a written handout to group members and to post a copy in the group room.

GROUP RULES

The group is member oriented, but there are a number of rules which everyone must follow for the safety of members and therapists, and to maximize the likelihood that all members will feel comfortable attending and have every opportunity to be successful. Having explicit rules also helps to avoid being overly critical when members are behaving inappropriately. For example, saying, "Matt, I know you have something you want to say but please remember that our rule is only one person speaks at a time," is much less harsh and critical than, "Matt, let Judy finish." The rules are presented on a handout and explained after everyone has been introduced and the general format has been explained.

Guidelines for Group Members

- The purpose of group is to help you reduce or stop your drug use. If you need to talk about other problems, tell the therapist before or after group.
- Only one person should speak at a time.
- Please no name-calling or swearing.
- Please no criticizing or making fun of others.
- Please no eating or drinking.
- Please always come to group sober.
- Please always respect privacy and confidentiality. What we say here should stay here.
- Please try to stay in group. You may be asked to leave if you are not sober or if your behavior makes people feel uncomfortable.
- You must participate in group for at least 30 minutes to get paid for attending. We can't pay you if you come very late or leave early.

When first presenting the rules therapists should also discuss confidentiality vis-à-vis other group members, members of the clinical team, other agencies, and law enforcement. Policies will vary by state, agency, whether the treatment is being implemented as part of a research project or as a clinical application, and if it is protected by a federal Confidentiality Certificate. Generally, BTSAS will be incorporated into a broader system of care and patients should know what may be put in the clinical record or shared with other clinicians.

SUMMARY

This chapter has provided an overview of issues involved in conducting BTSAS. We first described the treatment components, and then discussed the treatment philosophy and clinical stance with which therapists need to approach BTSAS groups. The emphasis throughout is on teaching rather than discussing, providing structure in a warm, positively reinforcing context, avoiding criticism or censure, and tailoring the treatment to the needs and level of functioning of each group member. BTSAS therapists must always keep in mind how difficult it is for anyone to change addictive behaviors, and that the difficulty is magnified for our dual disordered clients. We then discussed some general strategies employed in conducting BTSAS, including how to individualize treatment for members with different needs and levels of ability, and how to teach members how to be good group participants. Strategies for dealing with problems associated with specific components of the treatment will be presented in the broader discussion of each component. We concluded with a discussion of group rules that are helpful in providing structure and providing a useful way to deal with disruptive behavior.

Chapter 4

SOCIAL SKILLS TRAINING

Social dysfunction, an inability to fulfill expected social rolls (e.g., spouse, worker, parent), is one of the defining characteristics of schizophrenia (Bellack & Blanchard, 1993). It is relatively independent of other domains of the illness, such as psychotic and negative symptoms, and is associated with the course and outcome of the illness. While not as widespread perhaps in other disorders, social dysfunction is still among the most important factors contributing to disability among people with SPMI. There have been a variety of hypotheses to explain the basis of social dysfunction, but the most empirically supported perspective has been the *social skills model* (Meier & Hope, 1998; Mueser & Bellack, 1998). This model hypothesizes that social competence is based on a set of three component skills: (1) social perception or *receiving* skills; (2) social cognition or *processing* skills; and (3) behavioral response or *expressive* skills. Social perception is the ability to accurately read or decode social inputs. This includes such things as accurate detection of cues related to emotion (e.g., facial expressions and nuances of voice, gesture, and body posture), as well as verbal content (what the other person says). Social cognition involves effective analysis of the social stimulus or context (e.g., a job interview versus a casual social encounter); integration of current information with historical information (e.g., What has the other person done in previous interactions? What is one's experience in similar social situations?), and planning of an effective response. This domain is also referred to as social problem solving. Finally, behavioral response or expressive skills include the ability to produce effective verbal content (i.e., to say the right thing, or provide relevant information), to speak with appropriate paralinguistic characteristics (e.g., appropriate voice tone and inflection), and to use suitable nonverbal behaviors such as facial expressions, gestures, and posture. Effective social behavior requires the smooth integration of these three component processes in a way that meets the demands of the specific social interaction. For example, interactions with a supervisor at work require more formality and overt signs of respect than interactions with friends or family members. Moreover, the level of formality and respect that is required will vary with the particular supervisor, how long one has been on the job, and the nature of the organization. Effective social behavior also involves more dynamic or *macro* level response styles, including taking turns to speak, and providing social reinforcement (e.g., head nods, smiles, saying uh-huh while the other person speaks).

The term *skill* is used very pointedly to emphasize that social competence is comprised of a set of *learned* abilities, rather than traits, needs, or other mental processes. Conversely, faulty or ineffective social behavior is often the result of social skills *deficits*. Many basic aspects of social skill, such as smiling, listening attentively, and taking turns, are learned in childhood. More complex behavioral routines, such as dating and job interview skills, are generally acquired in adolescence and young adulthood. Still other skills may be learned later in life as one faces different challenges, such as interacting effectively with physicians and expressing condolences. Some elements of social competence, such as the perception of facial expressions of affect, are not learned, but appear to be genetically *hard wired* at birth. Nevertheless, research suggests that regardless of when or how they were acquired, virtually all social behaviors are *learnable*; that is, they can be modified by experience or training. For example, facial expressions of affect (emotion) are fairly universal, suggesting these responses may have a genetic component. However, cultures vary in when, where, and how intensely affect may be displayed, suggesting that both the cultural rules for expressing and interpreting affect are acquired.

It has been hypothesized that social dysfunction results from three circumstances: (1) when the person does not know how to perform important behaviors appropriately; (2) when the person does not use skills in her behavioral repertoire at appropriate times; or (3) when appropriate behavior is undermined by socially inappropriate behavior (e.g., the person expresses condolences at a funeral, but is dressed for the beach). Each of these circumstances appears to be common in people with schizophrenia and other SPMIs. First, there is good reason to believe that many people with schizophrenia do not learn essential social skills. While the illness typically develops in late adolescence or adulthood, children who later develop schizophrenia have been shown to have subtle attention deficits in childhood that may interfere with the development of social relationships and the acquisition of basic social skills. In addition, retrospective reports often suggest they had a certain oddness during childhood. Second, late adolescence and young adulthood, when schizophrenia often becomes manifest, is a critical period for mastery of adult social roles and skills, such as dating and sexual behaviors, work related skills, and the ability to form and maintain adult relationships. In addition, many people with schizophrenia gradually develop isolated lives, which remove them from their "normal" peer group, provide few opportunities to engage in age appropriate social roles, and limit social contacts to mental health staff and other severely ill clients. This limits the opportunity to acquire and practice appropriate adult roles. Moreover, skills mastered earlier in life may be lost due to disuse or lack of reinforcement by the environment during periods of chronic illness. Third, cognitive impairment, especially including deficits in social cognition and executive processes, interferes with both social perception and social problem solving. One area of cognitive dysfunction that is particularly relevant is difficulty integrating contextual information: the ability to see the relevance of previous experience to current events and to use experience to guide future behavior.

SKILLS TRAINING PROCEDURES

Improving social role functioning and quality of life for people with schizophrenia and other SPMIs has been a major goal of treatment programs for some time. Social skills training (SST) has proven to be one of the most effective approaches to increase social skills and enhance social functioning. The basic technology for teaching social skills was developed in the 1970s and has not changed substantially in the intervening years (Bellack, 2004; Drake & Bellack, 2005). Readers who are not familiar with SST are referred to *Social Skills Training for People with Schizophrenia* (Bellack, Mueser, Gingerich, & Agresta, 2004). This book is a detailed guide for conducting skills training and it is an excellent partner to the current volume.

Social Learning Theory

Social learning theory (SST) is based on social learning principles (Bandura, 1969). It emphasizes the role of behavioral rehearsal in skill development rather than conversational interactions between therapist and consumer. The process is conceptualized as *teaching*, rather than psychotherapy, and is analogous to the way a motor skill would be taught. Five principles derived from social learning theory are incorporated into social skills training, and are essential components of BTSAS: modeling, reinforcement, shaping, overlearning, and generalization.

Modeling

A central tenet of social learning theory is that people learn by observing others, or *modeling*. SST includes two forms of modeling: (1) directed modeling, in which therapists explicitly demonstrate how to perform appropriate behavior when introducing new skills; and (2) indirect modeling, which occurs when group members observe therapists and peers engaging in desired behavior without being directed to learn anything. For example, members will observe and learn from therapists who provide positive feedback to other group members and are not critical of members who provide dirty urine samples. It also occurs when members observe one another role-playing, struggling to solve problems, and being successful in doing so. Modeling is particularly valuable in working with dual disordered clients because they often have difficulty changing their behavior in reaction to admonitions to change or discussion about change.

Reinforcement

An important premise of social learning theory is that behavior is a function of its consequences: behavior followed by positive consequences tends to increase in frequency, and behavior followed by negative consequences tends to decrease in frequency. In regard to SST, the two consequences that are most relevant are positive reinforcement and punishment. Positive reinforcement is provided liberally in the form of verbal praise from the leaders and group members, and is used to reinforce both effort and the performance of specific components of social skill. Positive reinforcement also plays a central role in the urinalysis contingency employed in BTSAS. Punishment is the provision of negative consequences after a behavior; it is strictly proscribed in SST and BTSAS. No form of therapy promotes the use of punishment, but it often occurs subtly in the form of verbal criticism, negative facial expressions, and comments that imply dissatisfaction or failure. People with schizophrenia and other forms of SPMI seem to be especially sensitive to negative feedback, possibly because they have received so much criticism and failed so often in their lives. Punishment, albeit subtle and indirect, is counterproductive, and leads clients to avoid group, as well as to be noncompliant when they do come.

Shaping

Shaping is the reinforcement of successive steps toward a desired goal, including skilled performance of a particular behavior. Most skills that are taught in SST are too complex and difficult for clients to learn in a single trial. By breaking down complex behavioral routines into simpler steps and teaching the steps one at a time over multiple trials, complex social skills can be *shaped* over time. Similarly, performance can be improved by reinforcing progressively more polished (i.e., skilled) performance. BTSAS therapists use shaping to gradually increase motivation to reduce drug use, and to encourage members to abstain for longer periods of time or in more difficult situations, as well as using it in skills training segments of treatment.

Overlearning

The term *overlearning* refers to the process of repeatedly practicing a skill to the point where it becomes relatively automatic. Clients in SST repeatedly practice targeted social skills in role-plays in the group as well as in homework assignments outside of the group. It is common for new SST therapists to assume that once a group member can perform a behavior in a role-play that the skill is acquired and no more training is required. Nothing could be further from the truth. Clients invariably mimic the therapists during the first one or two role-plays. Only with repeated trials do they try to personalize the skill, and that is when problems become apparent. Moreover, it is much easier to perform a behavior in a structured situation with a supportive therapist than in an unpredicted situation in the community. Skills quickly break down under stress, as evident by the way that professional athletes screw up when the game is on the line, or musicians and actors who are great in rehearsal make errors in front of live audiences. There is also a good deal of forgetting or skill loss between treatment sessions. The essential solution to this problem is repeated practice until the response is so *overlearned* that it can be performed well even in difficult and unexpected situations, and can be maintained without additional practice over time.

Generalization

Generalization is the transfer of skills acquired in one setting to a different setting in which no training was provided. Clearly, training cannot cover every situation the person might encounter in the community. In order for SST to be useful, clients must be able to extrapolate what they have learned in group and use their new skills in community situations. The generalization of social skills is the ultimate test of skills training. There is an old maxim in behavior therapy that generalization should be *programmed*, not *expected*. In other words, the therapists must plan for it. Generalization in SST is programmed in part by giving members homework assignments to practice new skills outside the session in the natural environment. Homework assignments are then reviewed in the subsequent skills training session. In BTSAS homework is subsumed within goal setting and goal review at the beginning of each session, as well as being an explicit part of skills training.

Steps of Social Skills Training

SST requires a considerable amount of work on the part of therapists both before and during skills training groups. A critical first step is to develop a training plan, including a curriculum. Once it is determined what area of social skill will be taught (e.g., conversation skills), complex behavioral repertoires, such as making friends and going on a job interview, are broken down into discrete steps or component elements, similar to the way a music teacher would break a difficult piece of music into simpler segments. Each step is comprised of behaviors: verbal responses, nonverbal responses, and paralinguistic responses. For example, to start a start a conversation you must first gain the other person's attention via introductory remarks ("Hi, is this seat taken?" "Excuse me, does the number 2 bus stop here?"); orienting your body to the person you are addressing; making eye contact; and ending the question with a voice inflection. Maintaining the conversation requires asking general questions (e.g., "How have you been?" "Do you come here often?"); following up on responses with specific questions (e.g., "Did you see the game last night?"); and sharing information with *I* statements (e.g., "I think...," "I feel...," "I like..."). Nonverbal and paralinguistic behaviors are similarly segmented (e.g., make eye contact, shake hands, nod your head). In SST, the person is first taught to perform the elements, and then gradually learns to smoothly combine them through shaping and reinforcement of successive approximations. Behavioral rehearsal is conducted in the form of simulated conversations, or *role-plays*, which are repeated as necessary until the person can perform the response adequately. In keeping with the motor skill metaphor, role-plays are akin to going to the driving range to practice one's golf swing, or playing scales over and over on a musical instrument. Training consists of seven components, which are outlined in Table 4.1. The components are administered in standard sequence, as follows:

Table 4.1 Steps in Social Skills Training

1. Provide a rationale for the skill.
2. Describe the steps of the skill.
3. Model the skill in a role-play.
4. Engage group members in a role-play.
5. Provide positive feedback.
6. Repeat role-plays.
7. Assign homework.

Provide a Rationale For the Skill.

In order to motivate group members to learn a new skill, it is important to provide a justification or rationale for why it is important. This is accomplished in two ways: (1) The therapist provides a brief introduction explaining in simple terms why the behavior is important; and (2) examples are solicited from group members of how lack of the skill led to problems, or how the skill was used effectively to help the person achieve a goal. With most groups, a combination of both strategies is most effective. The rationale provided by therapists should focus on pragmatic issues that are relevant for group members, not on abstractions or moral arguments. For example, "When you want someone to stop asking you to get high with them it is most effective to be direct and tell them clearly that you do not want to use. Today we are going to work on how to say 'No' when someone asks you to use with them." Rationales should also be relatively brief: long winded lectures, let alone sermons, are useless at best, and counterproductive at worst.

Reasons for learning a new skill can be elicited from group members by asking leading questions about the importance of the skill. For example, when teaching the skill "Starting Conversations," the leader can pose questions such as: "Why is it important to be able to start a conversation?" In some groups throwing this type of question out to group members will elicit responses. In other groups such questions are greeted by silence, and it is more effective to direct questions to individual members, as with, "Raphael, can you think of why it is important to learn how to start conversations with other people?" When using this approach it is important that members not feel put on the spot. Therapists should turn to other members if the person seems to be uncomfortable or unable to provide a response. In addition, it is important to provide social reinforcement for effort, even if a response is not helpful. It can also be helpful to ask questions regarding the disadvantages of *not* using a specific skill. For example, when developing a rationale for saying "Thank you," the therapist might ask, "What do you think would happen if someone you know did you several favors and you never said anything to him about it? How would that make him feel?" Asking group members about the disadvantages of not using a skill is another way of helping them see the advantages of learning that skill.

Describe the Steps of the Skill

Once the group has a general understanding of what the skill is and why it is important, the leader describes each step of the skill. Every skill that is taught in SST is broken down into a series of discrete steps, as illustrated in Table 4.2. There are typically four to six steps, the first being "Make eye contact," and the last being a way to end the interaction; for example, "Give a reason and say goodbye." The steps of the skill are written on a poster or whiteboard so members can easily refer to them while role-playing. Members also receive a handout with the same information, which they can take with them or keep in a

Table 4.2 Steps in the Skill, Starting a Conversation

1. Look at the person.
2. Say hello and introduce yourself if you do not know the person.
3. Ask a general question:
   e.g., "Hi, how are you doing?"
   "Hi Tom, what's new?"
   "Hey Mary, how have you been?"
4. Ask a specific question related to what the person has said.
5. Give a reason for leaving and say goodbye
   e.g., "Well, I have to go to group now. See you later."

loose-leaf binder for future reference. As with providing the initial rationale for the skill, the leader briefly discusses each step of the skill, eliciting from group members the importance of each step or directly explaining it. When discussing the steps, the leader points to the step on the poster or flip chart.

Model the Skill in a Role-Play

Once the steps of the skill are described, the therapist demonstrates, or *models* the skill in a role-play. We customarily conduct SST groups (and BTSAS groups) with two therapists, in which case they do the modeling demonstration with one another. If there is only one therapist, she can invite one of the group members to help. The modeling demonstration is intended to help participants see how the different components of the skill fit together into an overall response that is socially effective. This helps translate the abstract steps of the skill into a concrete reality. The role-play situations selected for modeling should have high relevance to most group members. Notably, these role-plays should be brief and to the point. Often neophyte therapists get a bit carried away and role-play an extended social encounter, rather than demonstrating the steps of the skill in a simple and straightforward manner. These extended demonstrations are counterproductive because members lose track of what they are supposed to be observing. More extended role-play, which demonstrates nuances, should be reserved for later in the process, after members have mastered the basic steps of the skill. Before beginning the role-play, the therapist prompts the group members to look for the steps of the skill, and after the demonstration she reviews the steps. It is often useful to ask individual members if they observed particular steps; for example, "Shawn, did I ask a general question? What question did I ask?"

Engage Group Members in Role-Play

After the therapists model the skill the focus shifts to group members, who begin taking turns role-playing and getting feedback on their performance. When a skill is first introduced, it is preferable for participants to practice the skill using the same role-play situation that was modeled by the leaders. The purpose of these initial role-plays is to familiarize participants with the specific steps of the skill; variations are introduced after they develop some proficiency. Of course, it is always desirable to tailor situations to the individual member to insure that the training is relevant. Consequently, minor alterations, such as having the participant identify a specific person with whom the situation might occur or a specific question she would like to practice asking, are appropriate.

The first role-plays should be conducted with a group member from whom the therapist can anticipate cooperation and who will be able to perform the skill. This enables more skilled group members to serve as role-models for less skilled group members. The therapists should invite a specific member to role-play, rather than offering the open-ended question, "Who wants to do a role-play?" Making a direct request is usually more effective at engaging clients than waiting for a volunteer. Participants in role-plays are requested to stand up or move their chair to the center of the group, rather than role-playing from their seat. This increases the likelihood that the role-play will seem like a real behavioral interaction. The person role-playing then returns to her seat after the role-play is completed. Thus, a specific physical space in the group is reserved for active role-playing. The strategy of repositioning role-play participants has the added advantage of introducing an element of theater or drama. By increasing the theatrical quality of role-plays, the leader can attract the attention of less interested or more cognitively impaired clients.

Before beginning, the therapist asks the person to review what the role-play scenario will be, and then has him repeat the steps of the skill (usually by reading from the whiteboard). It is helpful to have the whiteboard in the person's view during the role-play in case he forgets one of the steps. Group members are prompted to see if the role-player performs each step. As with modeling displays, the therapist should stick close to the script, and not make the task more difficult by improvising. The goal of the role-play is to have the person be successful, even if the performance is imperfect. If the person gets stuck, the therapist should provide a prompt by referring to the whiteboard. In all situations the therapist should respond in a cooperative manner within the role (e.g., agree to a request; accept an apology), so the person is reinforced for effort.

Role-play does not always work smoothly. Problems are especially likely to arise with group members who have very poor skills or who have significant cognitive impairment. These individuals often get stuck or lost during role-plays, losing track of what they are supposed to be doing, or being unable to get past particular steps of the skill. Two strategies are especially useful in these situations: coaching and prompting.

Coaching

Coaching refers to the use of verbal prompts during role-plays to provide guidance about how the specific components of a skill should be performed, or to give suggestions when the person is stuck. Coaching is most often used when verbal instructions before the role-play are unsuccessful in producing the desired response. Rather than simply providing additional verbal instructions and hoping that the participant will be able to do better in the next role-play, the therapist helps the person through the role-play by providing verbal prompts during the interaction. This works best when the group is directed by two therapists. One therapist serves as role-play partner, and the other stands next to the group member and whispers instructions to her as needed. A coach might whisper something like, "Remember to tell him how you feel," or "Now ask him a question." The goal of coaching is to enable the person to have some success, rather than continued failure experiences. Coaching is gradually *faded out* (systematically decreased across role-plays), until the person can perform the skill without help.

Prompting

Prompting is a form of coaching that is used when all the person needs to perform a response effectively is a reminder. Rather than whispering instructions in the person's ear or giving him a suggestion about what to say next, prompting is a simple reminder or cue. It is often used for changing nonverbal and paralinguistic features of social skill, such as eye contact and voice volume. Typically, the therapist will work out signals with the person before the role-play, such as pointing to his or her eye to indicate that the participant should increase eye contact. Written signs can also be used, such as holding up a piece of paper saying "Louder" or "Softer," for members who need help with voice volume. As with coaching, prompting is faded out across role-plays.

Provide Positive Feedback

Role-play rehearsals are always followed by positive feedback. Ideally, the person did well and enthusiastic positive comments will come naturally. However, feedback must always positive, even if the performance was markedly flawed. Feedback should not be dishonest or disingenuous. Something positive can always be found, even in the poorest role-play performance. At a minimum, the person can be reinforced for effort; for example, "Good try Tom, I saw you looking at the board and trying to get the steps in." It is typical for the person to have included some steps, even if they could not do them all, so feedback might be, "Nice job. You had good eye contact and I could tell you had something important to say." It is also frequently possible to reinforce improvement; for example, "Good job Susan, you definitely spoke louder that time." Whether performance was marginal or excellent, feedback should be specific as well as positive.

Positive feedback should also be elicited from other group members. This keeps all members involved because they pay more attention when they know they may be called on to provide input. Also, the value of positive comments from peers differs from the value of positive comments by therapists. Useful questions to ask in order to elicit positive feedback take the form, "Mina, what did you like about the way—did that skill just now?" and Juan, which steps of the skill did you see—doing?" The therapists should be vigilant to ensure that all feedback given at this stage is positive. Negative or corrective feedback is quickly interrupted as the goal is to reinforce the member's effort in the role-play and to prove some specific feedback about what was done well. Members soon learn that positive feedback always precedes corrective feedback, and this rapidly becomes accepted as a group norm.

The feedback provided by group members is usually supplemented by additional comments from the leader in order to highlight important points. Feedback should be as specific as possible. It may pertain to the specific steps of the skill identified on the board, or other specific nonverbal and paralinguistic skills. At this point corrective feedback may be introduced to begin improving the participant's performance. Corrective feedback should be as noncritical and as behaviorally specific as possible. It also should not include an exhaustive list of all the problems in the person's performance. The aim is to identify the most essential aspects of the role-play interaction that need to be changed in order to enhance overall performance. Typically, it should focus on one, or at most two, steps of the skill at a time. Examples of appropriate corrective feedback include, "Anna, I noticed that you had good eye contact but it was hard to hear what you were saying. It would be better if you could speak more loudly"; or "Nice job Mark. You got most of the steps in. Let's do it again, and this time try to remember to give a reason before you say goodbye." Subtle changes or refinements are left for a later stage, after the basics are mastered, or are omitted entirely. A key criterion for the therapists to use in providing corrective feedback is: what is the minimal level of skill required for the person to achieve her goal in the situation? What do they need to add (or subtract) to achieve their goal? It is counterproductive to focus on social nuances with most people with SPMI, who often have difficulty having basic needs met in social interactions.

Repeat Role-Plays

Following corrective feedback (or positive feedback if no correction is required) the participant is engaged in another role-play of the same situation. The person is prompted to focus on behavioral elements needing correction. The role-play is followed by positive and corrective feedback, as with the first rehearsal. A third role-play then generally follows. If the person is making progress, the therapist can indicate that she will make the task a bit more difficult; for example, by initially refusing a request. Alternatively, the scenario might be modified. If the person continues to have difficulty, the same situation is repeated and the therapist does not do anything to make the interaction more difficult.

At this juncture the leader must make a decision about whether to engage the individual in additional role-plays of the same situation, to change the scenario, or to move on to the next group member. Several factors enter into this decision. The first and most critical factor is how the person is responding to the procedure. If she appears to be frustrated or fatigued it is best to move on to another group member. If no improvement has taken place, or if the person has done extremely well, it is also reasonable to move to another member. Conversely, if the person has shown modest progress and may benefit from consolidation of gains with another trial, then a fourth role-play is warranted. The therapist should also consider the rest of the group in making this decision. If other members appear bored or distracted, or if there is not much time left in group, it might be wise to move on so everyone gets at least some opportunity to role-play.

The training format is established with the first group member and continues with each of the other members of the group, in turn. The same principles of role-play, feedback, and praise for even small improvements are applied with each group member. It is typical that members enter group with different skill levels. Just as the content of role-plays is adjusted to individual needs, the level of difficulty is adjusted. Some members may need work on basic skills and others in the same group can role-play very sophisticated interactions. The task for the therapists is to make sure that everyone has an opportunity to participate and to learn. No one should be slighted due to too little or too much skill.

Assign Homework

At the end of each session, the therapist assigns homework to each group member to practice the skill covered in that session. The importance of homework cannot be overemphasized. While role-playing during group gives members the opportunity to practice new social skills, generalizing these skills to real-world settings is crucial to the success of training. That will only happen if members practice their newly developed skills in the community. In order to maximize the chances that a homework assignment will be completed, it is important that it be clear, as specific as possible, and within the realm of the person's ability. Individualizing homework assignments is essential in order to facilitate follow-through. Group members should be asked to identify specific situations in which they could practice the skill, rather than instructing them in a general way to practice the skill on their own. The assignment includes when and where the behavior will be practiced, as well as what the behavior is. The assignment is written down and each member leaves group with a personalized homework sheet.

SST sessions begin with a review of the homework assignment given at the end of the previous session. The therapist asks each member in turn to report on their experience with homework: if they tried to do it, and how it went. Sufficient information is elicited to determine if the person actually did the assignment or is merely reporting success. If the therapist concludes that the person actually did the homework she provides social reinforcement. If the person did not complete the assignment the therapist attempts to determine why not, and engages in problem solving to help circumvent problems that might recur. The group member is then invited to role-play the assignment with the therapist, and the importance of doing homework is underscored. In any case, the person should not be censured for failure to complete assignments.

GROUP STRUCTURE

SST groups are limited to six to eight members. The small-group format is essential so that each participant has an adequate opportunity to rehearse. Larger groups may appear to be cost efficient in many clinical centers, but they are counterproductive for people with SPMI because in large groups those clients do not receive enough individualized practice and coaching. Teaching must be tailored to the individual: the content of role-plays, pace of training, and criteria for progress each vary according to ability. For example, one group member might role-play saying no to a simple request, while a less impaired peer might learn to negotiate and compromise. One member may need three role-plays to reach an adequate level, while another member might need 10. One member might need special assistance remembering what to say, while another might have more difficulty with nonverbal or paralinguistic parameters, such as making eye contact or speaking loudly enough to be heard.

The content of skills training programs is organized into *curricula*, analogous to courses in school.

Examples include: conversational skills, job interview skills, medication management (how to communicate with health care providers), dating skills, and safe sex skills. Each curriculum is divided into teaching units or classes. For example, the program on conversation skills includes: starting conversations, maintaining conversations, ending conversations, making requests, refusing unreasonable requests, negotiation, and compromise. Each skill to be taught is broken down into specific steps or elements, as illustrated in Table 4.2 for the steps in the skill "Starting a Conversation."

The steps in Table 4.2 represent the minimum required for a brief conversation, and even this simple sequence often proves difficult for impaired people with SPMI. Once the person can perform these steps adequately, more complexity is added, and the interactions are extended through more back and forth responses. Higher functioning members may begin training at a more sophisticated level.

The duration of a group can range from four to eight sessions for a very circumscribed skill, to six months to two years for a comprehensive program. BTSAS lasts for six months, of which four to five months are devoted to training skills needed to decrease drug use. Regardless of duration, training sessions are typically held three to five times per week. Training is structured so as to minimize demands on neurocognitive capacity, especially attention and memory. Extensive use is made of visual aides. Instructions are presented in handouts and on flip charts or whiteboards as well as delivered orally. Material is presented in brief units, and there is frequent repetition and review. Group members are regularly required to verbalize what is being taught and what they are supposed to do during role-plays (e.g., the steps of a skill, what the person will say), rather than simply being allowed to provide minimal responses to yes-no questions. For example, "Joan, can you tell us why it is good to ask general questions?" as opposed to, "Joan do you understand why we need to ask general questions?"

EMPIRICAL SUPPORT FOR SOCIAL SKILLS TRAINING

There have been at least eight narrative reviews and four meta-analyses of the empirical literature on SST published in peer reviewed (English language) journals since 1990; see Bellack for a review of this literature (2004). These reviews employed different inclusion criteria, and did not all cover the same papers. One review concluded that SST was not substantially effective, but the others were all quite positive. The positive reviews each reached relatively similar conclusions. First, SST is not effective for reducing symptoms or preventing relapse. Second, SST has a reliable and significant effect on behavioral skills. Third, SST has a positive impact on social role functioning, although the findings in this area are not entirely consistent. The results are better for specific skills areas such as conversation skills or medication management, than for more general measures of social functioning. Fourth, SST has a positive impact on consumer satisfaction and self-efficacy: people in skills training feel more self-confident in (targeted) social situations after training. These general findings are reflected in the 2002 PORT recommendation for treatment of schizophrenia (Lehman, 2002): Patients with schizophrenia should be offered skills training, the key elements of which include behaviorally based instruction, modeling, corrective feedback, contingent social reinforcement, and homework assignments.

SUMMARY

This chapter provided an overview of social skills training, a treatment strategy that forms the basis of BTSAS. SST is a well-established treatment approach that was developed in the 1970s. It is based on social learning theory, and emphasizes teaching rather than conversation to change behavior. Complex social behaviors are broken down into component elements, including verbal responses, nonverbal responses, and paralinguistic responses. These elements are then taught in a model analogous to motor skills, such as playing a sport or learning to play a musical instrument. Key elements of training include instructions, modeling, role-play rehearsal, feedback, and homework. As with motor behavior, repetitive practice is essential if behavior is to be mastered. Practice in SST is conducted through role-play, in which group members enact simulated social encounters with a therapist or another group member. Many people with SPMI are sensitive to negative feedback, so a key premise of SST is to couch all feedback in positive terms. Difficult behaviors are gradually *shaped* by reinforcing successive approximations of the complete behavioral repertoire. There is an extensive empirical literature in support of SST. It is one of the most effective treatments available and has been recommended as an evidence-based practice by the Schizophrenia PORT.

Chapter **5**

ASSESSMENT STRATEGIES

INTRODUCTION

BTSAS is designed for clients with SPMI who abuse substances. In addition to the treatment strategies that make up BTSAS, another critical component of this intervention is assessment. Substance use and abuse, substance-related consequences, motivation to change, and treatment utilization are important areas of change within the BTSAS program. Accurate assessment of these domains is critical both clinically and empirically. Clinically, assessment allows us to monitor progress over the course of a client's involvement in BTSAS and to keep current with the successes a client makes as well as new areas of difficulty that emerge over time. Empirically, accurate assessment is integral to the study of how BTSAS works and to a determination of which components are most effective for which types of clients.

There are numerous challenges that we face in attempting to perform accurate assessment of substance abuse and related constructs in clients with SPMI. Consequently, there are to date few measures designed specifically to assess substance use patients with SPMI.

ISSUES IN THE ASSESSMENT OF SUBSTANCE ABUSE IN SPMI

There are a number of issues related to SPMI, the assessor, and the measures that make assessment of substance use in SPMI patients challenging.

Illness Related Factors

Assessment of substance use disorders and related domains in SPMI is difficult due to factors associated with SPMI. Diagnosis is especially difficult because substance use and withdrawal can resemble psychiatric disorders (Schuckit, 1983). For example, long-term alcohol use and withdrawal can lead to psychotic symptoms, and abuse of amphetamines often results in psychotic symptoms that are identical to schizophrenia. People experiencing withdrawal from cocaine often report severe depression. Because symptoms of substance use and withdrawal can resemble SPMI symptoms, differential diagnosis can be confounded. In addition, there is overlap of diagnostic criteria between substance use disorders and

SPMI. For example, DSM-IV lists problems in social functioning as symptoms of both schizophrenia and substance use disorders (American Psychiatric Association, 1994). That some criteria can count toward multiple diagnoses can potentially increase comorbidity rates and can make diagnosis of substance use disorders difficult. Importantly, it is hard to apply DSM-IV criteria to substance use disorder in SPMI. To meet a diagnosis of dependence, a client must report three of nine mostly behaviorally based criteria (trying to quit, use despite knowledge of consequences, give up or decrease important activities, lots of time spent obtaining drugs or using or recovering). Abuse is also a pattern of behavioral involvement (use in risky situations, use despite its effects on social, occupational, or physical functioning). Many SPMI patients don't meet these diagnoses because they don't have jobs, activities, or relationships that are disturbed by their substance use. It is also difficult to determine the impact of substance use and abuse when SPMI profoundly affects most areas of functioning. Clients with SPMI have a range of impairments in social, cognitive, occupational, and psychological functioning, and it is difficult to evaluate the negative impact of substance use disorders on patients whose functioning is so poor to begin with. Finally, it can be very difficult for SPMI patients to participate in and concentrate on a lengthy assessment of substance abuse, and there is evidence that clients with SPMI may underreport substance use and abuse. Patients with substance abuse and SPMI experience a range of cognitive and social deficits that can result in their providing unreliable or inaccurate information, or minimizing their substance use, especially if they have much to lose by admitting to or honestly discussing their substance use, such as services, benefits, or child custody (Ridgely, Goldman, & Willenbring, 1990).

Assessor Related Factors

Assessment is also affected by the interviewer and the treatment system in which assessment occurs. Patients with SPMI and substance abuse experience numerous points of entry to the treatment system, including emergency rooms, mental health clinics, substance abuse treatment centers, and other community care facilities, making it difficult to obtain information on substance abuse in any standardized fashion. For example, a patient presenting at an ER for psychotic symptoms will get a different assessment from a patient presenting at an outpatient mental health clinic, and a patient presenting for intake at a substance abuse treatment facility would get still another assessment. In addition, SPMI patients show high rates of treatment nonattendance, dropout, and sporadic attendance, making it difficult to obtain complete information. Importantly, substance abuse and mental illness historically have been viewed as separate problems, and the service systems designed to address these disorders developed relatively independently (Grella, 1996; Polcin, 1992; Ridgely, Lambert, Goodman, Chichester, & Ralph, 1998). Consequently, mental health treatment providers are often not trained to assess substance abuse, and often fail to detect substance abuse among SPMI patients (Albanese, Bartel, Bruno, Morgenbesser, & Schatzberg, 1994; Breakey, Calabrese, Rosenblatt, & Crum, 1998; Drake et al., 1990; Wilkins, Shaner, Patterson, Setoda, & Gorelick, 1991). Importantly, studies find that when mental health staff are properly trained, they are competent in assessing and identifying alcohol and drug use and associated problems, and often have access to more detailed and valuable information than can be gathered with a brief self-report measure (Drake et al., 1990).

Measures Related Factors

Most measures of substance use were developed with higher functioning populations. It is unclear how relevant these measures are to clients with SPMI. Although some studies have found these measures to perform adequately in psychiatric populations (Appleby, Dyson, Altman, McGovern, & Luchins, 1996; Appleby, Dyson, Altman, & Luchins, 1997; Cocco & Carey, 1998), others have found that some of the measures most widely used in primary substance abusing populations perform poorly in dually diagnosed samples (Carey, Cocco, & Correia, 1997; Lehman, Myers, Dixon, & Johnson, 1996; Toland & Moss, 1989; Zanis, McLellan, & Corse, 1997). Measures developed on less impaired populations can be problematic both in the information that they gather and in the language that is used to gather it. In terms of content, such assessments may fail to tap domains or experiences that are relevant to patients with SPMI, but may not impact other populations of substance abusers. For example, issues related to medications, side effects, and psychotic symptoms are often intimately related to substance use and abuse in SPMI patients and yet are not widely included in assessment measures. Corse and colleagues (Corse, Herschinger, & Zanis, 1995) found that measures designed for primary substance abusers may fail to capture the severity of problems experienced by patients with SPMI, and may focus on certain substance-related problems that are more pertinent to a higher functioning population (family or social conflicts) and neglect others that are more relevant to lower functioning patients (using substances to relieve social isolation). In addition, existing measures may fail to tap patterns of use and abuse that are uniquely relevant to SPMI patients. Generally, people with SPMI use and abuse lower quantities of drugs than other populations of substance abusers, yet experience comparable levels of negative consequences related to this use (Lehman, Myers, Dixon, & Johnson, 1994, 1996; Mueser et al., 1990). Measures designed for primary substance abusing populations may not have the flexibility to capture patterns of use that are clearly problematic for SPMI patients. Relatedly, most measures are designed to be used cross-sectionally and to assess whether problems have ever occurred in a patient's life or over some long period of time such as the last year. However, SPMI patients tend to cycle in and out of use, heavy use, and abuse; thus a measurement at one point may not accurately reflect substance use over a longer period.

In terms of language, the cognitive and neurological deficits that are commonly seen in SPMI patients may preclude their understanding measures that were designed for less impaired individuals. SPMI patients have deficits in attention, memory, and higher level cognitive processes, such as abstract reasoning and other "executive" functions (Bellack, Gold, & Buchanan, 1999) that undoubtedly impact their ability to understand measures that were developed for patients without cognitive impairment. For example, some measures utilize complex, open-ended questions or use fairly sophisticated language, both qualities that will make for difficulties when using them with patients with cognitive impairment. Some measures also incorporate shifting time-frames, asking patients to remember use or treatment involvement in any number of periods, some of which can be fairly removed in time from the actual assessment. Given the cognitive and memory limitations of many patients with SPMI, shifting assessment time-frames and asking patients to report on information that occurred months or years before can make accurate assessment difficult.

Implications

Given these challenges, selecting the points in treatment when assessments are done, as well as the measures that are used, is extremely important. Ideally assessments would be done frequently and by professionals who have some background knowledge in working with SPMI clients. In addition, the measures used should either be ones that are designed for the SPMI population or show relevance and utility with these clients. Measures should also take into account the unique domains and patterns seen in SPMI substance abusers as well as use language that is simple and easy to understand.

Use of Assessment in BTSAS

Assessment is used at different points in the BTSAS program and for different purposes. We consider there to be four main points of assessment during the six months of BTSAS: (1) Referral to BTSAS; (2) start of treatment/first motivational interview; (3) during treatment; and (4) end of treatment. Table 5.1 summarizes options for assessment at each of these points.

Table 5.1 Recommended Assessment Points and Options

Time point	Domains to assess	Interview options	Self-report options	Other options
Referral to BTSAS	SPMI diagnosis; Substance use disorder diagnosis Recent use Recent consequences DALI	SCID DIS Clinical interview Intake interview ASI	TLFB MAST DAST	Urinalysis Collateral reports Chart review
Start of treatment; First MI	General functioning Motivation to change	SUESS BQOL Abstinence self-efficacy scale Readiness ruler	URICA Decisional balance	Collateral reports
Assessment during treatment	Drug use Attendance group participation		Ask client during group	Urinalysis at each session Ratings of participation
End of treatment and follow-up	Recent use Recent consequences General functioning Motivation to change	ASI DALI SUESS BQOL Decisional balance Abstinence Self-efficacy scale Readiness ruler	TLFB MAST DAST URICA	Urinalysis Collateral reports

REFERRAL TO BTSAS

Assessment truly begins when a client is referred to the BTSAS program. The assessment at this point is geared toward ensuring that a client is appropriate for the BTSAS program. Because BTSAS is designed for clients with both SPMI and substance use disorders, it is important to ensure that clients who are referred to the program in fact have some form of SPMI and some substance use disorder. Clients in BTSAS are generally lower functioning than primary substance abusers. While a primary substance abuser will certainly not be harmed by attending BTSAS, it is important to be sure that clients in the BTSAS program are those for whom the program is intended. While criteria for entry into the BTSAS program will differ by treatment setting, several of the most important characteristics of appropriate BTSAS clients are: (1) some form of SPMI; (2) some substance use disorder (abuse or dependence); (3) recent substance use and consequences; and (4) ability and willingness to participate in the intervention. Clients do not have to accept that they have a problem or express a desire to stop using drugs in order to participate in BTSAS. Many clients will be ambivalent about changing their drug use. Others may be referred due to legal troubles or at the insistence of their mental health treatment team and so may not even be considering any changes in their drug use. While clients must be able and willing to attend groups, they do not have to be ready to change their patterns of drug use.

ASSESSMENT OF SPMI AND SUBSTANCE USE DISORDERS

SPMI can be defined in many different ways. We use a definition based on criteria developed by Lehman and colleagues (1997) that includes: (1) a diagnosis of schizophrenia, schizoaffective disorder, or other severe mental disorder including bipolar disorder, major depression, or severe anxiety disorder; (2) the patient has worked 25% or less of the past year; or (3) the patient receives payment for mental disability (SSI, SSDI, VA disability benefits). Adherence to these criteria ensure that clients not only meet diagnostic criteria for a disorder, but also that the disorder has some impact on his or her functioning. It is important that clients have a true SPMI, rather than some transient SPMI-like symptoms due to substance use or withdrawal that will remit once acute withdrawal symptoms are gone.

There are several methods and measures for assessing SPMI and substance use disorder diagnoses. Structured clinical interviews such as the Structured Clinical Interview for DSM-IV (First, Spitzer, Gibbon, & Williams, 1994) are the most reliable way to gather diagnostic information on both SPMI and substance use disorders. These sorts of interviews, which are linked to DSM criteria, have undergone extensive standardization and revision and so are highly reliable when done well. These features make structured clinical interviews a good option for intervention research, as well as in cases in which there are precise and limited criteria for entry into the BTSAS program. However, structured clinical interviews are time consuming and require highly trained interviewers for administration rather than lay professionals—a big disadvantage in real-world clinical settings.

In situations where exact and specific inclusion criteria are not an issue, use of a less structured clinical or intake interview to establish SPMI and substance use disorder diagnoses is preferable. This is fairly straightforward in terms of SPMI diagnoses. For example, referring patients to a BTSAS group at a community mental health center requires only that someone talk with the client and gather information on symptom type and duration that can be used to generate a DSM diagnosis. As this is standard practice at most clinics and settings that serve patients with SPMI, using information gained from the admission interview and other contents of the client's medical record is likely to be sufficient to establish an SPMI diagnosis. However, the medical record often is less precise when it comes to determining a substance use disorder diagnosis. Although chart reviews have the advantage of using collateral sources of information (records from other treatment settings, information from other treatment providers and family members), the information in the medical record is subject to variation depending on what is actually placed in the chart. Oftentimes SPMI patients, who typically enter treatment with a number of pressing issues, are not asked about their substance use at intake. Because not all information is recorded in the medical record, reviews can underestimate rates of substance abuse among SPMI clients.

Assessment of Recent Use

BTSAS is designed for clients who are current drug users. "Current" can mean different things to different people, depending on the treatment setting and the nature of drug use among the clients. It is important to figure out what substance use behavior you as the therapist are most interested in treating, and the time-frame that is most important to you, and to tailor the assessment accordingly. For example, is any drug use problematic in a particular client population, or is the focus on drug use that has negative consequences associated with it? If the latter, is the therapist only interested in those clients with the most severe substance-related problems (substance dependence), or is he or she also interested in those who show less severe but still regular consequences of drug use (substance abuse)? Is the interest focused on clients who are using every day, or is a client also of interest who has monthly binges that are tied to receiving money at the start of each month? Some clients may have achieved some block of abstinence, but that abstinence is fragile and triggers for relapse are substantial. All of these sorts of factors need to be considered when setting up a BTSAS program and selecting measures for assessment.

Based on our experience in developing and administering the BTSAS program, we can provide some guidelines regarding the degree of current use and consequences that is appropriate for a BTSAS referral. First, we have found that among SPMI clients, most use is problematic use. That is, there is less variation than one would find among non-SPMI individuals in terms of degree of harm associated with drug use. Few SPMI clients use drugs recreationally; most use drugs to cope with symptoms, negative affect, or cravings. While there are SPMI clients who may smoke marijuana occasionally and without great consequence, our experience has been that the majority of crack, powder cocaine, long-term marijuana, and heroin use among SPMI clients generates a range of problems including poor illness management, failure to regularly take neuroleptic medications, and instability of housing and other forms of support. Second, we have found that a six-month window for current use with some consequences is a good one in terms of capturing a large group of clients for whom substance use is problematic. Clients who use drugs daily would clearly be captured in this group, as would clients whose pattern of use is more sporadic but problematic nonetheless. For example, many SPMI clients have little or no money most of the time but engage in drug binges at the beginning of the month when they receive SSI or SSDI payments. Such a regular and harmful pattern of use (all money for the month is gone; bingeing is a particularly dangerous form of drug use) would be captured within a six-month definition of "current" use. Third, clients who have not used in six months could be considered stably abstinent. While these clients may benefit from ongoing support and problem solving in order to assist them in maintaining their abstinence, a focused and intensive group such as BTSAS is not appropriate in such cases.

There are several ways to assess recent drug use. It is important to remember that clients may minimize or be untruthful about the full extent of their use. As discussed earlier, reasons for minimizing use range from symptoms of SPMI that impact memory or cause confusion to fears of losing housing or money. Whatever the case, it is important to ask questions regarding current use in a safe and non-judgmental manner, and to reassure clients that disclosure will not lead to punishment. Under such circumstances, it is often the most helpful to just ask the client a few simple questions about his or her recent use, such as:

What drugs to you use?
Which drug do you use the most often?
How often do you use this drug?
When was the last time you used this drug?

It is then useful to summarize the information the client has provided in response to these questions, to make sure that you are correct: "You have told me that you use crack, and that these days you are using crack about once per week. Also, you said that the last time you used crack was about two days ago. Does this all sound about right?"

A more standardized method for assessing recent substance use is the Time-Line Follow-Back method (TLFB; Sobell & Sobell, 1992). The TLFB requires the client to reconstruct his or her substance use on a day-to-day basis using a calendar, and can include assessment of multiple substances (drugs and alcohol) at the same time. This method allows for a summary of the primary dimensions of substance use: amount, frequency, pattern, and degree of variability. The TLFB has been shown to have good reliability and validity. Reports of the same period tend to be replicable over time, and generally good agreement has been found between self- and collaterals' reports of use and between self- and official reports of arrests and hospitalizations. Carey et al. (1997) have reported comparable results for psychiatric patients with psychotic disorders. A 30-day period is generally evaluated so as to provide an index of recent substance use behavior and to focus on a period of time that should enhance accuracy of recall. If the window for program entry is six months, it would be important to establish that the most recent month assessed with the TLFB is representative of the previous six months, and if not, in what ways use has changed over that period of time.

Other means of assessment, such as laboratory and urine tests and collateral reports, are also available to assess recent drug use. Biological tests can be extremely useful in promoting accurate self-report of use. That is, clients are more likely to report recent drug use if they know that they are receiving a urine test that will be positive for drugs. However, most substances stay in the system for one to three days, so that a client can have a negative test and still have used recently (false negative). Our experience is that biological testing is useful as a component of a comprehensive substance use assessment. Collateral reports, including information provided by family members or other treatment professionals, is also a good source of information about a client's behavior in the natural environment. Counselors and case managers in particular often have in-depth knowledge of clients and their substance use that can be especially helpful (see Carey & Correia, 1998, for a review), while information from relatives can contain biases due to relatives' attributions and feelings about a client's illness and substance use.

Assessment of Substance Related Negative Consequences

There are a number of relatively brief self-report measures that can be used to assess substance related negative consequences. Probably the most widely used assessments for substance use in SPMI are brief self-report measures, including the Michigan Alcoholism Screening Test (MAST; Selzer, 1971) and the Drug Abuse Screening Test (DAST; Skinner, 1982). Both are brief lists of consequences for alcohol and drug use (25–28 items); and clients are asked if they are ever experienced any of these problems. Both are easy to score, and studies have shown that a cutoff of 5 is indicative of problem use. Some research with the MAST has shown good sensitivity and specificity, and moderate psychometric properties with SPMI populations (Searles, Alterman, & Purtill, 1990), while others have found poorer psychometric functioning in SPMI clients (Drake et al., 1990). One study showed good psychometric properties of the DAST with psychiatric patients (Cocco & Carey, 1998). The Alcohol Use Disorders Identification Test (AUDIT; Saunders, Aasland, Babor, De La Fuente, & Grant, 1993) is another brief (10 items) measure that taps consumption, drinking behavior, and alcohol related problems. The AUDIT has shown good reliability and validity in SPMI clients (Dawe et al., 2000). Importantly, all of these self-report measures were developed and normed on less severe populations so their applicability to clients with SPMI, as well as their reliability and validity with this population, is not fully established. Also, some of these measures may be too complex for SPMI patients. For example, some clients are unable to read and so would be unable to complete these sorts of self-report instruments. Our practice is to read these questionnaires to our patients; however, we do not know if such procedural changes impact the performance of these measures in our SPMI clients.

INTERVIEW MEASURES OF RECENT USE AND CONSEQUENCES

There are several interview measures that assess both use and consequences. The most widely used of these is the Addiction Severity Index (ASI; McLellan, Luborsky, Woody, & O'Brien, 1980; McLellan, Kushner et al., 1992), a structured clinical interview designed to assess the severity of addiction-related problems experienced in seven areas: medical, legal, drug abuse, alcohol abuse, employment, family, and psychiatric that has been used extensively in substance abuse research (e.g., Carroll, Power, Bryant, & Rounsaville, 1993; McClellan et al., 1980; McClellan, Luborsky, Woody, O'Brien, & Druley, 1983). While the ASI has become the standard measure of substance use and consequences for most substance abuse treatment providers, there is evidence that it performs less well with SPMI clients. For example, Lehman et al. (1996) found that the ASI missed approximately 20% of cases of substance use disorder identified through structured diagnostic interview, and several other studies have similarly found that the ASI performs less well in psychiatrically impaired populations (Carey, Cocco, & Correia, 1997; Corse, Herschinger, & Zanis, 1995; Zanis, McLellan, & Corse, 1997).

There have been a few attempts to develop measures of alcohol and drug use designed for SPMI patients. Rosenberg and colleagues (1998) developed the Dartmouth Assessment of Lifestyle Instrument (DALI), a brief screen for substance use disorders in psychiatric patients. The DALI was developed by identifying, via logistic regression in samples of patients with psychiatric disorders, the most useful items for classification from many of the widely used substance use disorder screens that were developed for primary substance abusers, including the MAST and the DAST. The DALI is brief, can be used in a range of settings by different types of professionals, and shows a high degree of classification (Rosenberg et al., 1998). However, it cannot provide in-depth assessment of substance use and associated problems in SPMI patients: it assesses only alcohol, marijuana, and cocaine; it was designed on a rural and primarily Caucasian population; and its brevity limits the amount of information that can be gathered regarding quantity and frequency of use.

An Integrated Assessment for BTSAS Referrals

To sum up, the main domains to be assessed at referral to BTSAS are diagnoses of SPMI and substance use disorder to ensure appropriateness of referral, and recent drug use and consequences. In order to quickly determine SPMI and substance use disorder diagnoses, we recommend the following approach. First, the intake should include a discussion of symptoms of both SPMI and substance use disorders. Intake interviewers should be trained to assess the DSM criteria for substance use disorders (both abuse and dependence), and there should be some section of the intake evaluation to record this information. Of particular importance is to establish that clients have both SPMI and substance use disorder, and to pay special attention to making sure that symptoms of SPMI are not merely secondary to drug use. Second, it is useful to have both a discussion of recent use and consequences, as well as to have clients complete a brief questionnaire measure of drug-related negative consequences.

We find it particularly helpful to have clients first complete a brief questionnaire about consequences they have experienced, and then review the clients' responses as a way to generate discussion of substance-related negative consequences. The combination of measures is beneficial because a questionnaire can include a longer list of consequences than a clinician can remember to ask about, and clients are often more willing to report consequences when asked about them in a questionnaire format. In addition, a urinalysis test for drug use should accompany this assessment of recent use, both to objectively test use over the last few days, as well as to improve clients' report of their recent use. The BTSAS therapist should have some contact with the client's mental health treatment team and get their perspective on the client's substance use at the point when they make a referral to the BTSAS program.

START OF TREATMENT/FIRST MOTIVATIONAL INTERVIEW

Once it has been determined that the client has SPMI, substance use disorder, and recent drug use with consequences, and so is appropriate for BTSAS, the focus of assessment changes to evaluating the client's level of general functioning and to gauging his or her level of motivation to change. It is important to establish a baseline level of functioning that can be compared to how a client is doing both during and at the end of treatment. In addition, gaining some understanding about a client's level of readiness to change is useful both to frame the discussion that occurs in the first motivational interview, and also to provide important information about the client's goals for treatment and reasons for change.

Establishing a Baseline Level of Functioning

In addition to determining appropriateness for BTSAS participation, assessment at referral to BTSAS allows us to establish a baseline level of functioning in order to determine if a client's situation has improved at the end of treatment. As part of our work with SPMI clients we have developed a measure, the

Substance Use Event Survey for Severe Mental Illness (SUESS), to assess the important clinical issues that are most relevant to dually diagnosed SPMI patients. The SUESS covers both mental health and substance use domains, taps the experiences and domains that are especially relevant for patients with dual disorders, utilizes language that can be easily understood by highly impaired patients, and would be useful to a range of professionals. The SUESS contains two types of items: (1) items related to service use, and (2) items to gather descriptive information that may relate to service use in SMI patients. In combining these two types of items in one assessment, the SUESS collects service use data within the context of the treatment issues and life events that are highly relevant to this patient population. The format of the SUESS is based on the ASI—it assesses medical issues, alcohol use and treatment issues, drug use and treatment issues, family issues, and psychiatric issues—yet it also includes topics that are relevant to SMI patients, including psychotropic medication use, the experience of medication side effects, and victimization issues. In addition, we included items to assess factors related to motivation to change in dually diagnosed patients. For example, the SUESS includes an assessment of changes that the patient has made in his or her use in the last 90 days as well as what factors may have contributed to this change, including being arrested, health concerns, psychiatric illness, changes in psychiatric medication, the urging of a family member or a friend, a treatment program, financial issues, or negative affect such as being bored or lonely or sad. The SUESS also contains a Reasons for Seeking Treatment scale that includes possible motivators for seeking treatment that are relevant to this population, including experiencing a traumatic event, worsening of psychological problems, being warned by the doctor about using, and being referred from legal sources or from the case manager or therapist. Such information is a key to our understanding of what motivates SMI patients to seek treatment, and is relevant to designing services as well as outreach to those who need treatment but have not yet sought it on their own. We also wanted the SUESS to be useful in tracking service use in dually diagnosed patients. Items assess a range of inpatient and outpatient services to treat substance use and psychiatric problems that are highly relevant to an SMI population. For example, for both alcohol and drugs, patients are asked if they attended an inpatient program, participated in outpatient treatment (including self help and dual diagnosis groups), received medications for detoxification, received medications that block the effects of substances, received blood or urine tests, or had a serious discussion about their substance use. Similarly, the Psychological/Emotional Issues section includes items asking if the patient has been hospitalized; taken medication; seen a therapist, case manager, or social worker; or been in any treatment groups.

Another measure of general functioning that is useful with SPMI clients is the Brief Quality of Life interview (BQOL: Lehman et al., 1996). The BQOL takes about 15 minutes to administer and provides a global measure of satisfaction, as well as objective and subjective indicators of quality of life. Ratings cover a broad array of variables, including residential stability, daily activities, frequency of family and social contacts, availability of spending money and adequacy of financial supports, employment status, arrests, victimization, and health status. The BQOL is a shorter version of Lehman's Quality of Life interview, which has been found to have adequate reliability and validity (Lehman, 1988).

Finally, obtaining collateral information about a client's functioning is a good way to validate the client's report. People who have known the client for a long time, such as long-term clinicians and caregivers or family members are most able to provide a realistic picture of the client's functioning in treatment and in the community.

Evaluating Readiness to Change

Chapter 6 includes a description of the ways in which assessment is used during the first MI that is a part of BTSAS. Specifically, the first MI includes some aspect of feedback in which the client and the therapist discuss findings from pretreatment assessments, as well as information that was collected from other clinicians or family members concerning the client's substance use. There are many options for the sorts of information that can be included in this feedback, and the selection of feedback needs to match with the overall goals of the MI. We have found it most useful to focus the first MI on helping clients talk about the things that have happened to them because of their drug use, and on coaxing clients to make self-motivational statements that we can then reinforce. To this end, our first MI includes brief feedback on days of use and days of treatment attendance (both mental health and substance abuse treatment) in the last month and on clients' responses to items from a questionnaire on motivation to change that tap readiness to change.

There are a number of ways to assess days of drug use and days of treatment attendance in the last month. Most easily, the information collected at referral, either via the TLFB or the ASI, can be used. The TLFB is traditionally used to capture drug use over the last month, but can also be used to assess which days in the month the client attended treatment. In addition, the ASI contains items that ask about both drug use and treatment attendance in the last 30 days. If neither of these measures is being used, simply asking the client for the number of days of use and treatment attendance in the preceding month is also an option. While a client may underreport use and possibly overreport treatment attendance, we have found that when asked about their use in a nonjudgmental way, clients are generally honest in their responses. Coupling this self-report with information from the client's counselor or mental health treatment providers is usually sufficient to get a reasonable estimate of the client's current use and treatment attendance.

In terms of motivation to change, we recommend a simple and brief assessment. There are numerous measures of motivation to change and related constructs, most of which were not developed with SPMI clients and may be difficult for this population to understand and answer validly. Rather than a thorough assessment of motivation to change, we recommend selecting a measure with items that can generate discussion about change and change strategies, which links nicely with our MI goals. For example, we have clients complete the University of Rhode Island Change Assessment (URICA; DiClemente & Hughes, 1990), a 32-item questionnaire which assesses the client's stage of change. The URICA employs a 5-point Likert scale format by which respondents rate their degree of agreement (disagreement) with each item. The URICA has been found to have utility with a wide range of substance dependent individuals (Carbonari, DiClemente, & Zweben, 1994). Traditionally the URICA is used to place a respondent in a particular stage of change (precontemplation, contemplation, action, maintenance). In our MIs, we use select items from the URICA to generate discussion regarding interest in and readiness to change. As we will discuss more fully in chapter 6, several items from the URICA tap problem recognition and general change efforts, including: At times my problem (with illegal drug use) is difficult, but I'm working on it; I have a problem (with illegal drug use) and I really think I should work on it; Even though I'm not always successful in changing, at least I'm working on my problem (with illegal drug use); I wish I had some more ideas on how to solve my problem (with illegal drug use); and I am actively working on my problem (with illegal drug use). Feedback and discussion on these items can help professionals figure out where a client is in terms of motivation, and help in setting realistic goals.

There are other options for assessing thoughts about change. One construct that we have found useful for SPMI clients who are ambivalent about change is the decisional balance. Using the illustration of a see-saw, we discuss with clients the things that they like about using as well as the problems they have experienced from their drug use. A Decisional Balance measure was originally developed for use with smoking cessation studies and a variety of other health-related behaviors (Prochaska et al. 1994; Velicer, DiClemente, Prochaska, & Brandenberg, 1985). We have used drug and alcohol versions which include subscales measuring the perceived benefits ("pros") and perceived costs ("cons") of using drugs and drinking, respectively (LaForge, Maddock, & Rossi, 1999). In order to enhance the relevance of this scale for the SPMI clients we treat, we have added several items that have been identified as important in our pilot work (e.g., being on conditional release from jail, being evicted from a residence, court control of one's children).

We have also found it useful to understand the situations in which our clients use drugs and the level of difficulty clients would have in not using when they are in these situations. The Abstinence Self-Efficacy scale (ASES; DiClemente, Carbonari, Montgomery, & Hughes, 1994), a 20-item scale which assesses the degree to which subjects feel "tempted" to use drugs or drink in different situations, and the degree to which they feel confident in their ability to abstain from drug or alcohol use in the same situations. Clients rate their degree of temptation and self-efficacy using 5-point Likert scale formats. Scale scores for temptation and self-efficacy are computed separately for each of four subscales (Negative Affect, Social/Positive Influences, Physical and Other Concerns, and Withdrawal and Urges). Psychometric properties of these scales are strong across varied addictive behaviors (DiClemente, Fairhurst, & Biotrowski, 1995).

A brief way to get a snapshot of a client's thoughts and efforts regarding change of different substances is the Readiness Ruler; see Hesse (2006) for a review. The Readiness Ruler lists a range of substances, including alcohol, and asks clients to rate their change thoughts/efforts for each item on a 10-point scale tapping "Not ready to change," "Unsure," "Ready to Change," and "Trying to change." The Readiness Ruler is simple to understand and easy to use, and allows for a discussion of change and differing attitudes toward change as it relates to multiple substances.

An Integrated Assessment for General Functioning and Motivation to Change

To sum up, at the start of treatment it is useful to have some structured measure of general functioning as well as information on readiness to change. We think that using a semistructured interview like the SUESS or the BQOL is a good way to systematically assess general functioning (rather than asking open-ended questions about current functioning as part of a nonstandardized intake interview) and to provide a template of questions that can be repeated at the end of treatment in order to assess changes in functioning. There is a range of options for assessing readiness to change. Rather than use these measures to place clients within a particular stage, we find it more useful to use items from these sorts of measures to generate discussion about change and change efforts as a part of our first motivational interview.

ASSESSMENT DURING TREATMENT

Once clients have begun the BTSAS program, their progress in the program must be assessed. We gather information at each BTSAS session that describes the client's use and participation on that particular day. When data from all sessions are strung together, we can generate a picture of a client's progress within the program. We have developed a form for in-session data collection, called the Session Data Collection Form, which is provided here. This form includes the following domains that are assessed at each BTSAS session: (1) attendance; (2) drug use; and (3) group participation.

Assessing Attendance at Each BTSAS Session

Attendance at BTSAS sessions is tracked, both to enhance our understanding of how much BTSAS a client needs to meet substance use reduction goals, but also for practical reasons, such as to figure out when a person has dropped out or reached his or her 52-session mark and is ready to graduate from the program. Clients are listed as either having attended the session, having an excused absence, or having an unexcused absence. The distinction between excused and unexcused absences is relevant to the urinalysis contingency program (UCP) described in detail in chapter 7. In the UCP, unexcused absences result in the contingency being reset, with clients who miss a session having to work back into earning money for negative urine tests. In contrast, excused absences do not result in the contingency being reset, as clients can be excused for legitimate reasons (we require the client to bring some documentation of the reason for the absence).

Assessing Drug Use at each BTSAS Session

Since the goal of BTSAS is to reduce drug use, it is imperative to measure drug use at each session. We gather both self-report and objective information about between session drug use. At the start of each session, clients are asked whether or not they have used their goal drug and any other drugs since the last BTSAS session. The client's self-report of drug use is recorded on the Session Data Collection Form. This is followed for every client with a urinalysis test, the results of which are recorded on the Session Data Collection Form as well. Both self-report and objective results are provided separately for the three main goal drugs found in our SPMI population (cocaine, heroin, and marijuana), and the form also has an "Other Drug" category in the event that a urinalysis testing system provides testing of any additional substances.

We believe that it is important to gather both self-report and objective information on drug use between sessions. Use of the urinalysis is more objective, so it would seem that the self-report information is not needed. However, we want clients to talk honestly about their drug use. While the urinalysis helps to encourage honest reporting, we believe the actual reporting by clients is useful. Many SPMI clients will have had past substance abuse treatment that included harsh words, threats, and coercion as tactics to convince them to stop their drug use. As a result, many clients will have learned to downplay or misrepresent their use as a way of avoiding punishment. We want to show clients that honest reporting is important and beneficial to their reduction efforts, and that admitting and discussing periods of use can help us to learn ways to cope in the future. To this end, we praise and reinforce accurate self-reports of use, both when the client has used and when the client has remained abstinent.

Assessing Group Participation at each BTSAS Session

Most BTSAS session involve role-playing, and it can often be useful to track how many role-plays clients do while they are part of the program, as well as to rate more generally the quality of their participation in each session. One way this is useful is in examining whether clients who do more role-plays or who participate more in BTSAS sessions have better outcome than those who are less involved in the program. We record the numbers of role-plays clients complete, during both the goal-setting and training/planning components of the program. In addition, we have developed ratings for client participation and effort that are made for both the goal-setting and the training/planning components of each session. These ratings include: attentiveness, cooperation, performance, self-efficacy, and likelihood of success (goal setting only). Table 5.2 lists the descriptions and anchors for these ratings.

END OF TREATMENT AND FOLLOW-UP

At the end of treatment, it is useful to reassess clients to determine how their drug use and general functioning has changed during their participation in BTSAS. Assessments can also be done at different points following the end of treatment to determine if change is sustained over time, if clients who showed little change initially show some improvement later on, or if clients who were doing poorly continue to deteriorate. We recommend readministering measures that were used at the referral and start of treatment points, so that client responses to the same questions can be compared at the start and end of treatment. The end of treatment is also a good time to check in with treatment providers or family members who provided collateral information when the client began the BTSAS program.

Table 5.2 In-Session Ratings

	Attentiveness	Cooperation	Performance	Self-efficacy	Likelihood of success (goal setting only)
1	**Inattentive** Attending approximately 0–20% of the time. May at times know what is being discussed; usually self-absorbed or preoccupied.	**Uncooperative** Only minimally. preoccupied willing to participate. Openly defiant/ disruptive. Considerable time is taken encouraging client to participate.	**Poor** Requires tremendous amount of help. Shows little/no ability without extensive coaching.	**Unsure** Client expresses a total lack of confidence in self.	**Low** Therapist firmly believes that client will not even attempt the goal. Client chose goal only to be compliant.
2	**Somewhat inattentive** Attending approximately 20–40% of the time. Fades in and out of awareness, but on average is following half the time.	**Somewhat uncooperative** Rather reluctant to participate but shows some definite efforts. May answer some questions but refuses to answer others and refuses to do role-play when asked.	**Somewhat poor** Requires considerable coaching during role-play, but is able to demonstrate some skill spontaneously. With great help, can come up with some sort of goal. Is unable to engage in any independent problem solving.	**Somewhat unsure** Client reluctantly accepts the goal/skill. Expresses little optimism in his or her ability to achieve it.	**Somewhat low** Therapist believes it unlikely that client will attempt the goal. Client reluctant to name the goal.
3	**Neither attentive nor inattentive** Attending approximately 40–60% of the time. About half the time the client is following and the other half is distracted or acting bored.	**Neither cooperative nor uncooperative** Willing to do what is asked with no resistance. Answers questions and engages role-plays. Does not volunteer ideas.	**Neither poor nor good** Needs some help or redirection, but can come up with at least one goal and is able to problem solve around that goal with extensive therapist direction.	**Neither unsure nor sure** Client accepts the goal/skill but does not express confidence in being able to achieve or perform it. Client is willing to try but has reservations.	**Neither high nor low** Therapist thinks client will attempt the goal but is unsure if client will succeed.
4	**Somewhat attentive** Attending approximately 60–80% of the time. Most of the time the client is following although there may be a few lapses.	**Somewhat cooperative** Actively participates, at least partly without prompting. May start off hesitant, but warms up quickly and displays some enthusiasm.	**Somewhat good** Needs little corrective feedback. With some help, can come up with a mostly realistic goal/plan and can problem solve around that goal/plan with little direction. Needs help "fine-tuning."	**Somewhat sure** Client accepts the goal/skill and agrees to attempt it. Client has reservations his or her ability to be successful but expresses optimism.	**Somewhat high** Therapistpist thinks client will attempt the goal and has reasonable expectation of success.

(continued)

Table 5.2 In-Session Ratings (continued)

	Attentiveness	Cooperation	Performance	Self-efficacy	Likelihood of success (goal setting only)
5	Attentive Attending 80–100% of the time. Client follows and gives relevant and specific answers to questions.	Cooperative Easy to engage and enthusiastic. Volunteers information and ideas. May make spontaneous suggestions.	Good No assistance necessary. Can come up with a realistic and relevant goal/ plan and is able to independently problem solve around that goal/plan and discuss potential solutions.	Sure Client expresses confidence and states with certainty that he or she can achieve goal, skill, or plan.	Very high Therapist believes that client will attempt to achieve goal, cares about the goal, and will succeed.

SUMMARY

Assessment with dual diagnosis SPMI clients presents many challenges. Finding the right combination of measures for a particular clinic and goals is an important facet of implementing a BTSAS program.

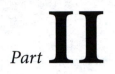

Part **II**

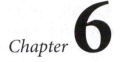

MOTIVATIONAL INTERVIEWING IN PEOPLE WITH SPMI

INTRODUCTION

Engagement and attendance in substance abuse treatment can be serious problems for people with SPMI. Their many significant problems in addition to substance abuse, which include unstable housing, medical problems, poor medication adherence, and a lack of community support for nonuse, can make it extremely difficult for them to get to treatment and to continue attending. It is important to help people with SPMI at the start of BTSAS to recognize the important reasons for attending substance abuse treatment, as well as to help them to increase internal motivation to change. An intervention that incorporates collaboration with clients and attention to client motivation is motivational interviewing (MI; Miller & Rollnick, 1991). MI is nonconfrontational and directive, and involves providing clear feedback and advice along with negotiating goals and problem solving to overcome barriers to treatment. MI combines the therapeutic elements that have been found to be successful components of brief interventions for substance abuse (Bien et al., 1993), including giving clear advice and feedback, utilizing an empathic counseling style, and addressing barriers to treatment. There have been numerous tests of MI as both a precursor to treatment and as an add-on to treatment-as-usual in both inpatient and outpatient settings, with a range of client populations (see Miller & Heather, 1998 for a review). Overall, the literature supports MI as an effective strategy for raising client motivation, increasing treatment attendance, and reducing substance use (Miller, 2000).

While we have used the term *motivational interviewing* in deference to Miller and Rollnick (1991), there are a number of important differences between our approach to MI and theirs. As indicated in chapter 1, people with SPMI have cognitive impairments that limit their ability to deal with abstraction, to draw relationships between past, present, and future events, and to develop and pursue self-directed behavioral plans over time. Hence, the client-centered style and stimulus for self-exploration central to Miller and Rollnick's approach is not likely to be useful for most people with SPMI. Consequently, we adopt a more directive style, leading clients toward recognition of one or a few key factors that can serve as motivators for decreased substance use. For the most part, these focal issues involve concrete, negative circumstances, such as avoiding arrest, getting back into a community residence, or regaining custody of children. More abstract goals (e.g., "taking control of one's life," or "regaining the respect of one's children"), and lifestyle goals (e.g., pursuing one's career) are generally not relevant for people with SPMI. Typically, the therapist is very active in reminding the client of problems identified during pretreatment assessments (e.g., Addiction Severity Index), rather than waiting for the client to come to his or her own realization of how substance abuse has been personally harmful.

The objective of motivational interviewing is to help clients mobilize and utilize internally generated motivation to change their drug use. These sessions are used to discuss the impact that the negative consequences of substance use has had on clients lives, for the therapist to acknowledge and reinforce internal motivation and any change efforts that the client has made, and to chart progress in decreasing or abstaining from substances over the course of the client's involvement in BTSAS.

MI sessions take place three times over the course of a client's participation in BTSAS: at the start of BTSAS, at the midpoint of the intervention (after three months of involvement), and at the end of BTSAS participation. Each session includes several parts: (1) an introductory discussion in which the client can tell the therapist about his or her use or progress in the group to date and in changing substance use; (2) discussion of negative consequences that have occurred as a result of substance use; (3) feedback on drug use and motivation for change from the research assessments; and (4) goal setting and plans for achieving the goal. The focus of each of these parts differs as a function of the time at which it takes place; that is, content differs at baseline from both the three- and six-month sessions, and of use status (abstinent from all substances vs. still using some substances but not goal substance vs. still using all substances). Ways to adapt to these variations at these different points in time, and use status, are outlined in the following sections.

INITIAL MI SESSION

The first MI session takes place as the client begins BTSAS. The goal of the initial MI is to help clients discuss their thoughts about changing their substance use, and to guide clients toward a positive view of change. Prior to the MI session, it is important to do a clinical assessment of the client's substance use and to determine the number of days of use in the last month, and the number of days the client has attended treatment (for substance abuse, mental illness, or both) in the last month. The MI discussion centers on the client's experiences over his or her lifetime.

Introduction to the Initial MI

The introduction is used to help the client feel comfortable talking to the therapist and to get the client talking about substance use. People with SPMI can find it difficult to talk with a new therapist and may need time to get acclimated to a new person, so it is important to explain what is going to happen in the MI session at the start and ask for questions. To get the MI started, the therapist can say,

> Today we are going to talk about your substance use and any changes you might be thinking about making in how much or how often you use. First we will talk about some of the things that may have happened to you as a result of using drugs, and then we will talk about some of the information that you gave during the assessments that you completed. Finally, we will come up with a substance use goal and talk about steps for achieving that goal. You will go over those goals during group as well as in the individual sessions that we will have together. My hope is to help you think about your drug use and make any changes that you want to make in how much or how often you use. This meeting should take about an hour. Do you have any questions before we begin?

Next, there are some basic questions to ask the client so that he or she will get used to and comfortable with talking about substance use. Appropriate questions include asking the client what drugs he uses and which drugs he uses most often; does the client use alone or with other people; has the client ever stopped using and if so when and why; and has the client ever attended substance abuse treatment before. In addition, the therapist can ask some simple questions about motivation to change that can help set the stage for talking about negative consequences in the next section. These include asking the client if she has thought at all about changing her drug use and what she has been thinking about changing, if anything. The purpose of these questions is to get the conversation flowing and get the client feeling comfortable with discussing substance use. The role of the therapist is to listen, summarize, and help the client feel comfortable.

Discussion of Negative Consequences

Following the Introduction, there is a discussion about the negative consequences of the client's substance use. The goal of this section is to have the client review and discuss the different problems he has encountered due to substance use. During this discussion, the therapist remains empathic and nonjudgmental, helping the client to talk about consequences without making him feel badly about what has occurred or hopeless regarding his ability to change. To start this section of the MI, the therapist can say:

> *Thank you for telling me a bit about your substance use. Now I want to get an idea of the things that have happened to you because of your drug use. We know that people who use drugs often experience problems that come from their drug use, like problems with their family or problems with the law. Can you tell me about any problems you have had because of your drug use?*

The client is first asked to list negative consequences that he has experienced due to substance use, and is then asked to elaborate on details of the experience and think about how they might change if he were no longer using. For example,

> *You have said that one problem that you have experienced from using drugs is that your symptoms get worse. What happens? How do they get worse? So one good thing about not using or using less is that your symptoms would not get worse. You also said that you are not allowed to see your children because their mother won't let you come visit when you are using drugs. It's clear from how you talk about them that you love your children very much and that you would like to see more of them. So another good thing about not using is that you might be able to see your children more often.*

Throughout this discussion, the therapist must reinforce any self-motivational statements. For example, if the client is talking about a consequence such as spending all her money on drugs and states that she would like to have money for other things, the therapist can say,

> *What I hear you saying is that you would like to spend your money on other things rather than drugs. What sorts of things would you buy if you didn't spend your money on drugs? It's great that you can think of things that you would do with your money other than buy drugs. That tells me that you have things that you would like to do with your money other than buy drugs.*

Assessment Feedback

The next section of the Initial MI focuses on providing feedback from any pretreatment assessment that was done, as well as information that was collected from other clinicians or family members concerning the client's substance use. Providing feedback regarding assessment and other clinical information is useful in several ways. First, it helps the therapist and the client start out on the same page in terms of what the client's problems are and identifies the important things to be addressed in treatment. By reviewing assessment and clinical data at the start of BTSAS, it is clear what the therapist knows about the client, allows the client to clarify anything that is incomplete or incorrect, and lets the client know if other people (clinicians, family members, home care providers) have provided information that is relevant to substance abuse treatment. Second, assessment information can provide important information to clients and help them to view their substance use differently. For example, reviewing information about days of use and years of regular use may help a client view his substance use as a more significant problem than he might have viewed it before.

The discussion of assessment feedback must be easy for participants to do and to understand. In order to promote a collaborative discussion, the therapist should provide a duplicate of the assessment information for the client to look at during the review, or should have a clipboard or some other way to hold the form so that both the therapist and the client can see it. The therapist can introduce this to the client by saying,

> *You might remember that you filled out a lot of forms before our meeting today. Those forms help us learn about people and what sorts of substance use issues they have. I have some information from those forms about your substance use over the last month and your responses to some questions about cutting down on your use. I want to go over this information with you.*

In more traditional MI approaches, feedback generally includes levels of drinking or drug use in comparison to national norms, comparison of levels of negative consequences in comparison to other clients entering treatment, results of medical testing of physical functioning (e.g., liver enzymes), and family history risk. In our experience with people with SPMI, these sorts of comparisons are generally too abstract and complex for most clients to understand. We have found it useful to discuss with clients simple information that helps them think more about their own substance use and changes they want to make, rather than comparing their use to the use of others. In this way, our "feedback" is really better described as our telling the client some of the important things we have learned about them and getting their thoughts on it. It is important to select information for feedback that is simple and easy to understand. In addition, information selected for feedback should be information that the client can provide with fair reliability. Importantly, feedback should be reinforcing and positive. We have found it most helpful to include feedback on current frequency of substance use, frequency of treatment attendance, and responses on measures of motivation to change. For example, the number of days of use in the last 30 days is fairly simple and easy for a client to understand, as is the number of days of treatment in the last month. Providing feedback on this information can happen in the following way:

> *In your assessment you said that your drug of choice is cocaine, is that correct? I have here that you used cocaine 10 days in the last month. Is that pretty standard for you or is 10 days less that you usually use? How many days do you usually use? That's great that 10 days is less days than you usually use. So you have used less cocaine this month than you usually do. Terrific! You also said that you went to treatment on three days this month. What sort of treatment was that? It's great that you got some treatment this month, and you used less cocaine that usual this month. That's a great start for you now that you are entering the drug treatment group!*

Another example involves providing feedback regarding responses on a measure of motivation to change. For example, the University of Rhode Island Change Assessment (DiClemente & Hughes, 1990) is a frequently used measure to assess motivation to change. Several items tap problem recognition and working on change, including: At times my problem (with illegal drug use) is difficult, but I'm working on it; I have a problem (with illegal drug use) and I really think I should work on it; Even though I'm not always successful in changing, at least I'm working on my problem (with illegal drug use); I wish

I had some more ideas on how to solve my problem (with illegal drug use); and I am actively working on my problem (with illegal drug use). Feedback and discussion on these items can help you figure out where a client is, motivationally speaking, and help you set realistic goals.

For example, suppose a client provided the following ratings for these items: At times my problem is difficult, but I'm working on it—disagree; I have a problem and I really think I should work on it—undecided; Even though I'm not always successful in changing, at least I'm working on my problem—disagree; I wish I had some more ideas on how to solve my problem—agree; I am actively working on my problem (with illegal drug use)—disagree. The therapist can say the following:

> *From what you said on this assessment, it looks like you're not yet working a lot on your drug use. However, you did say that you're unsure but you are starting to think that you have a problem with drugs and you would like some ideas on what to do to deal with your drug use. What that says to me is that you are starting to think that using less might be a good idea but you're not sure how to get started. Does that sound right? It's great that you are starting to think about using less. We know from working with other people who have stopped using drugs that it's pretty tough to decide to stop or to cut down, so it's great that you are starting to think about it. Why do you think it might be a good idea to stop using? Well, you said that when you use you spend all your money on drugs and you have no money left for the other things you want to get. So you could use your money for other things if you weren't doing drugs. That's great. I'm going to help you come up with some ideas about how to work on your drug problem.*

As another example, suppose a client provided the following ratings for the same items: At times my problem is difficult, but I'm working on it—agree; I have a problem and I really think I should work on it—agree; Even though I'm not always successful in changing, at least I'm working on my problem—agree; I wish I had some more ideas on how to solve my problem—strongly agree; I am actively working on my problem (with illegal drug use)—agree. Therapist feedback could go something like:

> *I see from your assessment that you are really trying to change your drug use. What sorts of things have you been doing to change your drug use? That's great! You seem to be really motivated to stop using. We know from working with other people who are trying to stop using drugs that when you are motivated to stop it is easier to stop. You also said that you would really like suggestions and help with stopping your drug use. That's what I can help you with, along with the group that you are going to be attending.*

This section can be used in a similar way with clients who are not currently using or who have recently stopped using. Such clients are clearly motivated and will be particularly easy to reinforce. Since the client has already begun to make changes in substance use, the purpose of the MI is to help him clarify and concretize his goals. The interviewer must reinforce the fact that the client has already started to make changes in his substance use. Whenever possible, this type of reinforcement should be worked in throughout the entire session. For example, at the start of the MI session, the therapist should acknowledge that the client is not currently using and congratulate him on his progress. As the MI progresses, the therapist will want to ask questions that help the client to talk about his nonuse and the strategies he has used to be successful. Questions that can be asked in order to elicit self-motivational statements include: What made you decide to do something about your substance use problem? What was bad about using drugs? What has improved in your life since you stopped using drugs? If the client has difficulty answering, the therapist can get more specific and ask the client what has been good about not using this week (or today, if the client lacks the ability to think about any time other than the present). The therapist can even offer examples such as, "Have you had a little more money in your pocket since you stopped using drugs?"

Goal Setting

The final section of the Initial MI involves goal setting, in which the therapist and the client collaborate in developing a concrete, short-term goal that the client can work on between the end of the Initial MI and the client's first group. Goal setting as part of the Initial MI has several purposes. First, goal setting is an integral part of the BTSAS intervention, and experiencing it during the Initial MI allows clients to get a feel for something that they will be doing in the group that it is hoped will serve as a draw for them to attend their first group session. Second, the aim of goal setting, whether during the Initial MI or during the group itself, is to help clients see that solutions to larger problems (such as reducing or stopping drug use) can be broken down into smaller, more manageable steps that can be accomplished one at a time. This is an important lesson for SPMI clients to learn—many have tried and failed many times to stop drug use, and the process of reducing or stopping use often seems so huge as to be impossible to achieve. Goal setting is a way to help clients develop small goals that they can achieve, and provide reinforcement for these smaller achievements, with the hope that continued reinforcement will lead to continued small successes. It is stressed in goal setting that these small achievements will add up and will eventually lead to the client accomplishing reduction or quitting goals.

It is important to remember to design a goal that a client is willing and able to do, rather than the goal that *you* want him or her to do. Oftentimes a therapist is ready for a client to change long before the client himself is ready. Do not set the therapist's goal; set a goal that will fit with how a client is thinking about his or her use right now. Remember that the Initial MI is aimed at getting clients to engage in treatment. Once the client starts attending BTSAS, the therapist has many opportunities to help the client consider change as a goal.

The therapist can introduce goal setting to the client by saying,

The information that we just reviewed tells me that you are thinking about changing your drug use and considering being clean or cutting back on your use. That is a tough thing to think about and I think you did a great job talking to me about it. Now I want us to do something called setting a goal. This means that since we know that you are thinking about changing your drug use, we work together to come up with a goal that will get you started. We know from working with other people who have changed their drug use that setting a goal helps a person get started when they want to make a change. It doesn't have to be a big goal, only something that will help you try out using less and something that you think you can do.

It is important to remember that goal setting involves concrete, short-term goals. Goals should be generated in collaboration with the client, and a goal that is decided on in the Initial MI should be something that the client finds easy to do (as we will discuss in chapter 7, goals that are formed as part of the goal setting that takes place during the BTSAS groups can get more challenging, depending on the client's progress and length of time in the group). Keeping the goal easy during the initial MI is important because at this point, the therapist does not know the client very well, and the client may come to the intervention without a real commitment to change. If a client who is unsure about change is met with a goal that he perceives as too difficult, such as staying clean until the first group, the client may become turned off to the intervention altogether. Keeping the goal concrete, small, and relatively easy will allow the client to achieve some immediate success, with the hope that the positive feelings brought about by this success will lead the client to think positively about the intervention and to attend the first group. Often the goals developed in the goal-setting component of the Initial MI involve making an attempt to reduce use between the Initial MI and the first group. Other times clients who are not ready or able to commit to reduced drug use will develop goals such as attending a self-help meeting prior to attending their first group, or simply attending their first BTSAS session.

As an example, consider the first hypothetical client who was unsure if he wanted to change his drug use and hadn't started working on any strategies yet. For this sort of a client, goal setting during the Initial MI can go something like this:

OK, you said that you are starting to think about reducing you drug use but you're not sure how to go about doing it. What we need to do is to come up with a small goal that you can do over the next few days that will get you started on changing your drug use. It has to be a goal that you think you can do, and something that can get you started with reducing your drug use so you can see if cutting down is right for you. Once you try out this small goal, we can discuss how it went during your first group meeting, and we can figure out other goals that are right for you. What do you think a good, small goal might be that you could do and might help you figure out if reducing your drug use would be good for you?

As another example, take the second hypothetical client who is working on reducing drug use and is highly motivated. In this case, goal setting may go something like this:

We have talked about how you have already started doing some things to reduce your drug use and that you want more ideas on other things that you can do to stop using. What we need to do is come up with a goal that you can do over the next few days that will keep you going in your work to stop using drugs. What do you think would be a good goal?

Throughout goal setting, the therapist should reinforce any self-motivational statements, while keeping a realistic view of what the client can accomplish. For example, if a client who is a recent and fairly heavy drug user says that she wants her goal to be stopping drug use immediately, the therapist can respond,

It is great that you really want to stop using drugs. I can tell how serious you are about wanting to stop using and how important it is to you to totally stop using drugs. That high motivation is going to be important as you make your way through this intervention. One thing that we have learned from other people who have stopped using drugs is that they have an easier time of it if they make their goals small and work their way up to bigger ones. Since you are just starting out with group, maybe we can think of a goal that involves not using drugs and will help you totally stop using drugs, maybe a goal of not using drugs for the next few days. After all, if you stop for a few days, it will be easier to stop for a few days after that and so on. How does that sound to you?

As with the section on "Assessment Feedback," goal setting can be done the same way for clients who are not using or who have recently stopped their drug use. The goals such clients set might be somewhat different. For example, if the client has achieved some clean time from his drug of choice, the therapist can suggest that the goal be to stay clean until the first group, reduce use of alcohol or some other substance of abuse, or to do some other task that would support a nonusing lifestyle (reconnect with mental health treatment, open a bank account, attend a self-help meeting, etc).

FOLLOW-UP MI SESSIONS

The BTSAS intervention includes two follow-up MI sessions at three- and six months from the start of treatment. The follow-up MI sessions focus on charting client progress with their goals, as well as providing a setting in which clients can be reinforced for motivational statements and progress can be used in a motivational way. As such, follow-up MI sessions include an introduction and review of use and treatment attendance; a brief discussion of any negative consequences that have happened in the last three months; a discussion of things that have improved in the last three months; feedback on frequency of use, frequency of treatment, and other items; a discussion of helpful strategies used in the last three months, and goal setting.

Introduction and Feedback

The first section of the follow-up MI is designed to remind the client of the purpose of the MI meetings and to gather information from the client concerning recent use and substance abuse treatment attendance. We then compare this information to figures that the client provided at the Initial MI session. Remember that in contrast to more traditional MI approaches, we utilize information in our MIs that is simple and applies to the client very currently and concretely. Information such as days of use in the last month and number of days of treatment in the last month are things that most SPMI clients can accurately report and can be used to track progress and provide motivational content. This information can be collected before the Follow-up MI session, but we often collect it right at the start of the MI session. So at the start of the Follow-up MI session, the therapist should have, written down, both the number of days of use of drug of choice in the last month and number of days of treatment attendance from the Initial MI.

The therapist can start off this section by saying:

Today we are going to talk about your substance use over the last three months and see how you are doing in terms of making the changes that you wanted to make in your drug use. We will talk about some of the things that may have happened to you as a result of using drugs over the last three months, and then we will talk about how your drug use and treatment attendance have been during that time. We will end by doing a quick goal setting, just as we do in group, and talk about steps for achieving that goal. Do you have any questions before we begin?

The therapist should then ask the client to report the number of days she used her goal drug in the last month, as well as the number of days she attended any kind of outpatient substance abuse treatment in the last month. Use of a sheet with a one-month calendar printed on it can be helpful to the client in terms of recollecting days of use and days of treatment.

As an example of how this feedback can be delivered, we can use the following information: drug of choice is cocaine; number of days of use in last 30 = 5; number of days of use in last 30 at Initial MI=10; number of days of treatment in last 30 = 6; number of days of treatment in last 30 at Initial MI = 3. The therapist can say the following:

We know that your drug of choice is cocaine, and you said you used cocaine on five days in the past month. When we last met, you had told me that you used cocaine 10 days that month. So you have reduced your use by five days per month—that's great! That shows me that you are really working hard to reduce your cocaine use. You also got twice as much treatment this month— you attended treatment on six days this month, up from three days per month when we last met. Good for you!

Discussion of Negative Consequences.

This section of the Follow-up MI involves reviewing any negative drug-related consequences that have occurred in the three months since the Initial MI. The goal here is to be up to date on the client's drug-related consequences, use these as immediate prompts to enhance motivation to change, and to track whether the number and severity of consequences has decreased or increased in the intervening three months. This discussion is handled differently for currently using and nonusing clients. For clients who are currently using, it is likely that they have experienced some negative drug-related consequences in the last three months. It is also good for the therapist to review the previous MI, in order to be able to prompt clients about current negative consequences by reminding them of the consequences they reported earlier. The therapist can ask what sorts of negative consequences the client has experienced in the following way:

> You might remember that last time we met we talked about some of the problems that you have had as a result of your drug use, like spending all of your money on drugs so that you didn't have money left to buy other things. You also said that you were not allowed to see your children since you were doing drugs. Have any of these sorts of problems happened to you since we last met, in the last three months?

Some currently using clients will have experienced many consequences. If the client has experienced some negative consequences in the last three months, discuss them briefly, and also point out that he or she would not experience these negative consequences if the client were not using. For example:

> You have said that one problem that you have experienced from using drugs in the last three months is that your symptoms got worse when you were using. So one good thing about not using or using less would be that your symptoms would not get worse. What do you think about that?

Another example:

> So in the last three months you have spent money on drugs that you would have liked to use on other things. That's pretty common and I'm glad you told me about it. So one good thing about coming to group and continuing to try to reduce your drug use would be that you would be able to spend your money on other things that you need, like clothes or your rent.

Other clients may be currently using but have reduced their drug use since the last MI and so may be experiencing many fewer drug-related consequences than at the first MI, or have reduced their use to the point where they are not experiencing any consequences at all. If there are no negative consequences that have happened in the last three months, then this is a very good place to reinforce the client's motivation—what better proof that reducing/stopping use is a good thing than having fewer/no problems related to drug use in three months. Similarly if there is a drastically reduced number of consequences due to reduced drug use, this can be highlighted and reinforced in the following way:

> When we first met you told me about a lot of problems you were having because of your drug use. You said you were having arguments with your family, you were having a lot of trouble getting to your treatment appointments, and you weren't taking your medication regularly. You are now telling me that since you have reduced your use, your family is not yelling at you about your use, you have been able to get to most of your appointments, and you are taking your medication every time you are supposed to. That is terrific! You have made a big change.

Discussion of Things That Have Improved

If a client has stopped or cut down his or her use since the first MI, you can then review some of the things that have improved over the last three months since the client has cut down or stopped using drugs. The goal here is to help the client make the link between cutting down or stopping drug use and resulting improvements in the way things are going. Here is an example of how to discuss this with clients:

We have talked about how you have really cut your drug use over the last three months. That's great! Tell me what that has been like for you. We find that when people cut down or stop using drugs, oftentimes things in their lives get better as a result. What are some things in your life that have been better lately since you have cut down on your use?

The therapist should inquire about physical health (most clients feel better physically when they cut down or stop using), relationships, financial issues (most clients have more money and are spending it on other things rather than drugs). The therapist should use information that he or she knows about the client to stress that the changes in drug use are directly related to improvements in functioning. For example:

One thing that I know has improved is that you were able to get a job! I remember you telling me when we last met that you really wanted to stop using and get a job, and now you are working! Congratulations!

or,

Lots of people say that when they stop using, they have more money to spend on things that they enjoy or they are able to save? Has this been the case with you over the last three months?

Listing of Helpful Strategies Used in the Last Three Months

As a further way to get the client thinking about and focused on the positive changes he or she has made in the last three months, it is useful to have a discussion of the strategies the client has used to reduce/stop use. The goal here, once again, is to get the client talking about anything that they have done that has led them to any sort of change in their use. The therapist can introduce this section by saying:

You have told me that you are using less cocaine than you were using three months ago. That's great! I want to get an idea of the things you have done that have helped you cut down on your use. What's one thing that you have done in the last three months that you think has helped you cut down on your drug use? Why was that helpful?

The therapist should continue to query the client about helpful strategies and ask for explanations for each, as well as propose strategies that the therapist has seen the client use that have likely been helpful. For example,

So staying busy and attending your treatment appointments are two things that you have found very helpful in terms of cutting down your drug use. That's great. You have also talked about spending more time with people who don't use, such as your mother and your daughter, because when you are with them you don't use. You have even told me that some weekends you have stayed at your mother's house so that you could help her out and also be away from the people in your building who use drugs. So it seems like spending time with nonusers has also been a useful strategy for you. What do you think?

Goal Setting

The follow-up MI also ends in goal setting. Now that the client has had some time in treatment, his or her goals may differ from those at the first MI. For example, someone might just be trying to get to treatment sessions at the first MI, but might be ready by the second MI to consider attempting nonuse for a few days. As always, it is important to design a goal that the client thinks he or she can achieve, and to keep the goal at the right level for each client. The goal should be decided by both the client and the therapist and should be something that the client perceives as beneficial and will try to do. For example, one client who has reduced his or her use might be ready to give temporary abstinence a try, while another client who has also reduced his use may not be ready to attempt abstinence, but may be willing to attend an AA meeting or to reduce his use even further. This is particularly important for clients who have not made any changes in their use since the first MI, or who may have even increased use or be experiencing the same or a greater number of drug-related problems. For such clients, developing a goal that is meaningful and useful is critical. A way to talk about this with a client is as follows:

We have now talked about some of the things that are going on with you over the last three months. You have been able to come to lot of BTSAS sessions and that's great. It sounds like you are still having a rough time in a lot of ways, so it's really especially good that you are continuing to come to treatment, and I am really glad that you have been able to do this. What we need to do now is think of a goal that you can work on between now and your next group. I know that you have talked a lot in group about wanting to cut down on your drug use, but you have had a tough time giving that a try. Can you think of something that you could work on that would get you more ready to give that a try?

SOME MORE EXAMPLES

The following are some additional examples of ways to conduct different section of the MI and tailor them to individual clients.

Example 1

The first is an example of an Initial MI for a client who is currently using, is attending treatment due to coercion ("My therapist said I had to come here"), and is not working toward change. His assessment information is as follows:

Drug of choice	Cocaine
Days of use in the last month	15
Days of treatment in the last month	0
URICA item: At times my problem is difficult, but I'm working on it.	Disagree
URICA item: I have a problem and I really think I should work on it.	Disagree
URICA item: Even though I'm not always successful in changing, at least I'm working on my problem.	Disagree
URICA item: I wish I had some more ideas on how to solve my problem.	Disagree
URICA item: I am actively working on my problem (with illegal drug use)	Disagree

This is a client who does not want to be doing the MI or any other substance abuse treatment. For this client, it is important to realize that the goal of the MI is not to change his mind, but rather to work with him, to acknowledge his uncertainties, to place the responsibility for change onto him, and to stress that you are here to talk and provide information but you will not tell him what to do. For example, getting started on the discussion of negative consequences section of the Initial MI could be done in the following way:

Thank you for telling me a bit about your drug use. It sounds like the things that brought you here today are that your therapist thinks it would be good for you, and if you didn't come, your therapist would tell your probation officer, and then you might have to go to jail. Those are good reasons to come, and I am glad you are here today. The goal of this meeting is to talk about your drug use, any changes you might want to make, and to talk about things from your point of view. I am not here to tell you what to do or what you have to do. Rather, my goal is to talk with you about your use, how you see things going these days with your use, and your thoughts about what you should be doing or changing or not changing. While I won't tell you what to do, I will tell you my thoughts about what's going on with you, and I will tell you about the sorts of things our treatment program teaches people. My hope is that you will find some of this information useful. The first thing I would like to do is to talk some about the sorts of things that have happened to you because of your drug use. Most people who use drugs and who have been using for a while have had some things happen to them because of their use, things like legal problems or health problems, things like that. Since you have a probation officer, does that mean that you have had legal problems associated with your drug use? Why don't you tell me something about that?

The nonjudgmental and uncritical tone should persist throughout the MI, especially in the section on Assessment Feedback. Remember that it is not the goal of the MI to directly convince a client that he is wrong and you are right. Rather, the interviewer wants to engage the client in a discussion in an effort to get the client to verbalize reasons for change. Based on the assessment information above, the feedback could go something like this:

I have here some of the information you provided during your assessment, and I would like for us to go over it together. First, you said that your drug of choice is cocaine, and that you used about 15 days in the last month. Does that sound about right? Is that pretty typical for you—to use about half the days in the month? So you were using every day, and in the last few months you have cut down to every other day. That is good news— you have been able to cut your use a lot on your own. Why did you start to use every other day instead of every day? So you had less money and you didn't have enough to use every day. Now, you also said that you did not go to any treatment in the last month, and I know from talking with you now that you have come to a few appointments here at the clinic because you don't want your probation officer to send you to jail. It sounds like you have a very good reason then for coming to your appointments—not wanting to go to jail. Why is it important for you to stay out of jail? So it sounds like for you, jail means keeping you locked up and you hate being locked up and not being able to do what you want. You really like to be free and make your own decisions—is that right? I can understand wanting to make decisions for myself. So for you, keeping out of jail means having freedom and making your own decisions. That sounds to me like an excellent reason to attend your clinic appointments.

Further discussion of the URICA motivational items can go as follows:

When you did your assessments, you were asked a bunch of questions about your thoughts on doing something to change your drug use. You might remember you were asked if you agreed or disagreed with statements like these: "At times my problem is difficult, but I'm working on it," and "I have a problem and I really think I should work on it," and "Even though I'm not always successful in changing, at least I'm working on my problem," and "I am actively working on my problem (with illegal drug use)." You said that you disagree with these statements. Tell me something about that—why do you disagree? Sounds like all of these things refer to drug use as a problem, and you don't see your drug use as a problem. And since you don't see your use as a problem, you don't see it as something you need to change. Is that right? I'm not here to tell you whether or not you have a problem with your drug use. You yourself are the best one to know about your use. One thing we have talked a lot about today though is the problems that using drugs have caused you, especially the chance of going back to jail. Whether or not your drug use is a problem, we can agree that you don't want to go to jail. And given that you are here today and have come to a few of your clinic appointments, it seems like you are trying really hard to do what you need to do to stay out of jail. I see that as some really hard work you are doing to stay out of jail. What do you think of that? So my view is that we should start where we agree, which is that neither of us wants you to go to jail. In this treatment program, we work very hard to help clients achieve their goals by teaching them strategies that they can use to talk to people, to reduce or stop their drug use if that's what they want to do, and to accomplish things like attending treatment and staying out of jail. So you don't have to think you have a problem with drugs to come to these groups. What we hope is to help you think about your goals and help you learn skills to achieve those goals. What do you think of that?

It is important to remember to talk with clients about their goals and their ideas, rather than try to convince them of yours. That is, if a client only wants to attend a group because it will keep him out of jail, that is a fine reason for a client to begin attending a group. The rest of the BTSAS intervention is designed to get clients hooked into the treatment process, to think positively about change, and eventually to attempt change.

In wrapping up the Initial MI for this client with goal setting, it is important to focus on what the client is willing to do. He is unlikely to sign on to stopping his drug use at the Initial MI. However, he is motivated to attend sessions in order to stay out of jail, so attending the first BTSAS session seems like something he would be willing and able to do. The focus of goal setting, then, can be on accomplishing the goal of attending the first BTSAS session, and problem solving can focus on things that might get in the way of the client getting to the first session.

Example 2

The next example is a Follow-Up MI with a client who has reduced her use from the Initial MI to the follow-up. This client has successfully cut down her use, and she has not used any drugs for the two weeks prior to her Follow-up MI. Remember that the Follow-up MI is an opportunity to reinforce the client for successes she has achieved, and to increase self-efficacy by making links between her behavior (reduced drug use) and any positive changes in her life. Getting starting with the feedback can go as follows:

It is great to see you again. Since we have been working together in group, I have seen you cut down your drug use a lot, and you haven't used any drugs for the past couple of weeks! I think that is fantastic! You are really working hard to change. What do you think about what you have been able to do in the last few weeks? That's right— you have made a big change. You might remember that we met for a meeting like this right when you started the BTSAS program. At that time, we asked you lots of questions and you said that you were using cocaine several times a week when you started and you told us that in the month before you came to see us you had used about 10 days, and you were only going to treatment once per month to see your psychiatrist. That has changed a lot hasn't it! How many days would you say you have used in the last month? So, maybe two days, since you haven't used at all in the last two weeks, and before that you had really cut down on your use. That is just great— that's a huge change! And I see you in treatment so I know you come to our groups twice per week, you see your therapist every other week, and you see your psychiatrist once per month. So you are coming to your treatment regularly and keeping your appointments—that's another great accomplishment! Congratulations!

The Follow-up MI includes discussions of any negative consequences that have occurred since the Initial MI, as well as a discussion of the things that have improved over that time. In this case, the client is doing so well that the time spent on these sections should be skewed—little time should be spent on negative consequences and the status of consequences that were discussed during the Initial MI, as well as on any continuing consequences that can serve as further motivators for change. Instead, a lot of time should be spent on the discussion of how life has improved since the client has reduced/stopped use. This can be done as follows:

When we first met a few months ago, you told me about lots of problems you had because of your drug use. At that time two of the main problems were that your mental illness was really bad because you weren't taking your medications, and you weren't able to see your kids because of your drug use. Have those things changed in the last few months? So, your mental illness is much better controlled because you are going to your treatment appointments and taking your medication regularly— that's terrific! How about seeing your kids? You haven't been able to see your kids yet because you haven't finished the program and you haven't been clean for very long. So it sounds like one important thing that we need to focus on now as you keep coming to the program is getting you through the program and building up your clean time so that you will be able to see your kids. You are on you way since you have stopped using for the last two weeks. We need to make sure we keep it up. So your mental illness has improved since you stopped using drugs, and you are now able to work toward seeing your kids since you stopped using. Those are really important accomplishments. Tell me what other things have improved in your life over the last few weeks as you stopped using drugs?

Next comes the section of the Follow-up MI in which the client and therapist list the strategies that have been helpful to the client as she has reduced and stopped her drug use. The therapist needs to emphasize the connection between the client's behavior change (actual substance use reduction), and the things that the client has done differently to achieve this change. The purpose of this is to help build the participant's confidence not only in her ability to efficaciously change behavior, but to also help her realize that the strategies that she used lead to positive results. The following exchange is an example of how to discuss the things that have worked as a way to increase a sense of self-efficacy:

Therapist: You have made a really big change in your drug use, going from regular use to not using at all in the last two weeks. What is something you think has helped you to do that?

Client: Well, I told my friend that I didn't want to use because I was afraid I wouldn't ever get to see my kids again.

Therapist: Why do you think that worked for you?

Client: I had to tell her a lot of times. After telling her over and over I think it finally sunk in—she has kids too so I think she can understand not wanting to lose them.

Therapist: Excellent. So telling your friend no and giving her a good reason why you didn't want to use has helped you stay clean for several weeks. That's wonderful! What else have you done in the last few weeks that has helped you to stay clean?

Client: Well, I have really tried to stay away from the corner where I used to buy drugs.

Therapist: Great. So in addition to giving your friend a good reason why you don't want to use, you have avoided the place where you used to buy your drugs (we call that a high-risk situation in group, remember?), you were able to stay off drugs for two weeks.

The idea is to keep linking the specific behavior change with the positive outcome and to help the client identify any other behaviors that may have been useful. The aim is to simply help the client link specific behaviors with successful goal attainment.

Example 3

As a final example, consider the Follow-up MI for a client who is having difficulty achieving his goals in the BTSAS groups, continues to use drugs, and continues to experience negative consequences of his use. In this case, the goal of the Follow-up MI is to help the client figure out what obstacles remain on the way to achieving his goal, without being critical or judgmental. If obstacles can be readily identified, then the therapist needs to help the individual develop new strategies for overcoming them. For some individuals, however, less ambitious goals may need to be set. For example, instead of suggesting that the client "stay clean," perhaps sampling clean time for a day or reducing weekly so that the client has one clean day per week would be appropriate goals. The purpose of the Follow-up MI in this case is to start to build success experiences for the client and to simultaneously build confidence in his ability to change. The most challenging sections of the Follow-up MI in such a case are likely to be the discussion of negative consequences and goal setting. Let us first give an example of how the discussion of negative consequences section can go:

> So at this point you are using about as often as you were using when you started the BTSAS program. While we are still figuring out what's going to be helpful for you in terms of reducing your use, you have accomplished several important things since we first met. One thing that you are doing really well is you are coming to group regularly—that's great! We really count on you as an important part of the group, you have shown a lot of support to the other group members, and you are doing great when you practice the skills we teach in the group. You are a really great role player and you know all the steps by heart—that's terrific. You are coming to group and you are really working hard when you are there—we notice it and appreciate it and it will help you and it helps the other group members. The other thing you are doing very well is you are being honest in group—you are talking about how hard it is for you to cut down your drug use and being honest when you do use. Being honest can be really tough and it is great that when you come to group, you tell us honestly what's going on with you. I know that since you have been using over the last few months, you have had some problems from your use. I remember that in group you talked about getting into a fight with your roommate because of your drug use, and now he is threatening to get you kicked out of your housing. What else is happening to you because of your drug use these days? So in addition to fights with your roommate, you continue to have problems paying your bills because you are using your money to buy drugs. It sounds like we need to remember that two things that would be better for you if you cut down or stopping using drugs would be that you wouldn't have fights with your roommate and risk losing your housing, and you would have enough money to pay for the things you needed because you wouldn't be spending your money on drugs. That's important for us to remember as we try to figure out ways to help you cut down your drug use.

It is important to remember that this discussion should not be a listing of all the ways the client is continuing to mess up, but rather should focus on the problems the client is having as a way to increase motivation to change. Stressing at the start any positive steps the client has made (in this case, attending BTSAS groups and working hard during the groups) sets the stage for a discussion that is not accusatory or negative.

For a client who is struggling to achieve his goals, goal setting can be difficult. Here is an example of how this section can be carried out for this type of client:

Therapist: Your goals in group have been to stop using crack. It seems that you are having some difficulty with this goal. What do you think has been making it difficult for you to stop using?

Client: Well, I don't know, well I guess whenever my friend comes over he smells like crack and always has some ready to fire up.

Therapist: So it is difficult for you not to use and to say no to your friend when he has drugs on him and even smells like crack.

Client: Yeah.

Therapist: Well, maybe we can change your goal a bit to focus on reducing your use. After all, reducing can eventually lead to stopping, and maybe focusing on cutting down will be helpful to you. When people try to cut down, it is helpful to think about a situation in which they always use (remember in group we call this a high-risk situation) and then to think of how to escape or avoid that situation so that they won't be faced with that temptation. This is often a good way to start cutting down on using. Sounds like this situation with your friend coming over might be a good place to start. Let's think of an escape strategy or a way to avoid him all together when he has crack on him or smells like crack. What time does he usually come by your house?

Client: Around 5:00 on Saturday or Sunday afternoon before dinner.

Therapist: Is there some place else you can be during that time?

Client: Sometimes I can go to my mom's house. No one uses there.

Therapist: OK, so one thing you could do this Saturday is before 5, maybe at 4:30, you can go to your mom's house. Do you have transportation to get there and will your mom be OK with your visiting?

Client: I can get there. But sometimes she doesn't want me to come over or she is out and I can't go there when she is out.

Therapist: OK, so this Saturday you will see about going to your mom's house so that you won't be home at 5 when your friend comes over to use. If you can't go to your mom's, what else could you do to achieve your goal of not using on Saturday?

Client: I don't know.

Therapist: Would you feel comfortable not opening or answering the door if your friend comes over at 5?

Client: Yeah, I could just pretend I'm not home. It might be hard to ignore the knocking on the door though.

Therapist: Has there ever been a time when you were able to ignore the knocking on the door?

Client: Yeah—one time my friend came over but I didn't hear him knocking because I was in my bedroom on the phone.

Therapist: Well, how about trying that this Saturday. If you can't go to your mom's, go in your bedroom and make a call—who could you talk to that would distract you from your friend knocking on the door?

Client: I could call my sister and ask her how the kids are.

Therapist: That's great!

The therapist should continue to problem solve with the client until they arrive at an agreeable solution.

SUMMARY

The MI procedure described here is adapted for the needs of an SPMI population. As such, it is more focused, more concrete, and more directive than a traditional MI would be. However, we have preserved the philosophy of MI in our procedure, which involves collaborating with the client rather than telling him or her what to do, showing support and caring while communicating that the client's thoughts and ideas are important, and eliciting the client's own reasons for and thoughts about change rather than lecturing about how the client's life is bad and would be good without drugs. The goals of our MIs, both the Initial MI and the Follow-up MI, are to have an individual discussion about reasons for change, and to help the client see the benefits of continued work and treatment attendance. It a client continues to be engaged in the BTSAS program, there is a greater chance of change.

Chapter 7

URINALYSIS CONTINGENCY AND GOAL SETTING

INTRODUCTION

The urinalysis contingency procedures (UCP) and goal setting are integral components of the BTSAS program. The UCP is designed to provide immediate reinforcement, both financial and social, for reductions in drug use. Specifically, clients provide a urine sample at each session, the sample is immediately tested, and clients with a sample that is clean for a self-selected goal drug receive a small sum of money as a reinforcer. Specifically, the financial reinforcement for clean urinalysis testing starts at $1.50 and increases by $0.50 whenever the client provides negative samples in two consecutive scheduled sessions (e.g., twice within a one-week period), up to a maximum of $3.50. So, the progression of payments is as follows: $1.50 for the first two consecutive clean samples; $2.00 for samples 3 to 4; $2.50 for samples 5 to 6; $3.00 for samples 7 to 8; and $3.50 for samples 9 to 10. If the client produces a positive urine sample at any time or is absent from a group session, the payment is reset back to $1.50, and the value increases in units of $0.50 again after two consecutive clean samples. Positive samples are met with discussion and problem solving. The immediate nature of this feedback is very important with SPMI clients. Most individuals with SPMI experience cognitive deficits that impact the ability to anticipate high-risk situations, see the connection between substance use and negative consequences over time, and impede the ability to develop realistic goals. In addition, often the goals that most clients are working toward are long term and difficult to achieve (staying out of jail, seeing one's children, getting better housing). Providing immediate feedback reinforces the connection between even a small amount of reduced drug use and a tangible reward, right in the here and now. The fact that the reinforcement is both financial and social is important as well. The financial reinforcement serves as a concrete reward for a job well done.

The social aspect of the contingency (attention and praise from the therapist, applause and good wishes from other group members) serves an important function for people with SPMI who experience varying degrees of social impairment. They often have difficulty developing social relationships with individuals who do not use drugs and difficulty developing a social support system to assist them in reducing their drug use. The social component of the reinforcement gives clients the sense that a community of people is there to help them meet their goals and support them when they achieve some success. Our experience has shown that the applause, cheering, and good wishes that make up the social reinforcement is highly rewarding to clients, who typically smile, laugh, and thank group members for their help.

The goal-setting component of BTSAS is designed to help clients establish and achieve concrete, short-term abstinence or reduction goals. Goal setting occurs at the start of each group session. Clients collaborate with the therapist to create a concrete goal to work on between sessions. Often these goals involve reducing or abstaining from drug use from one group session to the next. Other times clients who are not yet ready or able to commit to reduced drug use will develop goals such as attending a self-help meeting, saving money rather than spending it on drugs, or simply attending the next BTSAS session. Goals are written down in a formal "contract" that is signed by both parties and the client is given a copy to keep. Goals are reviewed at the start of each group session, success is reinforced, and failures are responded to with problem solving and encouragement.

GENERAL ISSUES IN THE URINALYSIS CONTINGENCY PROCEDURES IN BTSAS

Clients with SPMI who meet DSM-IV (American Psychiatric Association, 1994) criteria for a substance use disorder often abuse multiple substances. While it would be desirable for them to achieve abstinence for all drugs of abuse, that is an unrealistic initial goal for most clients. Consequently, we employ a harm reduction model in which we shape reduced use of a primary substance of abuse first, and then target use of other substances of abuse as use of the primary substance is drastically cut or stopped.

UCP and the Selection of the Goal Drug

The primary substance of abuse, referred to in the BTSAS program as the goal drug, is identified by the client and the therapist. It is typically the substance that causes the most harm, whether or not it is the substance used most frequently. For example, many clients use alcohol or cannabis frequently, but select cocaine as the goal drug because it increases symptomatology or causes more disruption in their lives than the other substances. In deciding on the goal drug, it is also important to take into account which substance the client is likely to have some initial success with in terms of cutting down or stopping. For some clients, the drug that is used less frequently, and is perhaps less of an issue for the client, can be a good place to start because it is relatively easy to stop use of that drug. For example, a client might use marijuana, heroin, and cocaine, with her use of heroin being less frequent than her use of cocaine. The client might be willing to select heroin as her goal drug and be unwilling at this point to stop using cocaine, even though she is using cocaine more frequently and cocaine might, in reality, be the bigger problem for her. Remember: start where the client is willing to start. If a client is willing to attend treatment and to work on stopping her heroin use, this is a good starting point, and can provide some initial success that can be reinforced, and as attendance at BTSAS increases and heroin use decreases or stops, there will be time to address the cocaine use. In such a case, once a client has had success stopping heroin, she might be more willing to address her cocaine use, and might even go so far at some point as to change her goal drug and the focus of her work in BTSAS to cocaine.

UCP and Financial Reinforcement

In developing the UCP and deciding on the amount of money to be offered for negative urinalysis tests, it was important to strike a balance between an amount that was meaningful to clients and at the same time not cost prohibitive for treatment centers and clinics to offer in the real world settings in which people with SPMI receive care. As described above, clients with a clean sample earn small sums of money starting at $1.50, which increases by $0.50 with every two successive clean tests to a cap of

$3.50. We believe that this level of financial reinforcement achieves the desired balance. Most people with SPMI are unemployed and often have *no* cash between welfare or SSI payments; consequently, $1.50 to $3.50 is a noticeable amount of money for these individuals. It is not a powerful enough incentive to drive behavior change on its own, but the combination of money coupled with regular urine checks, social reinforcement, and public attention to drug use is intended to provide a tangible reward for (even modest) success, and increase the salience of goals for reduced use.

CONDUCTING THE UCP

The UCP begins in the third BTSAS session. New clients observe the UCP for their first two sessions, and are informed that they will be asked to provide a sample during their third group.

Getting Started

SPMI clients require early and rapid reinforcement in order for treatment to be experienced as rewarding. To this end, we wanted clients to be able to earn money for nonuse of their goal drug as soon as possible. We have found that at least some clients who begin the BTSAS program are willing and ready to give abstinence on their goal drug a try at the start, and we wanted clients to get immediate reinforcement for this behavior, rather than have them reduce drug use or try out abstinence, only to have to wait for financial incentives. Beginning the urinalysis in session 3 rather than immediately at the start of treatment gives clients time to get acclimated to group, to learn some basic social skills, and to contemplate a change in drug use before actually having to make such a change. Many clients are actively using when they begin BTSAS. We felt that collecting urine before clients know the goals of the program would result in those who have recently used drugs not earning financial reinforcement at the first session, perhaps setting the stage for continued "failure" or reduced motivation to attend.

Documenting Self-Report of Use and Doing the Urinalysis Test

When a client attends a BTSAS group, they are asked if they have used their goal drug since the last meeting. It is important that, at first, the therapist ask only if a subject has used his or her goal drug, in order to maintain the reinforcing nature of the group. The subject may lose focus on being clean for his goal drug if he has used another substance. The client is then given a urine cup and goes to a restroom near the BTSAS room and provides a urine sample in private. We do not observe urination as there is little incentive for clients to bring clean urines with them (e.g., there are no legal consequences for using, and the reinforcement is modest), and few clients with SPMI are cognitively organized enough to plan and carry out a dissimulation. Nevertheless, clients are not permitted to bring a coat, purse, or package into the restroom, and urine samples are checked for temperature. Invalid (e.g., cold) samples and missing samples (e.g., client cannot void) are assumed to be positive and the client does not earn a reinforcer. However, clients who cannot void are offered water during the group and invited to try again to provide a sample, in which case a negative sample is reinforced.

Providing Immediate Feedback and Reinforcement if the Urinalysis Test is Negative

When all subjects have voided and testing is complete, the results for each client are announced in the group. Clients who have negative samples receive immediate social reinforcement. Generally the therapist will applaud and group members will follow this example and applaud as well. A typical example of how this is done is as follows:

Bob, you told us that you did not use cocaine since the last group, and your test was negative. That's great! You were able to achieve your goal from the last group, and this means that you have had three clean tests in a row. Here is your $2.00 for your hard work—congratulations!

For a client who provides a clean test for the first time, the therapist can say:

Sue reported that she did not use heroin and Sue, your test is clean! That is your first clean test—congratulations! Here's your $1.50 and now you are on board and starting to earn some money. That is great!

Other group members are also encouraged to be reinforcing (e.g., "Let's all congratulate Juan on being clean for three weeks now!").

There are two important things to remember about providing this feedback. First, you cannot be too reinforcing. This is a chance to have fun and reward clients for their hard work. Make sure your words, tone, and actions are all extremely positive. Keep in mind that people with SPMI and substance use disorders have few occasions to be praised by anyone, and oftentimes the other substance abuse treatments that they have been in or are attending in conjunction with BTSAS do not recognize incremental reductions in use as a success. Thus the BTSAS group is, for many clients, the only source of praise they have. Second, both the financial and the social reinforcement must be immediate. Remember that the goal is to link the clean test with a tangible reward. The closer the test result and the reward are in time, the better. This typically takes the form of the therapist giving the test result, followed by congratulations and applause, followed by the therapist handing the client the money earned in the UCP. Each client is provided the feedback and reinforcement in full before the therapist moves on to the next client in the group.

Discussion If Test Is Positive

Most of the time, clients who have used their drug of choice are honest about their use and report using even before the urinalysis test is completed. Other times, clients will be unsure if their use was within the window to be picked up by the test. New BTSAS therapists are at first often uncomfortable providing UCP results when the urinalysis test comes back positive. However, the goal of the UCP and its feedback is to celebrate success and treat positive tests not as treatment failures but as an opportunity to learn about how to better handle a situation next time it is encountered. Feedback for positive tests can also be, at first, difficult for clients, who may be used to disappointed, frustrated, or frankly angry and judgmental reactions to their use from treatment providers. The expectation of being criticized or yelled at following a positive test is, we believe, one reason why some SPMI clients have difficulty engaging in substance abuse treatment—they expect negative feedback and prefer to not show up rather than have yet another person criticize them.

Thus it is very important that BTSAS therapists understand that the feedback we provide following a positive test is not critical or judgmental. Rather, this feedback has three main components. First, feedback is delivered in a straightforward and calm manner. The goal is to show that this is a component of the treatment program but that success or failure in treatment is not determined by any single positive test. We do not express anger or hostility; rather the client is told how the test turned out, and the discussion moves on from there. Second, in providing feedback following a positive sample, the therapist should be empathic and supportive. The key here is to remember that, even for a client who has yet to make any real reductions in use, SPMI clients would much prefer to change their drug use and to stop using. The positive test is typically as disappointing to the client as it is to the clinician, and the client should be treated with support and encouragement. Finally, this feedback involves immediate problem solving in which the client and therapist identify the high-risk situations that lead to use and plan for how the client might better cope in these situations between now and the next group. If substance use has occurred in a social situation (e.g., social pressure or temptation due to someone else using), the therapist can conduct a role-play. This allows the client to practice the skill that might be used to avoid or cope with this situation in the future. Coping strategies for nonsocial risk situations (e.g., boredom, craving) will be more variable, and need to be tailored to the individual client's needs and abilities.

These three aspects of this feedback are evident in this example:

Joe, your urine test came back positive for cocaine today (straightforward and calm). *I realize that you have been trying to cut down and you were hoping for a clean test today and I'm sorry you're disappointed* (supportive). *Let's go right to your goal setting now and figure out what situation led to your drug use and how you might better deal with that in the next few days. So, since our last group, when did you use cocaine and what was going on when you decided to use?* (start of immediate problem solving).

In cases in which the client has already reported drug use and so a positive urinalysis result is not a surprise, feedback can be much the same: straightforward, supportive, and focused on problem solving the situation in which the use occurred. The feedback in this case could go something like this:

Sam, you reported using cocaine this week, so it's no surprise that your urine test is positive. I'm glad that you were able to be honest with us—that is really great. What was the situation in which you used? Let's see if we can role-play that and practice a strategy that would keep you from using in that situation in the future. So your friend came over and asked you to use, and after a couple of times of his asking you said yes and you used. This sounds like a good situation to role-play your drug refusal skills. Let's review the steps of drug refusal skills.

The therapist would then proceed with a quick review of the steps in drug refusal skills, and then set up the role-play and have the client do the role-play. The following is an example of how the therapist could set up a role-play:

Therapist: So Marie, you goal was to stay clean between the last group and today. You told us that you used on Saturday night. What was going on when you used?

Client: My sister came over with crack and we smoked it.

Therapist: It sounds like being able to tell your sister that you don't want to use would have helped in this situation. Is that right?

Client: Yeah, but she says it over and over until I give in.

Therapist: OK, let's set up a role-play so we can practice using drug refusal skills to tell your sister that you don't want to smoke crack with her. The first and second steps in drug refusal skills are to make eye contact and to say "No, I don't want to use" in a firm voice. Why do you think making eye contact and using a firm voice are important?

Client: So the person knows you are serious.

Therapist: That's exactly right! Great! If you look at someone and speak firmly, she will know that you mean what you are saying. The third step is to give a reason why you don't want to use. What reason could you give your sister?

Client: I could tell her I'm trying to stay clean.

Therapist: OK, that's a great reason not to use. So you will make eye contact, tell her you don't want to use in a firm voice, and then tell her that you are trying to stay clean. Step 4 is to tell your sister to stop asking you to use with her. How would you like to say that?

Client: I could tell her could she stop bothering me about using?

Therapist: Great! You can see that we wrote all the steps and what you are going to say on the board. Let's do our role-play now. I'll be your sister and I'll knock on the door and tell you I have some crack and you'll use these drug refusal skills to tell me you don't want to use. Ready?

If the person did not use drugs as a result of an interpersonal problem, the therapist should focus a brief discussion on a coping skill that might circumvent the problem in the future. The emphasis is on simple behavioral plans that are rehearsed immediately and require minimal emphasis on "will power" or sophisticated planning and problem solving. Common problems and potential coping strategies include:

1. Being home alone and bored: Leave the house and go for a walk; call a friend or significant other; plan an activity for when you can anticipate being alone and tempted to use; attend an AA/NA meeting.
2. Having money (e.g., SSI paydays): Get a representative payee or have someone hold your money; bring someone with you who doesn't use when you go to get your check; do not walk home past the dealer on days you get paid.
3. Bothered by symptoms/side effects: Medication management skills for explaining problem to physician.

Clients will often report that they simply had an urge to use. If avoidance/escape is not feasible or effective, the therapist can help the client to make a list of reasons for not using, or can teach the client a simple self-talk strategy, in which he or she reviews the one or two most powerful reasons for not using until the urge/craving has passed. An example of this technique is as follows.

Therapist: So Marcus, let's think of why it is so important to you to not use crack.

Client: 'Cause I'm on conditional release and I'll go back to jail if they catch me using.

Therapist: And why would that be so bad?

Client: It scares me. My voices get real bad when I'm locked up.

Therapist: OK. Now, I want you to close your eyes. OK? Good now imagine you're on your sofa and you start to think about crack. You are bored and you really feel like doing some. Can you imagine that?

Client: Yeah. I can imagine that.

Therapist: Good, now tell yourself why you don't want to use: about going back to jail and stuff.

Client: If I go buy some stuff I could get arrested and sent back to jail.

Therapist: OK, now tell yourself why that would be so bad.

Client: My voices get real bad when I'm locked up

Therapist: So should you go out and score some crack?

Client: No.

Therapist: Why not?

Client: Because I could go back to jail.

This process is repeated three to four times until the client can quickly enumerate his or her primary reasons for not using. Simultaneously, the cotherapist writes the basic question and the key responses on a 3 × 5-inch index card that is then given to the client. The client is instructed to carry it in his or her wallet/pocket/purse, and take it out and read it whenever he or she feels very tempted and may give in. This strategy should be rehearsed in the next few sessions, even if the client has a clean urine sample. The key is repetition of one or a few simple statements that carry considerable weight for the client and are likely to motivate restraint or be an effective distraction until the craving subsides.

Difficult Issues

There are two situations in which the UCP feedback can be especially challenging. The first is when a client reports that he did not use his goal drug since the last session and the urinalysis test comes up positive. In this situation, there is always a tendency for the therapist to want the client to admit he or she really used, and most of the time the client is not going to admit this. This has the potential to set up a conflict between the therapist and the client over the urine results. In BTSAS, we strongly believe that having conflicts with clients, arguing over who is right, and getting clients to admit use is both not reinforcing and counterproductive. Our approach is to deliver test results in a straightforward and calm manner, provide support if a client is upset over test results, shift the focus to what might go wrong between today and the next session, and use potential problems for a role-play. The following example illustrates the matter-of-fact way this is done:

> *I'm sorry Bob, you tested positive for—(client's goal drug). You do not get $1.50 because you used. Let's try to figure out how to deal with the situation that led to your use, so that next time you are in that situation you will be able to get through it without using. What was the situation in which you used?*

There are infrequent times when the client will insist that the test must be incorrect and that he or she did not use. Engaging in a long debate runs the risk of sidelining the entire session with this client and his or her dissatisfaction with the urinalysis test. Again, we do not argue with clients or get them to see that the test is positive and so they must admit that they used. Rather, in the spirit of motivational interviewing (Miller & Rollnick, 1991), we find it more helpful to "roll with resistance"—use the client's anger or insistence as a cue to move on. The following is the typical way we respond to a client who is insisting that the urinalysis test is incorrect:

Client: I know you say that my test was positive, but I didn't use cocaine. The test is wrong.

Therapist: You have been working really hard in group and out to try to cut down your cocaine use, and I can tell that you are disappointed that you test came back positive. These tests pick up cocaine for three to four days after use and heroin for about three days after use.

Client: Well I know I haven't used in the last four days. The test is wrong.

Therapist: We have found that this system is very good. But the really important thing for us to do here is to get on with a goal and figure out what we can do so that you can achieve that goal. You goals over the last several groups have been to stay clean from one group to the next? Do you want that to be your goal for this group?

Client: I don't care about making a goal. I want to get paid for today because I didn't use and the test is wrong.

Therapist: You have worked very hard and have been really focused on having negative urine tests and that is great. You have also been coming to groups regularly and I can tell that you are giving it your all to try to stop using cocaine. We all see the hard work that you are doing here. What I want to do is get going on goal setting so that we can talk some about how to help you with your goal of staying clean between now and the next group. Let's get going with that and if you want we can talk more about this after group.

GOAL SETTING

Upon completion of the urinalysis protocol and problem solving for positive tests, the therapist engages group members in goal setting. Goal setting proceeds for each client individually, with the therapist asking for ideas and participation from other clients as the need arises. The purpose of goal setting is to identify a specific goal, have the client verbalize a few personal reasons for staying clean, and problem solving a few important barriers to achieving the goal. Generally, the goal drug is the target of the goal. Working with the goal drug increases the likelihood that the person will have some success in being clean, and links goal setting to the UCP (the goal is to stay clean from the goal drug, the UCP documents whether or not this goal has been achieved). After success is achieved with the goal drug, another drug can be added to the goal, provided it could be objectively measured in a drug panel. We feel that shaping new behavior and gradually expanding the scope of goals increases engagement and the chances for success. For clients who are not yet ready to attempt abstinence, goals can focus on reductions in use (using only $5 per day, selecting a day in the week to stay clean, etc). Clients who are not yet ready or able to commit to reduced drug use can develop goals such as attending a self-help meeting, saving money rather than spending it on drugs, or simply attending the next treatment session. Goals must be reviewed each session to see if the client wants to make any changes, but the therapists should appraise the chances for success and tailor goals accordingly.

Goal setting has several parts: (1) developing a goal; (2) review of reasons for staying clean or cutting down; (3) problem-solving barriers to achieving the goal; and (4) reviewing the goal between sessions.

Developing a Goal

There are several important things to remember when helping clients develop a goal. First, goals should be realistic and set to minimize the chances of failure. Clients, especially at the beginning of their BT-SAS program, will often be unrealistic in what they propose to try. Sensible but unrealistic goals (e.g., "I don't want to use cocaine anymore") should not be rejected, but should be praised as evidence that the client is very serious about stopping his drug use. However, therapists need to help clients create a realistic goal, one that can be achieved and that moves the client toward the more superordinate goal (e.g., "How about if this week we try to use only on weekends?" or "How about trying to stay away from cocaine between today and our next group?"). Of course, the therapist must use his or her knowledge of the client, the specific situation, and what he or she knows about behavior change in general in order to determine what is realistic and what is not. The general rule of thumb is to be conservative. Second, if the client continually fails to achieve her goal, the therapist should help her to generate an intermediate goal that is more attainable (e.g., if the client can't avoid using crack all week perhaps she can try to restrict use to one or two days). It is critical to remember that behavior change is difficult and must be shaped by gradual approximations. Third, it is important that the therapist not imply that the client is being foolish or naive or that it is the client's inadequacy or lack of competence that makes the goal unsatisfactory. Be reinforcing and encouraging, always couch feedback in positive terms. For example, rather than, "I think that's too much for you to take on," or "I don't think you're being realistic here," try something like,

That's a good goal, and it shows that you are really serious about stopping your drug use. That's what I like to hear. But one thing I have learned from working with people with mental illness and substance abuse is that sometimes you need to start small in order to get going. Staying clean for an entire week is a pretty big jump from where you are now. How about if we try...

Or

I'm glad you want to make such a big change, but it might be hard to not use if your brother keeps bringing stuff home to use with friends. How about if you plan on leaving the house [escape] when he comes up with his friends to use?

Review of Reasons for Staying Clean or Cutting Down

When a client selects staying clean between sessions or reducing use as the goal, he or she is next asked for two reasons for staying clean/cutting down. We do this in order to give the client an opportunity to say, in his own words, the things that are motivating him to reduce or stop using. It is a good idea when discussing clients' reasons to remain clean or cut down to frame reasons in *I* statements that reflect negative consequences of behavior. Clients are more likely to refrain from using when their motivation is to avoid something negative (e.g. "I will go back to jail if I use") as opposed to a more abstract, positive reason (e.g. "I want the respect of my family").

Problem-Solving Barriers to Achieving the Goal

At this point group therapists should shift to a means-ends problem-solving approach for goal setting, including identifying what could go wrong or what the client might do next, with other group members providing input and feedback about possible problems and solutions. A simple 5-step means-ends problem-solving strategy is employed for goal setting, anticipating, and coping with high-risk situations that might interfere with achieving the goal. The steps of the procedure are as follows:

1. The client is first asked: What could keep you from meeting your goal?
2. After a problem is identified, the client is asked: What could you do so that wouldn't happen?
3. After a reasonable solution is suggested, the client is asked: And what could go wrong with that or why might that not work?
4. After a likely problem is identified, the client is asked: OK, what could you do if that happened?
5. After a reasonable solution is suggested the therapist says: That sounds like a good strategy; let's role-play that so you get some practice

The strategy is illustrated in this prototypical dialogue:

Therapist: So Raul, your goal this week is not to use crack on Wednesday or Thursday. What do you think might make it hard to meet your goal?

Client: Anita might come over with some good stuff and ask if I want to party with her.

Therapist: What could you do if Anita comes over wanting to use?

Client: I could tell her I don't want to use.

Therapist: That's good—you could use your drug refusal skills and tell her you don't want to use. What if you tell her but she doesn't listen to you. Then what could you do?

Client: Maybe I could tell her to leave and come back when she doesn't have any stuff with her?

Therapist: That's a great idea! You could tell her to leave and come back later without the drugs. What could go wrong with that?

Client: She could say we could have sex if she stays.

Therapist: OK, then what could you do?

Client: I could tell her I don't care. She should come back later.

Therapist: OK. That sounds great. I think we should role-play this to give you some practice.

In general, the therapist should try to have the client generate and evaluate two to three alternatives. Many clients will not be able to generate more than two reasonable options, and the goal should be two choices that the client is likely to be able to use, that have a reasonable chance of working, and that are socially appropriate. If the client is stuck or cannot generate viable solutions, the therapist should ask group members if they can help come up with some ideas.

Reviewing the Goal Between Sessions

Whenever possible, the client should be encouraged to make a public statement to a significant other (parent, case manager, sibling, etc.) about his goal and what he can do to achieve the goal. The person, time, and place in which the commitment will be made should be identified, and the client can role-play what he will say to the person if need be. The therapist can portray initial skepticism, followed by enthusiastic support. For example:

Therapist: (portraying significant other) Hi. Wanda. What's up?

Wanda: My goal in group is to stay clean this week.

Therapist: I've heard that before.

Wanda: No man, I am serious this time.

Therapist: Well that's great. How can I help?

Some clients will report that they have no one with whom they can review the goal between sessions. In these instances, the therapist should be creative in identifying different strategies, and the best method for reviewing the goal needs to be selected for each client. If group cohesiveness exists and the client appears to benefit from a public statement of his goal, he can publicly review his goal with the group. Often, it may appear that the client is just reading the goal statement without any apparent investment or commitment in the plan. In this case, ask the client to choose another member of the group and paraphrase his goal to that person. Remember that the client should get something out of publicly reviewing his goal, regardless of the method. If reviewing the goal is nothing more than a "task" to the client, and other members appear bored, do not have the client review the goal during the session. Rather, encourage the client to review the goal himself between sessions. Another option is to have the client call you to review the goal.

Goal-Setting Form

A goal-setting form is used to record the goal, two or three possible barriers to achieving this goal, and ways to overcome these barriers so that the client can be successful. The new goal should be written on the goal sheet and signed by both the client and therapist. The client should be directed to save the goal sheet and to put it somewhere where he will see it during the time between sessions.

Sample Goal Setting

The following is a sample goal setting.

Therapist: So Marie, what would you like your goal to be between now and our next group?

Client: To stay clean.

Therapist: That's a great goal! I know that you have been working really hard to stay clean, and I think having that as your goal is a great idea. So your goal will be to stay clean from cocaine between now and our next group. What are some reasons why you want to stay clean?

Client: I want to stay out of jail.

Therapist: That's a really good reason to stay clean. What's one other reason?

Client: Using messes me up and I want to be OK and not be messed up.

Therapist: OK—so two reasons why you want to stay clean are because you don't want to go to jail and you want to feel good and not feel messed up: Terrific. What's one thing that could get in the way of you achieving your goal of staying clean between now and our next group?

Client: I could get a craving.

Therapist: What could you do if you got a craving so that you wouldn't give in to it and use?

Client: Last week when I had a craving I watched TV and then took a walk and it went away.

Therapist: That's really great! Remember that a craving only lasts for 7 to 10 minutes, so if you can distract yourself for that long, most of the time it will go away. Sounds like when you watched TV and then took a walk, you distracted yourself and got through the craving. Great job!

Client: Thanks.

Therapist: So one thing that could get in the way of you meeting your goal of staying clean is if you have a craving. If you get a craving you can watch TV and take a walk—or really do anything that could distract you for about 10 minutes. Now, what's another thing that could get in your way of staying clean between now and the next group?

Client: My boyfriend could bring some with him when he comes over.

Therapist: So what is something you could do if your boyfriend brings drugs when he comes over so that you won't use and you will be able to achieve your goal of staying clean?

Client: I guess I could ask him not to bring any over.

Therapist: That's a great idea. That's a good way to make sure you never even see the drugs or have them near you—telling him to not even bring them over in the first place. Great job! How do you think you could tell him not to bring drugs over.

Client: I could call him and tell him to not bring it over.

Therapist: Why don't we role-play that so you can get some practice. I'll be your boyfriend. You call me and tell me not to bring drugs over. What do you think your boyfriend would say if you told him not to bring drugs over?

Client: He would probably get mad. He comes over to use and he likes to use at my place because it's comfortable.

Therapist: Is there any chance you both could do something else when you are together? Or will he just want to use drugs?

Client: He likes to go out to eat.

Therapist: OK, you call me on the phone and tell me you don't want me to bring drugs over. Remember to speak in a firm voice and tell me you don't want to use drugs. Also, you need to give a reason why you don't want to use. What reason could you give?

Client: I could tell him because of my drug test.

Therapist: That's a great reason to stay clean. So you are going to tell me in a firm voice that you don't want to use because you are getting drug tested, and you are going to offer me an alternative of going out to eat. Ready?

SUMMARY

UCP and goal setting are strategies to help make the benefits and aims of treatment more concrete and understandable for SPMI clients. Through UCP, clients receive immediate and tangible rewards for any reductions in drug use. Through goal setting, clients are able to develop short-term goals that are within their ability to achieve, and are helped to think about the things they need to do to be successful. Both strategies are delivered in a positive, reinforcing, and supportive way that communicates to the client that he is welcome and valued in the group no matter what stage of motivation or use he is at. Both UCP and goal setting reflect the adaptations needed for substance abuse treatment to be meaningful and engaging for SPMI clients.

Chapter 8

SOCIAL SKILLS AND DRUG REFUSAL SKILLS TRAINING

INTRODUCTION

The skills training component of BTSAS has two basic sections. The first includes three sessions (sessions 1–3) of general social skills training. The skills that are taught in the general social skills training section are making small talk, making plans with a friend, and general refusal skills. The second section involves training in drug refusal skills and lasts for the duration of the skills training component of the group (sessions 4–22). There are three basic skills that are taught and then practiced repeatedly: (1) refusing drugs and offering an alternative; (2) refusing drugs and asking that the person not ask you to use anymore; and (3) refusing drugs and escaping the situation.

Both general social skills and drug refusal skills are important components of BTSAS. Clients with SPMI often experience situations that pose challenges to substance abuse treatment. First, they show marked social impairment. They frequently are unable to achieve goals or have their needs met in situations requiring social interaction. The result is that clients have great difficulty developing relationships with nonusing peers, resisting social pressure to use, and accessing a support system for reduced drug use. In addition, most substance abuse in clients with SPMI occurs in a social context (Dixon, Haas, Weiden, Sweeney, & Frances, 1990). This suggests that substance use may be associated with social-affiliative needs, including the desire to seem "normal" and be accepted by peers, as well as help to reduce social anxiety and compensate for social skill deficits. Clients themselves often report substance use in order to socialize and feel normal around other people. In addition, clients with SPMI often lack a supportive environment, and have few or no positive and rewarding activities that make life without using both possible and reinforcing. People with SPMI have few opportunities to experience pleasure in their environments, and substance use may provide one of the only pleasurable experiences clients regularly have. When surveyed about their reasons for use, clients with SPMI often identify social facilitation and relief of boredom as some of their reasons for their use (Dixon et al., 1991; Test, Wallisch, Allness, & Ripp, 1989). In addition, clients with SPMI often find themselves doing things that they do not want to be doing (i.e., giving money to others, running errands for family members). SPMI clients often lack the ability to say no to requests, a situation that can provide an ongoing source of stress and anger.

In light of these deficits, the general social skills segment of BTSAS is designed to help clients learn new skills for engaging with other people and making new social contacts. Skills such as making small talk and making plans with someone are needed in order for clients to begin to build new drug-free support systems and try out new activities that do not involve drug use. BTSAS also includes a session on general refusal skills, designed both to help clients learn to say no to nondrug requests, but also to get them comfortable saying no in nondrug situations as a prelude to learning to say no in the high-stress situation of refusing offers of drugs. Following some preliminary training in general social skills, the remainder of the skills training sessions focus on key drug refusal skills that clients are taught and then practice repeatedly in an effort to have the steps of these skills become automatic. It is such familiarity in the safe context of a BTSAS group that will help clients learn drug refusal skills that can then be utilized in high-stress situations.

As you can see from the number of sessions devoted to each type of skill (general vs. refusal), the skills training focuses almost entirely on drug refusal skills. This structure was developed in response to client feedback regarding early versions of BTSAS. Originally we incorporated significantly more general social skills training sessions. However, we changed the focus to an almost exclusive emphasis on drug refusal skills in response to reports from clients that use most often occurred following pressure to use by significant others or a failure to refuse drugs when offered by other people. We had initially planned to teach clients a variety of coping skills to help manage negative affect states and cravings, but few subjects reported that negative affect or cravings were primary factors in their substance use (Gearon, Bellack, Rachbeisel, & Dixon, 2001). The coping skills unit was then reformulated to focus on training in avoidance and escape skills for use when other people were pressuring them to use or had drugs with them and were offering drugs to the client.

GENERAL SOCIAL SKILLS TRAINING

Social skills training (SST; Bellack, Mueser, Gingerich, & Agresta, 1997) is a behavioral approach for rehabilitation of SPMI clients that has been successfully employed since 1980. SST is a highly structured educational procedure that employs instruction, modeling, role-playing, and social reinforcement.

Rationale and Structure of Social Skills Training

In social skills training, complex social repertoires, such as making friends, are broken down into component elements such as maintaining eye contact and providing social reinforcers. Clients are first taught to perform the elements, and then gradually learn to smoothly combine them. There is a strong emphasis on behavioral rehearsal and overlearning of a few specific and relatively narrow skills that can be used automatically, thereby minimizing the cognitive load during stressful interactions.

Each general social skills session takes a similar format. Following the urinalysis contingency and goal setting, therapists review content from the previous session, teach a new skill, including the steps of the skill, and then clients and therapists develop and engage in role-plays. As discussed previously, each skill is broken down into steps, and during the skills training segment of each session, each step is reviewed and clients are asked to discuss the content and reason for each one. The steps do not differ much, so clients quickly become competent at explaining the reason for each step, which provides the therapist with excellent opportunities for reinforcement. In addition, we try to enhance realism in the role-plays so that situations are as close as possible to real life. For the general social skills component, this means designing role-play situations that reflect situations that clients actually encounter in their lives; using topics and language that clients would use and feel comfortable with; and making the role-plays harder as clients become more adept at following the steps.

The BTSAS social skills training curriculum is geared to relatively low functioning clients. However, therapists can tailor the material for clients with better skills by introducing more complex situations or by conducting more extended role-plays. The most common error is to progress too rapidly or to present too complex (e.g., abstract) material. It is almost always better to err on the side of oversimplification than overreaching. High functioning clients will tell you when you are being too simple; in contrast, low functioning clients will not tell you when the material is over their heads.

In the following sections of this chapter, we will discuss each BTSAS social skill session, and then provide Skills Sheets for each one. These sheets each contain an introduction to the teaching unit (rationale); a series of training steps; suggested responses for clients (e.g., examples of general questions so they do not get stuck because they are unable to generate ideas about what to say); sample scenes for role-plays, and general directions. The sheets are designed for therapists to take into sessions. The steps are provided to clients on handouts, as well as presented on flipcharts.

Introduction to Group Members

In the first general social skills session, clients are introduced to the concept of social skills and the rationale for teaching general social skills in an intervention for drug abuse. The main reason for providing this introduction is to inform clients of what they will be doing in the upcoming sessions, as well as to get them to understand the reason for learning and practicing social skills. Another reason to start with general social skills is that generally clients find these skills a bit easier to learn (in comparison to the upcoming drug refusal skills), and so these sessions provide some time for clients to get acclimated to the group and to role-playing.

As you can see on the Skills Sheet (p. 109), the introduction begins by providing a definition of social skills and a rationale for why learning social skills is important. Finally, the introduction informs clients about role-playing and what they can expect from these general social skills sessions.

Making Small Talk

The first general social skill that is presented is making small talk. This skill is basic and provides the foundation for meeting new people and feeling comfortable engaging with others. Clients learn the steps for making small talk, which are as follows: (1) Make eye contact and say hello; (2) ask a general question; (3) ask questions about an appropriate topic; (4) give a reason and say goodbye. The therapist then sets up role-plays and practices these steps with clients in the group. The goal of teaching this skill is to have clients learn and practice how to make small talk and how to select topics that are appropriate for short conversations. Often, in otherwise casual conversations, clients with SPMI talk in inappropriate ways or disclose information that is too personal or sensitive for the situation. Here we are teaching clients the sorts of situations in which making small talk is useful, the sorts of topics of conversation that are typically part of small talk, and how to gracefully end a brief and friendly encounter.

Since the Skills Sheet provides the structure of the group, the following is an example of how a BTSAS therapist would introduce the rationale for the skills to group members:

Therapist: Today we are going to learn how to make small talk. Has anyone ever heard of that expression: "making small talk"? Can anyone tell me what that means?

Client 1: To talk a little bit?

Therapist: That's right, making small talk means to talk to someone a little bit. You would make small talk when you want to talk to someone for a short amount of time, maybe someone you see in the waiting room as you are waiting for your appointment, or maybe you might make small talk with someone as you are standing on line at the supermarket. Small talk is a way to talk to other people that is pleasant and brief. John, have you ever made small talk?

Client 2: Well, I asked someone for the time in the waiting room before group today.

Therapist: That's great—that's just what I mean when I say "small talk." When you make small talk, it's usually about something a bit more than asking for the time, but it's brief just like that. Why do you think it's important to know how to make small talk?

Client 3: So that you can talk to other people.

Therapist: That's right! In this program we are going to work a lot on cutting down or stopping drug use. One important thing to do when you cut down or stop using drugs is to find other people to talk to and maybe become friends with. The first step in being able to find other people to be around who don't use drugs is to feel comfortable talking just a little bit to people. Bob, why do you think that being comfortable talking to other people is important?

Client 4: Because you can't meet new people if you can't talk.

Therapist: Exactly. Great job! In order to meet new people, you have to be able to start a conversation or just chat with someone. That's what small talk is all about.

Making Plans with a Friend

The second social skill that is covered in BTSAS is making plans with a friend. This skill builds on making small talk by helping clients learn how to progress beyond making small talk to appropriately asking someone if they would like to get together. The steps involved in this skill are: (1) Make eye contact and say hello. (2) Ask a general question. (3) Ask the person to do something fun with you. (4) Confirm the plans, give a reason why you have to go, and say goodbye. Again, the focus of this skill is on teaching clients appropriate situations in which to make plans, and to learn and practice skillful ways of making plans with other people.

Since the Skills Sheet provides the structure of the group, the following is an example of how a BTSAS therapist would teach the steps involved in this skill.

Therapist: As I said in the introduction, there are four steps for making plans with a friend. Everyone look at the handout—the steps for these skills are on the handout. Joe, can you please read the first step.

Client 1: Make eye contact and say hello.

Therapist: Great. You might remember that we talked about eye contact when we learned how to make small talk, and here it is again in today's skill of making plans with a friend. Now, why is it important to make eye contact when you are talking to someone?

Client 2: So they know you are talking to them.

Therapist: That's exactly right. When you look at someone and make eye contact, that person knows that you are talking to them. It is also a polite thing to do. If I am talking to you but I am staring at my feet, it's not going to make you feel very good about talking to me. So eye contact is polite and it lets the other person know that you are talking to them. Jane, can you please read step 2.

Client 2: Ask a general question.

Therapist: Great. Can someone give me an example of a general question?

Client 3: Maybe "How are you?"

Therapist: Great job! A general question is just one that will get a conversation going, like "How are you?" or "How ya doing?" or "What's up?" Last group Joe said that his general question that he likes to ask is, "What's going on?" Why do we start a conversation with a general question?

Client 4: It's a good way to start talking.

Therapist: Exactly. A general question gets things going and gets the person to start talking to you. Great. Now, can someone read step 3?

Client 1: Ask the person to do something fun with you.

Therapist: Great. One thing that it's important for us to do is to make sure we all know some fun things to do. Now, I know this may sound strange to have a talk about fun things to do. But what we have learned from working with people who use drugs a lot is that many times they forget what it's like to do something fun without using, and they sometimes have trouble thinking of non-drug-use things to do. Look on your handouts at the one called "Fun Things to Do"—we have made a list of things you can suggest to someone that you do together. Let's go over the list now. Jane, what is one thing on the list that you think would be fun to do with someone?

Client 2: I like to go to the movies.

Therapist: Excellent! So you could ask someone if she wants to go to a movie. Great idea. What about you Joe?

Client 1: Eat out.

Therapist: That's a really good thing to do with someone—eat out. Great job! Bob, can you read a few of the other fun things to do on the list?

Client 3: Go to a meeting, go for a walk, have coffee, go to a bookstore, go to church.

Therapist: Thanks Bob! Can any of you think of other things that are fun to do that we can put on the list?

Client 1: I like baseball games.

Therapist: Excellent idea! In the spring and summer, catching an Orioles game is really fun! Anything else?

Client 4: Sometimes I rent movies.

Therapist: Another great idea! I'm going to have to update my list. OK, so it seems like you all get the hang of suggesting something fun to do. The last step, step 4, is confirm the plans, a reason why you have to go, and say good bye. Why do you think it's important to confirm the plans?

Client 3: So that you both know what the plans are.

Therapist: That's exactly it! Great job. Confirming the plans makes it clear to you and the person you are making plans with just what the plans are and what you will be doing, so you are both thinking the same thing. And Jane, why do you think it's important to give a reason why you have to go?

Client 2: Because you don't want to be rude. Just leaving is rude.

Therapist: That's right. Great job! You give a reason because it's rude to just turn and walk away. What are some reasons you could give for having to end a conversation?

Client 1: "I have to catch my bus."

Therapist: Great. What's another one?

Client 3: How about "I have an appointment."

Therapist: Terrific! You really get the hang of this. Any others?

Client 2: "I have to go. See you later."

Therapist: That's a really great one—it combines the reason for leaving with saying good-bye. Great. So just to review, the steps are: Make eye contact and say hello, ask a general question, ask the person to do something fun, and confirm the plans, give a reason, and say good-bye. Let's try some role-plays now.

General Refusal Skills

The third social skill that is covered in BTSAS is general refusal skills. This skill is intended to give clients practice saying no to other people in everyday situations. SMI clients often have difficulty refusing requests, and as a result they often wind up doing things they don't want to do. Helping clients refuse requests can help them reduce a major source of stress in their lives. Teaching SMI clients to do this appropriately will help ensure that clients actually use this skill in their lives, and it has the intended result of clients not doing things that they cannot or do not want to do. In addition, teaching general refusal skills is a good way to set the stage for learning to say no to offers of drugs, which will be the focus of upcoming drug refusal skills training sessions. The steps involved in this skill are: (1) Make eye contact and use a firm voice. (2) Tell the person you cannot do what they ask. (3) Give a reason. (4) Offer an alternative. The focus of this skill is to teach clients appropriate ways to say no and how to provide a good alternative so that the client has improved interactions with other people.

Since the Skills Sheet provides the structure of this session, the following is an example of how a BTSAS therapist would set up a role-play to practice this skill:

Therapist: OK Joe, how about if we start with you. What is a situation in which you find yourself doing something you don't want to do, or where you find it hard to say no to someone?

Client: My sister always asks me for money and I don't want to give it to her because she doesn't ever pay it back.

Therapist: That's an excellent situation. When is the last time your sister asked you for money?

Client: Two days ago. I gave her the money I had and now I don't have any money.

Therapist: So this is something that is happening to you right now. And it sounds like it is important to you to be able to tell your sister no when she asks you for money. OK, let's set up the role-play. How does your sister ask you for money? Does she call you or come over?

Client: She comes to my house. She asks me for money.

Therapist: OK, so your sister comes to your house. Does she come over only to ask you for money, or does she come over to visit and sometimes ask you for money?

Client: She says she wants to see me, but she always asks for money.

Therapist: And what does she say when she asks you for money?

Client: She says "I don't have any money? Can you give me some?"

Therapist: OK, now let's go through the steps and figure out what you can say to her. So step 1 is to make eye contact and use a firm voice. Jane, can you remind us why this is important?

Client 2: So that the person knows you are serious.

Therapist: That's right! Great. Now Joe, step 2 is to tell the person you cannot do what they ask. How can tell your sister that you can't lend her money? What can you say to her?

Client: I can't lend you money.

Therapist: Great! That's short and to the point. Excellent. So you say, "I can't lend you money." Now you need to do step 3—give her a reason. What reason can you give her?

Client: I don't know.

Therapist: Can anyone help Joe out here? What's a reason he can tell his sister to explain why he can't lend her money?

Client 3: He could say he needs his money so that he can take the bus to his appointments.

Therapist: Great idea! You could tell your sister that you need your money for other things. What's something that you need your money for?

Client: I need to get food and I need to take the bus.

Therapist: Great! So the reason you can tell your sister could be, "I need my money for food and for the bus." Excellent job! Now step 4 is offer an alternative. Bob, can you remind us what an "alternative" is?

Client 4: It's another thing the person can do.

Therapist: That's exactly right! Let's offer you sister another thing that she can do since you can't give her money. What can you offer as an alternative, Joe?

Client: I could tell her to ask someone else for money. I could also give her just $5 to help her out.

Therapist: So you would give her a little money, just to help her out. Or you could tell her to ask someone else for money. Both of those are terrific alternatives. Which one would you like to offer in your role-play?

Client: I would like to offer the $5, since she's my sister.

Therapist: That sounds great. This seems like a situation in which you want to help a little, but you can't give her all of your money. So, look on the board—the steps are up there and what you are going to do for each one. First you are going to make eye contact and use a firm voice. Then you are going to say that you can't give her your money. Next you are going to tell your sister that you need your money for food and for the bus. You will then offer an alternative of giving her $5. Are you ready to practice?

Providing Feedback

After each role-play, the client is provided feedback on his performance, how he progressed through the steps, and directed to make any necessary changes for the next role-play that is done. There are a few important features of feedback in BTSAS. First, feedback always takes a positive tone. Clients are praised for the skills they performed correctly, reinforced for displaying partial skills as a way to bring them up to the point where they are successful with the full skill, and given feedback in a highly positive manner. Second, group members can provide feedback, but their feedback must be positive as well. Feedback can be solicited from group members via the use of leading questions that pull for the response you want the group member to provide (e.g., "Joe, what did you like about the role-play Bob just did?"). Another way to ensure some positive feedback from group members is to assign a group member a specific step to watch for, paying particular attention to assign the step that you know that client will easily demonstrate in the role-play (e.g., "Bob, as Joe is doing his role-play, watch and see if he makes eye contact. Jane, you listen to see if Bob uses a firm voice."). Then when asking group members for feedback, cue them so that their response is phrased positively ("Bob, I really liked how you spoke clearly and loudly in that role-play. Jane, you were listening for the firm voice. Bob's voice was pretty firm wasn't it?").

Third, feedback should offer a suggestion that the client can incorporate into the next role-play that would improve his or her performance. The suggestion could be to pay special attention to a step that was missed ("Let's do that role-play again and this time I really want to hear you say "No" in a firm voice), to stick to the script of the role-play ("This time keep your reason short and sweet—we have your reason written on the board and I want you to follow what's there when you do the role-play"), or to repeat the role-play the same way for additional practice ("Your role-play was terrific. Let's do it again the exact same way so that you get really good at these steps."). Finally, feedback should never involve criticism, portray a therapist's frustration, or take an otherwise negative tone. Remember that the goal here is to provide a supportive, positive, and nonjudgmental atmosphere. If clients are not great during their role–plays, it is because they are not good at refusing requests to use drugs—the exact reason they are in the group in the first place.

DRUG REFUSAL SKILLS

Drug refusal skills sessions have the same format as general social skills sessions, and the skills training segments are done in the same way.

General Rationale and Procedures

It is particularly important to make these role-play situations very personally relevant for group members. Clients should be asked to identify specific partners and situations where drug use is likely, and to indicate the specific language that would be used by the partner. Therapists must elicit information from clients when setting up the role-plays, including names of drug-using companions, locations in which their drug use is likely to occur, how the individual would ask the client to use, and what name the individual and the client would use to refer to the drug. We also put much more social pressure on participants than is ordinarily the case in treatments for schizophrenia clients. This practice of increasing the pressure during the role-plays was a response to consistent reports from clients that realism was enhanced when the therapists were very insistent and hostile in response to clients' attempts to refuse drugs. Therapists exert pressure by offering several reasons why the client should use, as well as using the client's own language and triggers as a means of persuasion.

There are several other issues that should be kept in mind before beginning the substance-related sessions. First, when beginning with new groups or integrating new members into an existing group, be sure to mention to members that you will be discussing substance use and asking individuals about their own use periodically. Substance use can be a difficult topic for SPMI clients to discuss; letting them know ahead of time that they will be asked questions about their use is a way to make sure clients understand the focus of the group and know what to expect. Second, in order for the therapist to understand a difficult situation, role-plays can be reversed with the group member playing the confederate (person who they are trying to refuse) This allows the therapist to gauge how that confederate would respond to the group member's refusal and create a more realistic role-play. *However* this may not be appropriate when the confederate is a user of the drug being offered because the goal of role-play is *not* to teach group members better drug use persuasion skills. Third, the skill of "offering an alternative activity," may be used as a suggestion after refusing the confederate's invitation to use drugs, so long as the scene does not involve the confederate having the drugs on them at the time, and is someone that the client would want to do something with. It is too risky to invite someone carrying drugs to engage in another activity in the presence of drugs. Of course, the same would be true if a drug dealer made the offer. If the confederate *does* have drugs with him or her, an optimum decision would be for the group member to tell the confederate that they would get together some other time and leave the situation (escape).

Situations with Friends/Family versus Situations with Drug Dealers

We have found that clients generally have two situations in which they need drug refusal skills: situations in which they need to refuse to use drugs with family members or friends (i.e., people that they know), or situations in which they need to refuse offers of drugs or drug use from drug dealers or strangers (i.e., people that they don't know or don't know well). Some clients experience both situations (i.e., a family member or friend frequently pressures them to use, and they often encounter drug dealers who offer them drugs to buy or free samples). Others only experience one or the other. Clients have told us that these situations require somewhat different refusal skills. Clients report that they can use all of the steps outlined in the curriculum with people that they know, but that making eye contact or giving a reason are often irrelevant to interactions with strangers (especially dealers). Therapists need to discuss this with clients during the drug refusal skills sessions and help clients create plans for use with strangers and drug dealers if these situations are relevant to them. For example, when therapists suggested to a client that he just immediately leave a situation in which he was being approached by a drug dealer, the client told us that he would have to be polite and respectful to the drug dealer in refusing offers and he could not turn his back on the dealer and walk away unless he wanted to risk getting beaten up or shot. This client was helped to develop a plan in which he came up with a reason that he felt could be used with the drug dealer (I'm not using today because I have a urine test tomorrow and if I come up positive I'll have to go to jail) and role-played the situation.

While the goal is to get clients to come up with those drug-related situations that are most relevant to them, sometimes it is difficult to elicit role-plays from group members. Some appropriate situations to set up role-plays around include:

1. Having money/payday. This is a very relevant situation for many people who receive or interact with people who receive large monthly disability or biweekly welfare checks. There is an increased likelihood that the client may either treat a peer or be treated to drugs or alcohol at those times.
2. Running into or being approached by a drug dealer on the street.
3. Being asked to use by a family member with whom the client frequently uses.
4. Having a phone conversation with someone who calls asking for drugs or offering to share drugs with the client.
5. Being asked to use drugs by other clients at the clinic.

The overall message here is to be aware of the need to tailor plans and role-plays to different situations that clients face. We have provided somewhat different session content highlighting these different types of situations.

Refusing and Offering an Alternative

In these sessions, clients are taught to refuse offers to use drugs and to offer an alternative activity to drug use. It is worth repeating that not all situations and offers to use drugs are appropriately met by offering an alternative. As previously discussed, the skill of "offering an alternative activity," may be used as a suggestion after refusing the confederate's invitation to use drugs, so long as the scene does not involve the confederate having the drugs on him at the time, and is someone that the client would want to do something with. The therapist must always ask the client if this particular confederate typically has the drugs with him or her when the confederate makes the offer to use. If he or she *is* carrying drugs, we teach clients to immediately leave the situation (escape).

The steps of this skill are as follows: (1) Make eye contact and use a firm voice. (2) Say no. (3) Give a reason why you don't want to use drugs. (4) Offer an alternative. Notice that many of the steps of this skill are the same as those of the other social skills already covered. This is intentional, and clients are meant to review the importance of these steps in each session in order to understand that these steps apply to many different situations. Even in later drug refusal skills sessions when clients are becoming very good at role-playing the skills, the therapist should still briefly review the meaning and importance of each step. Since clients will, at that point, know the correct answers to these questions, this review provides a good opportunity to reinforce clients for their knowledge and hard work.

Refusing and Requesting that the Person Not Ask You to Use Drugs Anymore

Clients have told us that they are able to say no once, but that often they are worn down and relent because the person offering the drugs is very insistent and "won't take no for an answer." In response we developed sessions that teach clients how to handle this situation and allow them to practice asking an insistent person not to ask anymore. The steps of this skills are: (1) Make eye contact and use a firm voice. (2) Say no. (3) Give a reason why you don't want to use drugs. (4) Request that the person stop asking you to use.

Refusing and Leaving the Situation

In many if not most situations, clients would be best served by saying very little and immediately leaving the situation. Clients have reported that this is true, especially when they are offered drugs by drug dealers or others whom they do not know well. The steps of this skill are: (1) Make eye contact and use a firm voice. (2) Say no. (3) Give a reason why you don't want to use drugs. (4) Leave the situation.

Example of Tailoring Drug Refusal Skills to Different Clients within the Same Session

Once the three basic sets of skills are introduced and taught (offering an alternative, requesting that the person not ask you to use, leaving the situation), drug refusal skills sessions focus on clients practicing whichever skills are most relevant for them. Different clients may want to practice different skills sets within the same session, and it is the job of the BTSAS therapist to figure out what is most relevant to each client and have him or her practice that skill set. The following is an example of how these themes and steps are worked into the sessions and role-plays of different clients within the same group.

Therapist: So far we have reviewed how to refuse requests to use drugs. We have learned and practiced the steps, and the last step has changed depending on the situation. Sometimes we want to say no and offer an alternative. Other times we want to say no and request that someone stop asking us to use. Many times we want to say no and immediately leave the situation, usually because someone has drugs with them right there. Today we are going to set up role-plays and you will need to pick which step 4—offer an alternative, request that the person stop asking, or leave the situation—you want to use. We need to figure out a situation that is really hard for you and then use the step 4 that you need for that situation. Bob, how about if you go first. What's a situation that has come up recently where it's hard for you to not use?

Client: When my friend Al comes by to use with me.

Therapist: OK, tell me a little bit about that situation. When does Al come over and what does he say?

Client: He comes over after dinner at night and says he has some crack and asks me if I want to use with him.

Therapist: So he comes over with the drugs. Which step 4 should you use in that situation?

Client: Leave the situation.

Therapist: That's right! Excellent! Since he has the drugs on him you want to leave the situation immediately. Let's set up the role-play. First you make eye contact and speak in a firm voice. Then you say no—how are you going to say no in this situation?

Client: I'm going to say I don't want to use.

Therapist: Great. And what reason will you give?

Client: I have to have a urine test tomorrow.

Therapist: That's a great reason. And then what will you do?

Client: Leave.

Therapist: That's right. Just leave. Don't talk a lot or listen to what he has to say. Just leave. Let's try it. [They do role-play three times]. That was great. Jane, let's go to you next. What situation do you want to use for your role-play?

Client: When my sister calls me and asks me to get crack for her.

Therapist: And what happens in that situation?

Client: My sister calls and she keeps asking me to get her drugs. She won't stop until I do it.

Therapist: So it sounds like in this role-play you are going to pick as your step 4, request that the person stop asking.

Client: Yeah. First, I make eye contact and then use a firm voice.

Therapist: Great! You really know your steps. How will you say no and what will your reason be?

Client: I'll tell her that I don't want to get her drugs or do drugs because I want to stay clean so I can see my kids. Then I'll say: "Stop calling and asking me. If that's what you want to say then don't call me."

Therapist: Excellent! You really are serious about this and that's great—I think that will come through in your role-play and also when you really try to say this to your sister. We have the steps and what you are going to say on the board. Are you ready to role-play? [They do three role-plays]. That was great! Tom, you're next. What situation do you want to practice today?

Client: I don't know.

Therapist: Last time you were working on saying no to your best friend Ed. You said that Ed doesn't usually have drugs with him, but he comes over and says he wants to go out, and you know that means he wants to buy drugs and use. How about if we practice that situation again? Which step 4 option will you use with Ed? Is he someone you can do some other activity with, or do you only do drugs with him?

Client: We used to bowl.

Therapist: So why don't we practice you telling Ed that you don't want to use but offer the alternative of going bowling. That's great! [Continue to set up and do role-plays].

OTHER IMPORTANT ISSUES IN SKILLS TRAINING
(BOTH GENERAL SOCIAL SKILLS AND DRUG REFUSAL SKILLS)

There will be SMI clients who are extremely low functioning. It is often difficult for such clients to come up with role-play situations, and to practice and become successful with the steps involved in these skills. There are several strategies to use in such situations. The main thing to remember is that the goal of the role-playing is to practice the steps of the different skills.

Working with Low Functioning and Symptomatic Clients

For low functioning clients, the goal is to come up with a situation that allows the client to practice the steps. It is our experience that some clients take longer than others, but the vast majority of clients will, eventually, be able to offer a suitable situation and participate in setting up a role-play. For some this happens right away, for others it may take almost the entire 22 skills training situations. This is why each Skills Sheet provides some sample situations that can be suggested by the therapist in the event the client is unable to provide one. For example, good situations for general social skills role-plays are making small talk with someone in the clinic waiting room or the hospital elevator, making small talk or plans with someone you know or met at an AA or NA meeting or at church, and refusing requests by others for money or cigarettes or to drive them places.

There are also cases in which a client is eager to develop a role-play situation, but the situation they suggest is too complicated, too difficult (this is relevant to early skills training sessions when clients are new to the skills; difficult situations are good during the later drug refusal skills training sessions when the client has had a lot of practice with the steps), or inappropriate for the skill that is being practiced. An example of this is a male client who suggests refusing an offer to do drugs with a woman with whom he often does drugs and has sex. This situation really requires that he say no to the woman's offers of both drugs and sex, but a client may want to practice refusing the drugs but still having sex with the woman. Another example is the client who suggests a drug refusal situation during the general refusal skills session. The goal of the general session is to get some brief practice with the steps before jumping into the difficult drug situations. A final example is a client suggesting a long and convoluted situation that may involve many people or many contexts and does not lend itself to being broken down into steps.

Other clients may have difficulty participating due to illness factors: they may not talk much, they may respond to symptoms of their mental illness, or (quite often) clients are recovering from the effects of use (fatigued due to lack of sleep the night before secondary to drug use, sleepy due to recent methadone dose, feeling ill due to being hung over, etc.). In such cases, the goal is to set up a role-play, even one that is simple, and have the client complete it as a way to start to practice the steps of these skills. For clients who are symptomatic or experiencing drug effects, this often involves repeating things to make sure the client has heard them, asking the client to stand or walk around while setting up the role-play so that he or she stays awake, and so on.

An example of how to set up a role-play with such a client is as follows.

Therapist: Bob, it looks like you are having a tough time today. Let's set up a role-play for you. Can you think of a situation where you need to say no to drugs?

Client: No.

Therapist: Has there been a time this week when someone offered you drugs?

Client: I don't know.

Therapist: OK. Let's say that you are getting on the bus, and someone approaches you and offers you drugs. Step 1 is make eye contact and use a firm voice. Next you need to say no and give a reason. How would you like to say no.

Client: No response.

Therapist: Bob, I know you are having a tough time today. Let's see if you can help me set up this role-play. Look at page 5 in your handouts—there is a list of ways to say no. Can you read the first one to me?

Client: "No, I don't want to use."

Therapist: Great! That's excellent. So you can say no by saying, "No, I don't want to use." Now we need to give a reason. You have said before that a reason for you to stay clean is to not get kicked out of your housing. That's a great reason to use in the role-play. The last step is to walk away. Let's give that a try now.

Keeping Drug Refusal Skills Interesting for 22 Sessions

A major challenge of the skills training sessions is keeping drug refusal skills training interesting for 22 sessions. There are several strategies to keep in mind that will help keep the sessions interesting and highlight the importance of these sessions to clients' efforts to reduce or stop use.

1. Clients with drug problems are not good at refusing offers of drugs. This may seem obvious, but it bears stating because it provides the basis for having 22 sessions of drug refusal skills. Clients with drug problems need to learn drug refusal skills and need to practice them repeatedly in order for them to use these skills effectively. We repeatedly remind clients that our goal is that they become very good at these skills within the group, such that clients find that they know the steps by heart and using the steps in role-plays becomes automatic. We stress that the reason for this overlearning is that when clients are out in the world facing actual people and actual offers of drugs, clients will experience stress and other sorts of discomforts, and will need to rely on knowing refusal skills so well that using them does not require a lot of thought when they are faced with an actual situation. We use the analogy of driving a car—you get so good at it you do not need to think about the different steps you take to get the car from one place to another—you just drive. Similarly, with drug refusal skills, if you know the steps of the skills very well, you don't have to think about it when you need it—you just refuse.

2. Each session is an opportunity for reinforcement. Most clients, after about three weeks of drug refusal skills, have memorized the steps, the reasons underlying the steps, and are pretty good at role-playing different high-risk situations. Rather than see this as a reason to be bored, it should be looked at as an opportunity to reinforce clients for their success. Clients who can easily answer questions about the steps or set up role-plays without difficulty should be noticed and reinforced for these accomplishments. They can be called on to help review the steps during each drug refusal skills session, to introduce newer members to the steps, and to provide input about how the steps apply to different situations. The following example illustrates how this can be done:

Therapist: Let's review the steps of drug refusal skills. Bob, you have really become an expert on these steps. Can you tell us what step 1 is and why it's important?

Client: It is make eye contact and use a firm voice. That's important so that the other person knows you are talking to them and they take you seriously.

Therapist: That's exactly right. I couldn't have said it better myself! Great job! Jane, you have also become really good at the steps—I think you even have them memorized! What's step 2?

Client: Say no.

Therapist: Great—and you didn't even need to look at your handout. And why is "saying no" important?

Client: Because then it's clear and you have said where you stand on it.

Therapist: Terrific! You hit the nail on the head— it's clear! Saying no means there's no confusion about anything. Jane, you really are doing great with this!

While the steps don't change, the sessions should not stay the same. Even though all 22 sessions are focused on learning and practicing drug refusal skills, it is important to understand that the role-playing should change over time such that clients are regularly getting new experiences using the steps. Role-plays should change in several ways. First, the situations that are selected for role-plays should start out relatively easy at the beginning of the 22 drug refusal sessions and get increasingly more difficult as the 22 sessions progress. Simple situations should be selected at the beginning of a client's involvement with BTSAS so that the client can learn the steps and have some success experiences with role-playing. Over time, topics for role-plays should increase in difficulty so that by the last several refusal skills sessions clients are practicing the situations that, for them, will be the most difficult in which to refuse drugs. For example, role-play topics to use in the first half of drug refusal sessions might include refusing offers of drugs from friends or family members who are supportive of the client's efforts to stop using or who will not pressure him or her to use, or situations in which the client is refusing only one person. More difficult situations might include refusing a group of people, refusing someone who is aggressively insistent, refusing people who are not supportive of the client's efforts to stop using, and refusing people who are offering sex along with drugs. Second, a client will have many situations in which it is difficult for him or her to refuse drugs. You need to ask clients what are difficult situations for them, and you need to reask this question every few sessions. Clients may practice refusing a family member for several sessions, and then when asked, may bring up a previously unknown situation with a drug dealer that needs to be reviewed and practiced. Clients may master the steps in one situation but forget them in another situation. The job of the BTSAS therapist is to select new situations while balancing the client's need to be successful and master the steps with the goals of getting practice in increasingly difficult situations. This requires a good relationship with and knowledge of each particular client. For example, Bob might master refusal skills in a situation in which he is refusing a friend, but fall apart when he has to refuse a drug dealer. Jane might be very good at telling a stranger that she doesn't want to use but be unable to tell her live-in boyfriend who pays her bills. By varying the situations and increasing their level of difficulty for all of the clients in a group, each of the 22 refusal skills sessions should be new or unique in some way.

SUMMARY

Skills training sessions, both general social skills and drug refusal skills training, form the core of BTSAS. The general social skills allow clients to learn strategies for meeting other people and feeling more comfortable in social situations. The drug refusal skills sessions allow clients to learn and practice steps for coping with high-risk drug situations in a positive, reinforcing atmosphere. These sessions operationalize the underlying theory that skills training and behavioral rehearsal are key components to behavior change for clients with SMI.

SKILLS SHEET: INTRODUCTION TO SOCIAL SKILLS

Goals

Group members will learn the definition of social skills and the importance of social skills in interacting with people. Review the format of social skills training via breaking down skills into steps.

Note to therapists: This introduction to social skills should be done with the session titled Making Small Talk and reviewed during each social skills training session. This is not a session by itself, but is used to help clients understand the rationale for social skills training.

What Are Social Skills And Why Are They Important?

[C]*Social skills involve learning to get along with and talk to other people. Lots of people have trouble making conversation and talking to others. In fact, in new or difficult or even exciting situations people often think less clearly. When people think less clearly, they may have difficulty knowing what to do or say. They may even say something they regret. Has that ever happened to you? Social skills help us talk to other people and feel comfortable talking so that we say what we want to say and have less of a chance of saying things that we regret.*

How You Will Learn Social Skills in This Group

We have found that it is easier to learn things in steps. When you break things down into steps, it's easier to learn what to do and remember what to do. Let's take an example. If someone was teaching you how to hit a baseball, he or she might break it down into steps. First she would show you how to hold the bat in your hands. Second she would show you how to stand at the plate. Next she would show you how to swing at the ball. The person probably would then have you practice swinging a couple of times before you even tried to hit an actual pitch. All that practice swinging helps you learn how the swing is supposed to go and helps the movement become familiar.

We have learned that the same is true when learning social skills—learning things in steps makes it easier to understand and to remember. So we have broken the social skills down into steps. We have also found through our research that just talking about a problem isn't enough. You need to figure out a plan and practice a lot so that you get good at it. If you can learn and plan and learn to talk about it in here, it will be easier to do out in the real world. That's why in this group we do a lot of role-playing—that's the way we practice the skills and plans that we learn so that you get really good at them. Have you ever heard the expression "Practice makes perfect"? Well that's true with social skills—the more you practice the easier the skills get. By practicing doing things in steps, people learn more effectively. Some of the steps we will practice will be easy and some will be hard. What we have learned is that the steps get much easier if you practice them. We will practice the steps by role-playing. Role-playing is acting out a scene the way you would if it were really happening to you. Acting out the steps can really help you learn each skill that we talk about.

Note to Therapist: You can use different metaphors for learning in steps. If baseball is not relevant to a particular client, find another metaphor that is relevant. Examples are learning a musical instrument (learn to hold the instrument, learn to play the different notes, then put notes together to make a song); riding a bike (start with training wheels to learn about steering, then ride with someone holding on to get the feel for how to balance, then try it on your own); etc.

In this group we will talk about and practice new ways of getting along with other people, making new friends, avoiding conflict, and learning how to compromise and negotiate. We will practice these skills by role-playing. Role-playing is pretending to be in a particular situation and acting it out. An example of a situation may be starting a conversation with a friend, or learning how to say "No." At first you might feel funny role-playing, but with time most people get used to it and find it a helpful way to practice these skills and get better at them.

SKILLS SHEET: MAKING SMALL TALK

Goals

Group members will learn the steps for maintaining a conversation by asking questions and making small talk. Group members will practice the steps for maintaining a conversation by asking questions and making small talk via role-plays.

Instructions to Therapists:

1. Conduct urinalysis and follow procedures in Urinalysis Contingency section (If this is the first group session, urinalysis is not done; urinalysis begins in the third session).
2. Review goals and complete goal setting (If this is the first group session, goal setting is not done; goal setting begins in the second session).
3. Brief review of last session (For some groups this will be the first session so there will not be anything to review).
4. Today's session: One reason we teach you conversational skills is because now that you are working on being clean, you need to make friends with people who don't use drugs or alcohol. You can use these skills to develop friendships with people you know who don't use drugs or alcohol. Sometimes you may want to keep a conversation going with someone because you like the person or are interested in what is being said. But, often, people don't know how to keep a conversation going, or they feel uncomfortable when having a conversation with someone they don't know very well. One way to keep a conversation going is to ask questions and make small talk with the other person. There are four steps to this skill.

Step 1: Make Eye Contact and Say Hello

Why is it important to make eye contact with someone when you are talking to them? This gets the person's attention. What if you were talking to someone but you were looking at their feet instead of their face? What do you think they would think of that? They wouldn't know that you were talking to them or they might not be able to hear you.

Step 2: Ask a General Question

This starts the conversation and gives the person a chance to talk with you. Some examples of general questions are listed on your handout:

How are you?   *How have you been?*
What's up? What's new?   *What do you think about this weather?*

These are all questions that get a conversation started:

Step 3: Make Small Talk by Asking Questions about an Appropriate Topic

Can you tell me what small talk is? Small talk is talking with someone about a very general subject—something you could talk about with anyone. Asking questions helps keep the conversation going. You have a handout that lists different topics for small talk and some questions you could ask about each topic (go over the list with clients). Can you think of any other questions that we could add? Are there any other topics that we should add to the list? What else could you make small talk about?

Movies/TV Programs.

What kind of movies do you like? Have you seen any good movies lately? What is your favorite TV program/movie?

Sports

What's your favorite sport? What do you think about Baltimore getting its own football team? Do you like the Baltimore Orioles?

Music

Who is your favorite band? What kind of music do you like?

Step 4: Give a Reason and Say Good-Bye

Why do you think it is important to give a reason why you have to go? That's right, it's a polite way to end the conversation. In your handouts there is a list of ways to say goodbye (go over handout with clients).

> *Well, I have to go. I have an appointment.*
> *I have to go meet a friend. It was good to see you.*
> *I have to go catch a bus. I'll see you later.*

Now let's do some role-plays showing how this skill works. First we will do a role-play and then you can do a few with us. In our role-play, we are going to pretend that I am sitting next to Tara in the waiting room before group and I want to start a conversation and make small talk with her. As we do the role-plays, you watch and see if we do all four steps.

Scenes to Use in the Role-Play

Note to Therapist: Talking with someone in the waiting room at the clinic; other relevant scenes identified by group members.

Lesson Plan

Note to Therapist: Coleaders perform a role-play with each other then with each group member. Have members role-play with each other during a second round of role-plays if appropriate.

SKILLS SHEET: MAKING PLANS WITH A FRIEND

Goals

Group members will learn the steps for making plans with a friend. Group members will practice the steps for making plans with a friend via role-plays.

Instructions to Therapists:

1. Conduct urinalysis and follow procedures in Urinalysis Contingency section (If this is the first group session, urinalysis is not done; urinalysis begins in the third session).
2. Review goals and complete goal setting (If this is the first group session, goal setting is not done; goal setting begins in the third session).
3. Brief review of last session.
4. Today's session: There are often times when you start a conversation with someone and ou find out you have something in common. As a result you may want to become friends with them. Remember, you are learning conversation skills so you can make friends with people who don't use drugs or alcohol. One way to start a friendship is to make plans to do something fun. Spending time with people who do not drink or take drugs makes it easier for you not to use, too.

Step 1: Make Eye Contact and Say Hello

Why is it important to make eye contact with someone when you are talking to them? This gets the person's attention. What if you were talking to someone but you were looking at their feet instead of their face? What do you think they would think of that? They wouldn't know that you were talking to them or they might not be able to hear you.

Step 2: Ask a General Question

This starts the conversation and gives the person a chance to talk with you. Some examples of general questions are listed on your handout: How are you? What's up? What's new? How have you been? What do you think about this weather? These are all questions that get a conversation started:

How are you?	*How have you been?*
What's up? What's new?	*What do you think about this weather?*

Step 3: Invite the Person to Do Something Fun with You

*Now you need to ask the person to do something **with you**. There are many different things that you could ask a person to do. You should pick something that you would like to do and that you would find fun. Why is it important for you to pick something that you would like to do and something that you think is fun? What sorts of things would it be fun to do with someone? Well, you could go to a movie, get something to eat, or just have a cup or coffee, or just take a walk. On your handout are some ways to ask a person to do something fun with you. Can anyone think of any other fun activities that we could add?*

There are some really good movies out now. Would you like to go see one with me Saturday night?
Sometime this week would you like to come over and watch TV with me?
There are some really good places to eat around here, how about joining me for lunch sometime?

Step 4: Confirm the Invitation with the Person, then Give a Reason, and Say Good-Bye

*Why do you think it is important to confirm the invitation? That's right—just to make sure that the person knows what you are going to do and when you are going to do it. Why do you think it is important to give a reason why you have to go? That's right, it's a polite way to end the conversation. In your handouts there is a list of ways to confirm the plans and say goodbye (**go over the handout with clients**).*

> *Well, I have to go. I have an appointment. I'll see you Saturday for the movies.*
> *I have to go catch a bus. I'll see you sometime this week at my place.*

Now let's do some role-plays showing how this skill works. First we will do a role-play and then you can do a few with us. In our role-play, we are going to pretend that I know Tara from a group that we go to and I want to ask her if she wants to go get a cup of coffee after the group tomorrow. As we do the role-plays, you watch and see if we do all four steps.

Scenes to Use in the Role-Play

You can ask someone out for coffee after an AA/NA meeting, have lunch with someone from your group at the clinic, ask someone to have a cigarette with you.

Lesson Plan

Note to Therapist: Coleaders perform a role-play with each other, then with each group member. Have members role-play with each other during a second round of role-plays if appropriate. Progress through more extended interactions based on how well each group member can learn. Higher functioning clients can be taught more complex skills (e.g., expressing feelings, asking personal questions): refer to the Bellack et al. (1997) for additional skill sheets.

SKILLS SHEET: GENERAL REFUSAL SKILLS

Note to Therapist: Goal setting begins in this session

Goals

Clients will learn the steps to use for refusing requests and how to offer an alternative. Group members will then practice refusing requests and offering an alternative via role-plays.

Instructions to Therapists

1. **Conduct urinalysis before group and follow procedures in Urinalysis Contingency section.**
2. **Review goals and complete goal setting.** *Before we begin the new skill, we need to talk about goal setting. We will be doing goal setting at the beginning of every group from now on. Goal setting is when we come up with something that each person here can try to do between sessions to reduce drug use or stop using drugs. We will use goal setting to come up with things to work on in order to reduce or stop drug use. With your handouts we have included a Goal-Setting Form. Let's fill these out, starting with you Bob. What would you like to change about your drug use? What is something that you think you could work on now that would help you reduce or stop using drugs?*

Note to Therapist: Group therapists will review the goals from the motivational interview when agreeing to specific goals for the week. Therapists do this with each member, reinforcing any ideas of goals, and negotiating a goal that the member thinks he or she can reach. The goal can be to use less than usual in the days between the sessions or to remain drug-free between sessions.

OK Bob, remember that you said that when you use crack it makes your voices worse and that if you stopped using crack your voices wouldn't be as bad? What can we do this week to help you move toward that goal?

Note to Therapist: At this point therapists should shift to problem solving and goal setting, including identifying what could go wrong, what the client might do next, with other group members providing input and feedback about possible problems and solutions. The therapist asks the following questions in order to complete the Goal Setting Form: What could go wrong or what could keep you from meeting your goal? What could you do if that happened **or** what do you think you could do to keep that from happening? What could you do if that happened **or** what do you think you could do to keep that from happening? And what could go wrong with that **or** why might that not work? OK, what could you do if that happened?

3. **Brief review of last session.**
4. **Today's session.** *Sometimes, we can't always do what other people ask us to do. Sometimes we may be unable to help the person out because we are tired, may not feel capable, or we simply may be too busy. If we refuse in a rude or gruff manner, it can hurt somebody's feelings or make them angry. On the other hand, if we are not clear about refusing or if we speak in a hesitant way, it might lead to a misunderstanding or an argument. So, it is important to learn how to clearly and politely say "No" in order to avoid conflict and reduce stress. However, there may be times when we can offer the person an alternative. Today we are going to practice saying "no" to someone, but then offering an alternative.*

Note to Therapist: Make sure to clarify the meaning of the word alternative.

Step 1: Make Eye Contact

Why is it important to make eye contact when you are talking with someone? This gets the person's attention. What if you were talking to someone but you were looking at their feet instead of their face? What do you think they would think of that? They wouldn't know that you were talking to them or they might not be able to hear you.

Step 2: Tell the Person that You Cannot Do What He or She Asked You to Do

Telling the person straight out that you cannot do what he or she asked you to do helps make it clear that you cannot help the person. Why do you think that it's important to be clear when you are telling someone that you cannot do what he or she wants you to do? That's right: If you are not clear, the person might think that you are going to do something for them that you cannot do. They might try to convince you to do it because they think you will give in. If you are clear, the person will know that you are serious.

> *I'm sorry, but I cannot....*
> *I would like to help you out, but I can't....*

Step 3: Give a Reason Why You Cannot Do What Was Asked

Why do you think it's important to give a reason why you can't do what was asked? Giving a reason helps the person understand why you cannot help them and it is polite. Remember to keep reasons honest. Why do you think it's important to be honest? Well, we know that when people are not honest, they get nervous or stressed and they find it harder to talk and to keep up with the lie that they told. Has anyone ever not been honest and then gotten stressed out over trying to keep up the story they told and keep it straight? That's a lot of stress that can make you think less clearly. So, if you stay honest, you will have less stress while you are talking to the person and you will be able to think more clearly.

Note to Therapist: Steer members toward reasons that imply that the member has no money, cigarettes, etc., to lend to others.

> I have to save the cigarettes that I have left for later today.
> I have an appointment.
> I'm really tired and don't feel like doing that right now.
> I need to use the money for my bills.

Step 4: Offer an Alternative

Note to Therapist: In this step you suggest another activity or an alternative to the person. Remember that an alternative is giving another idea if you have to say no to something. Why do you think it's important to offer an alternative? An alternative helps you tell the person that while you cannot do what they asked, there are other options or other times that you might be able to help them out. Your handout lists a few alternatives that we came up with for when someone asks you for money, asks you to do something for him or her, or asks you to do something that you don't want to do.

> You could ask someone else for a cigarette.
> We could meet at 1:00 p.m. instead.

You could ask someone else for money.

I can pick up groceries tomorrow.

Now let's do some role-plays showing how this skill works. First we will do a role-play and then you can do a few with us. In our role-play, we are going to pretend that Tara asks me to lend her some money and I want to tell her that I can't lend her money because I need my money to pay for my bills and food. As we do the role-plays, you watch and see if we do all four steps.

Scenes to Use in the Role-Play

- Someone asks you for a cigarette, but you need to save those that you have.
- Someone asks to borrow money, but you need to use your money to buy food.
- Your therapist asks to meet with you at 3:00 p.m. but you already have an appointment.
- Your roommate or family member asks you to pick up groceries, but you are feeling tired.

Lesson Plan

Note to Therapist: As with the general social skills, the goal is to shape effective behavior. Coleaders first role-play with each other, then with each group member. For the first role-play, the confederate will only accept the alternative after two attempts. Members should be invited to role-play with each other if they are capable. Gradually increase resistance over trials, and demand more sophisticated responses from higher functioning clients.

SKILLS SHEET: REFUSING ALCOHOL AND DRUGS I—OFFERING AN ALTERNATIVE

Goals

Group members will learn the steps for refusing offers to use alcohol and drugs and offering an alternative. Group members will then practice refusing alcohol and drugs and offering an alternative via role-plays.

Instructions to Therapists

1. **Conduct urinalysis before group and follow procedures in Urinalysis Contingency section**
2. **Review goals and complete goal setting.**
3. **Brief review of last session.** *At our last session we talked about refusing requests. When is it a good time to refuse a request that someone makes of you? That's right – if you can't do what is requested, or you don't want to do what the person is asking you to do, you can refuse a request. Can anyone review the steps we learned for refusing a request? First we make eye contact and second we tell the person that we can't do what he/she asked. Then we give a reason and then offer an alternative. What were some of the situations we role-played to practice refusing requests?*
4. **Today's session:** *In our last meeting we talked about refusing requests. Who can tell me why it's important to refuse requests that you can't or don't want to do? That's right – Sometimes we may be unable to help a person out because we are tired or we may be too busy We practiced saying no in a polite manner and using steps to to the skill. Because so many people use drugs and alcohol, each of you is likely to be pressured by someone to get high or drink. Because it is sometimes difficult to say "No," it is important to practice saying "No" and to come up with reasons why you don't want to use drugs or drink. This can be really hard when the person is someone that you know well and a person with whom you like to spend time. Sometimes you want to spend time with the person but they want to do drugs and you do not want to do drugs. Has that ever happened—a family member or friend wants you to do drugs and you do just because you want to spend time with them? So you need a way to tell them that you don't want to use, but you might want to do something else with them. So today we will discuss how to tell someone you don't want to use drugs and offer an alternative—suggest another activity that you could do together instead of using. The following steps have been found helpful when refusing someone's request to get high or drunk.*

Step 1: Make Eye Contact

Why is it important to make eye contact with someone when you are talking to him or her? This gets the person's attention. What if you were talking to someone but you were looking at their feet instead of their face? What do you think they would think of that? They wouldn't know that you were talking to them or they might not be able to hear you.

Step 2: Using a Firm Voice, Tell the Person that You Don't Want to Use Drugs or Alcohol with Him or Her

Why is it important to use a firm voice? That's right—this helps make it clear that you do not want to use/drink with the person. When you are firm with someone they will know that you mean what you are saying. Sometimes it can be hard to tell someone that you don't want to use. Why is it hard to tell someone that you don't want to use? They might get mad or upset. Since it's a hard thing to tell people, we have come up with some ways that you could tell someone that you don't want to use. On your handout there are some ways that you can tell a person that you do not want to use drugs or alcohol with them:

No, I'm sorry, but I don't use.   No, I don't use (drink) anymore.
No, I'm really trying to quit/stay clean.   No, I'm trying to cut back.

Step 3: Give Reasons Why You Don't Want to Use

Note to Therapist: See additional handout: It is very important to help each individual come up with a few personal reasons why they can't pick up and use.

Why is this an important step? It helps the person understand why you don't want to use drugs or alcohol. It is important to remember to keep reasons honest—don't make up a reason that is untrue. Why is it important to be honest when you are giving a reason? We think it's important because if the reason isn't the truth, you can feel stressed or upset at telling a lie and that will not help you think clearly and get your point across. On the handout we have listed some examples of reasons to give a person if they ask you to do drugs or alcohol

Note to Therapist: It is very important to help each individual come up with a few personal reasons why they can't pick up and use.

Step 4: Suggest Something Else to Do Instead

Note to Therapist: See additional handout: Leave the situation (Use when confederate has substance on him or her)

There are times when you can tell the person that although you don't want to get high or drunk with them, you would like to do something else. Remember that this is called offering an alternative—another idea about something that you can do together. Your handout has a list of other things that you could suggest to do, like going to a meeting or going to get something to eat:

Why don't we go to the movies instead? Let's take a walk together. Let's have lunch together instead. Why don't we go to church instead? Why don't we go to an AA/NA meeting?

It is very important to remember that sometimes someone will ask you to get high or drunk and he or she will have drugs or alcohol with them. If that happens, then you really don't want to offer an alternative because it's clear that they are going to use drugs or alcohol right now. In that case, you want to just leave the situation without offering an alternative. When the person is asking you to use and he or she has drugs with them, you need to just get out of the situation as soon as you can. Your handouts list a few things that you can say to the person so that you can get out of the situation.

Now let's do some role-plays showing how this skill works. First we will do a role-play and then you can do a few with us. In our role-play, we are going to pretend that Tara is asking me to use alcohol and drugs with her. I want to say no because I am not using drugs and I want to stay clean. I also want to offer her an alternative. As we do the role-plays, you watch and see if we do all four steps.

Scenes to Use in the Role-Play

Note to Therapist: Get each member to identify the people in their lives who are likely to pressure them to use or people who will be hard to say no to. In this session, have clients identify people whom they know and want to spend time with (e.g., a family member or friend). The person role-playing with the group member plays this particular person. Use the information gathered from the motivational interview to help identify sensitive people, places, and substances for each member.

If the group member encounters a drug dealer he or she may not want to make eye contact. In this case, tell the group member not to make eye contact and to escape the situation.

Lesson Plan

Note to Therapist: Coleaders role-play with each other and then with each group member. During the *first* group of role-plays, the confederate will play a person with whom the member has or does use in the place where they would be most likely to use. In this session the coleaders should attempt two to three times to get the member to use with them. The leader/confederate should then agree with the member's suggested alternative to using drugs/alcohol and end the role-play. In the next session, Coleaders continue to role-play with members using specific people and places. The level of difficulty is increased. Confederate will agree with alternative after three attempts. **Confederates should not use personal attacks as a way to convince the member to use**—coleaders will have to carefully structure role-play for confederate as well.

SKILLS SHEET: REFUSING ALCOHOL AND DRUGS II—
REQUEST THAT PERSON STOP ASKING

Goals

Group members will learn the steps for refusing alcohol and drugs and requesting that someone stop asking them to use. Group members will then practice via role-plays refusing alcohol and drugs and requesting that the person stop asking.

Instructions to Therapists

1. **Conduct urinalysis before group and follow procedures in Urinalysis Contingency section.**
2. **Review goals and complete goal setting.**
3. **Brief review of last session.** In our last group we talked about refusing when someone offers us alcohol or drugs and giving that person an alternative activity to using. Who can tell me when it's a good to offer someone an alternative? That's right – we can offer an alternative when the person is someone we often do things with other than drinking or using drugs, and it's a person that we want to spend time with. Does anyone remember the situation in which we don't offer an alternative? That's right—if the person has the alcohol or drugs with them , we just want to get out of that situation.
4. **Today's session:** *Last group we talked about how to refuse drugs and offer an alternative to using when someone you know, maybe a family member or friend, wants to do drugs with you. We practiced giving a reason why we didn't want to use and offering an alternative like going for a cup of coffee or seeing a movie. Sometimes when you say no to drugs or alcohol people can give you a hard time. Sometimes they keep pressuring you or they make you feel bad. Lots of times it is someone you know, a family member or a friend, who is pressuring you to use drugs. Has that ever happened to anyone here—a friend comes over and wants to use and keeps asking you to use with him or her and they really turn the pressure on? For the next two sessions we will practice using the skills to say no under pressure. Today we will talk about what to do in this situation—when a family member or friend or someone you know keeps pressuring you to use drugs (discuss the difference in step 4).*

Step 1: Make Eye Contact

Why is it important to make eye contact with someone when you are talking to him or her? This gets the person's attention. What if you were talking to someone but you were looking at their feet instead of their face? What do you think they would think of that? They wouldn't know that you were talking to them or they might not be able to hear you.

Step 2: Using a Firm Voice, Tell the Person that You Don't Want to Use Drugs or Alcohol with Them

Why is it important to use a firm voice? That's right—this helps make it clear that you do not want to use/drink with the person. When you are firm with someone they will know that you mean what you are saying. Sometimes it can be hard to tell someone that you don't want to use. Why is it hard to tell someone that you don't want to use? So they might get mad or upset. Since it's a hard thing to tell people, we have come up with some ways that you could say to someone that you don't want to use. On your handout there are some ways that you can tell a person that you do not want to use drugs or alcohol with them:

No, I'm sorry, but I don't use.	No, I don't use (drink) anymore.
No, I'm really trying to quit/stay clean.	No, I'm trying to cut back.

Step 3: Give Reasons Why You Don't Want to Use

Note to Therapist: See additional handout: It is very important to help each individual come up with a few personalized reasons why they can't pick up and use.

Why is this an important step? It helps the person understand why you don't want to use drugs or alcohol. It is important to remember to keep reasons honest—don't make up a reason that is untrue. Why is it important to be honest when you are giving a reason? We think it's important because if the reason isn't the truth, you can feel stressed or upset at telling a lie and that will not help you think clearly and get your point across. On the handout we have listed some examples of reasons to give a person if they ask you to do drugs or alcohol.

Step 4: Request that the Person Not Ask You to Use/Drink

This step is where the skill gets a little different. When someone is pressuring you to use, you need to tell him or her that you don't want to, and you also need to tell them to stop asking you to use or drink. Why is it important to tell someone that you don't want them pressuring you to use alcohol or drugs? That's right—you want them to know that you don't want to have to keep saying no to them, that you want them to leave you alone. How could you tell someone not to ask you to use drugs or alcohol again?

Note to Therapist: Use handout as needed to give clients ideas of what they could say:

> Hey, I said I'm trying to stay clean, so don't ask me again.
> I told you I don't use/drink anymore so stop asking.
> I'm trying really hard to stay clean, please do not ask me to use/drink again.

Now let's do some role-plays showing how this skill works. First we will do a role-play and then you can do a few with us. In our role-play, we are going to pretend that Tara is asking me to use alcohol and drugs with her. Imagine that she has drugs with her and she is pressuring me to use and asking me several times to go and use with her. I want to say no because I am not using drugs and I want to stay clean. I also want to tell her to stop asking me to use and to stop pressuring me. As we do the role-plays, you watch and see if we do all four steps.

Scenes to Use in the Role-Play

Note to Therapist: Use the people and places identified by each member earlier. If members have more than one person or place that is risky, then vary the role-plays accordingly.

Lesson Plan

Note to Therapist: Coleaders perform a role-play with each other to demonstrate the steps and then with each member. Do not immediately give in to the member's request that you stop asking. Make **at least three** attempts to persuade the person to use—*then* stop asking. Examples are below:

- Oh come on, it will be fun.
- It will make you feel better.
- Just a little bit won't hurt you.
- Fine. I thought you were my friend!
- Do you think that you're better than me?
- So I'm not good enough for you now?
- Well then, go to hell! I'm leaving!

SKILLS SHEET: REFUSING ALCOHOL AND DRUGS III—TALKING TO A STRANGER OR A DRUG DEALER; LEAVE THE SITUATION

Goals

Group members will learn the steps for refusing alcohol and drugs and requesting that someone stop asking them to use when the person is a stranger or a drug dealer. Group members will practice refusing alcohol and drugs and requesting that the person stop asking when the person is a stranger or a drug dealer via role-plays.

Instructions to Therapists

1. **Conduct urinalysis before group and follow procedures in Urinalysis Contingency section.**
2. **Review goals and complete goal setting.**
3. **Brief review of last session.** In our last group, we talked about using drug refusal skills and requesting that a person stop asking you to drink or use drugs with them. Who can tell me why it's important to request that someone stop asking you to use? That's right – this lets the person know that you don't want to use drugs and you don't want them to keep talking to you about it and asking you to use drugs with them. We review steps for how to do this. What were the steps?
4. **Today's session:** *Over the last couple of groups we have learned and practiced how to use drug refusal skills with people that we know, like family members and friends. We have practiced making eye contact, telling the person we don't want to use drugs, giving them a reason why we don't want to use drugs, and offering an alternative to drug use if we want to spend time with the person. Last group we talked about what to do if the family member or friend keeps pressuring us and practiced ways to tell the person that you don't want them to ask you again. Today we are going to practice drug refusal skills in situations in which the person offering the drugs to you is not someone you know or someone you want to spend time with. Rather, the person is a stranger asking you to use or a drug dealer pressuring you to buy drugs. Other clients in our groups have told us that you have to talk differently to a drug dealer from how you talk to a family member or a friend. What do you think is different in situations when it's a stranger or a dealer who is asking you to buy drugs? Is it harder for your say no to a stranger or to a drug dealer?*

Note to Therapists: Steps of the skill are listed. However, you need to tailor the steps to each client. For example, some will not feel comfortable making eye contact with a drug dealer. Others will want to leave the situation without saying anything, rather than giving a reason. Others might feel that they need to explain why they don't want to use this one time (such as being out of money or needing to be clean for a urine test), with the idea that the dealer might leave them alone if he thinks that they will be back another day.

Step 1: Make Eye Contact

Note to Therapist: Things to discuss with the client: Do they want to make eye contact with a drug dealer.

Step 2: Tell the Person that You Don't Want to Use Drugs or Alcohol

Note to Therapist: Things to discuss with the client: Should they use a firm voice. Should they say a few words in saying no, say just no, or not say anything at all?

Step 3: Give Reasons Why You Don't Want to Use

Note to Therapist: See additional handout: It is very important to help each individual come up with a few personalized reasons why they can't pick up and use.

Things to discuss with the client: Should you give a reason or just leave without talking, what kind of reason would be satisfactory in talking to a drug dealer?

Step 4: Request that the Person Not Ask You to Use/Leave the Situation

Note to Therapist: Things to discuss with the client: Do you ask the drug dealer to stop asking or just leave, what sort of tone would you need to use with a drug dealer?

Now let's do some role-plays to practice using drug refusal skills with a drug dealer or another stranger. We are going to ask you to think about how you would use the refusal skills, and we will make a different plan for each of you. First we will do a role-play and then you can do a few with us. In our role-play, we are going to pretend that Tara is a drug dealer and she is asking me to buy drugs. Imagine that she has drugs with her and she is pressuring me to use and asking me several times to go and use with her. I want to say no because I am not using drugs and I want to stay clean. I also want to tell her to stop asking me to use and to stop pressuring me. As we do the role-plays, you watch and see if we do all four steps.

Scenes to Use in the Role-Play

Note to Therapist: Use the people and places identified by each member earlier. If members have more than one person or place that is risky, then vary the role-plays accordingly.

Chapter 9

EDUCATION AND COPING SKILLS TRAINING

INTRODUCTION

The education and coping skills section of BTSAS is intended to present clients with information that will increase their motivation to avoid drugs, and to teach coping skills that will increase their chances of success. Education is provided about the particular problems that clients with SPMI face when they use drugs. Clients learn the biological bases of SPMI, as well as how medications work to relieve their symptoms. They then learn how drug use affects the brain and impacts the effectiveness of their psychiatric medications. Clients also learn about HIV, how substance use contributes to greater risk of contracting HIV, how to use condoms to decrease risk, and they practice role-plays of high-risk situations that involve both drug use and sex in an effort to get clients familiar with strategies to reduce their risk of infection. In the coping skills sessions, clients learn the meaning of and how to identify triggers for craving and use and high-risk situations. Coping skills such as avoidance and escape are taught and practiced so that clients learn strategies for not entering high-risk situations, and getting out quickly without using should they find themselves exposed to multiple triggers.

The education and coping skills section is structured somewhat differently from the skills training component, with blocks of education sessions alternating with sessions focused on coping skills. For the purposes of this chapter, all of the education sessions will be discussed first, followed by the coping skills sessions. However, the Skills Sheets that are presented at the end of the chapter are provided in the order in which they would be administered in a BTSAS group. In addition, for ease of presentation, we describe each of the education and coping skills units in session-long blocks. However, each unit can be subdivided into coherent sections and delivered across successive sessions. Units should be divided so that any subtopic is presented in toto in a single session. Each session should include a review of didactic material presented in the previous session.

EDUCATION SESSIONS

Overview

The educational component of BTSAS includes seven sessions involving topics that are relevant to the connection between drug use and SPMI, as well as incorporating information that clients, from our clinical experience, tend to lack regarding the negative physiological effects of drug use on their mental illness. Emphasis is placed on providing information that is personally relevant to group members, rather than presenting a general admonition about the dangers of drug use. Clients are prompted to relate personal experiences with drug use and abuse in an effort to alter the perceived risk–benefit ratio of drug use. The information is adjusted to the attention and learning capacity of clients, and makes extensive use of audiovisual materials and handouts. Clients are asked to repeat and explain information in their own words across sessions. The topics included in the education component include: (1) the positive and negative consequences of drug use; (2) the biological bases of SPMI; (3) the impact of substance use on SPMI symptoms; (4) links between drug use and HIV/hepatitis C and training in HIV prevention skills.

GENERAL INSTRUCTIONS TO THERAPISTS

While it is necessary to use a didactic format to present information in the education sessions, clients will not respond well to a lecture. The therapist should not speak for more than about five minutes without involving clients in the discussion. In general, the more clients discuss the material in their own words, the more they will incorporate the key points. Useful strategies for breaking up didactic structure include:

1. Asking a member to summarize or repeat a segment (e.g., "So, Susan, can you tell us what dopamine is?" "That's right. It's a brain chemical that is a problem in schizophrenia.")
2. Asking for a personally relevant experience (e.g., "Rafael, can you think of a time when your voices got worse after you scored some crack?"): in doing so, therapists are seeking an example that the group member will closely identify with, perhaps even identify what specifically about his or her *own* drug and alcohol use *scares* that group member.
3. Using review of goals and elicitation of positive and negative consequences of substance abuse that were covered in individual MI sessions. Group therapists can have copies of lists created in MI sessions to refer to.
4. Do not ask questions that yield yes/no or one word answers (e.g. "Is that clear?" "Do you all understand that?" "Are there any questions about that?"). Try to ask leading questions that get clients to explain points in their own words (e.g., "So, Maurice, can you tell us why cocaine makes your schizophrenia worse?" or "Juan, can you show us on this diagram what happens when you take your medicine?" "OK, now what happens if you smoke a joint?"). Also, therapists can ask questions using a "fill-in-the-blank" (if that is too difficult for members, ask questions, and give multiple choice options).

Lesson plans make ample use of visual aids and handouts. Participants should not be expected to remember everything that is presented. The goal is to have them learn and retain any of several key points that will help motivate them and sustain reduced substance use. For example, one client might learn to use dopamine as a buzzword or prompt for the negative effects of cocaine, while another might simply remember that her neuroleptic won't work as well if she smokes crack.

PROS AND CONS OF SUBSTANCE USE

In the first education session we engage clients in a discussion of the pros and cons of substance use. While for many clinicians and clients, talking about the negative consequences of drug use seems fairly standard for substance abuse treatment, most question the value of discussing the positive aspects of use, based on the idea that if you acknowledge that substance use feels good or has other benefits, this will cause clients to continue using. We disagree. Clients use drugs because drugs are beneficial (reinforcing): use may feel good or help a client forget his problems, or using is something to do when he is bored or helps him cope with SPMI symptoms, or helps him go to sleep. What's more, clients know that in many ways drug use is good. Not to acknowledge this is to lose an opportunity both to talk about why clients use drugs and to problem solve other ways to experience the benefits (feel better, sleep better, cope with symptoms) without the actual drug use.

This session involves listing the pros and cons of drug use. This should be an actual list that is written on a flip chart or dry erase board. This is an excellent topic to pull quiet or resistant clients to participate, because clients have definite ideas regarding what they like about drug use, and all have experienced negative consequences as a result of their use. That is, this is a topic that applies to everyone and is a good session to get all clients involved. In addition, the hope is that the "visual" aspect of the list helps clients to further understand that drug use is on the whole more harmful than beneficial. The goal here is to construct a list in which the "cons" segment is visibly longer or larger than the "pros" segment. This visual difference should be part of the overall discussion once the pros and cons of drug use have been listed. The therapist can point out the difference in the length of the pros and cons portions of the list and direct the discussion to the realization that drug use causes more problems than it solves.

BIOLOGICAL BASES OF SPMI

The goal of the session on biological bases of SPMI is to provide background to clients on how the brain functions and how neuroleptics work to correct the deficits in brain functioning that underlie mental illness. While this particular session is not specifically drug related, it provides important information to dually diagnosed clients. First, it is always surprising to find how many clients with SPMI have no understanding of what underlies their mental illness or why they experience the symptoms they do. We have found that our basic education on brain functioning as it relates to mental illness is often the first time many clients have been taught anything about their illness. Second, this session provides the foundation for upcoming sessions that focus on the unique risks experienced by clients with SPMI when they use drugs. In order for clients to understand information on how substance use compromises the effectiveness of their neuroleptic medication, they first must learn how the brain works and what these medications do.

It is important to remember that this session is not meant to be a comprehensive course on neurobiology and neuropharmacology. The focus is on a few key ideas that are reviewed over the course of several sessions and provide a biological reason for the unique risks experienced by SPMI clients who use drugs. The key concepts of this session include: (1) Brain cells communicate via chemicals; (2) too much or too little of certain chemicals is central to SPMI; (3) medications correct the imbalance of these chemicals so that SPMI symptoms remit. Remember to keep language simple (for example, the word *chemicals* can be used in place of *neurotransmitters*), and tailor the language and content to particular group members. For example, you might use a more complex word (i.e., *neurotransmitters*) when directing a comment to a higher functioning client who has heard of some of the concepts you are discussing, but use a simpler word for another client who has difficulty following complicated language.

IMPACT OF SUBSTANCE USE ON SPMI SYMPTOMS

This session takes the content of the previous session a step further and connects substance use to worsening symptoms of SPMI and poorer functioning of SPMI clients. It is important to review the content of the previous session on biological bases of SPMI, and as part of the review to make sure clients understand the three main concepts (brain cells communicate via chemicals; too much or too little of certain chemicals is central to SPMI; medications correct the imbalance of these chemicals so that SPMI symptoms remit). Following this review, the aim of the session is to help group members understand that substance use alters neurotransmitter levels in the brain and can initiate/exacerbate symptoms of mental illness. As with the session on biological bases of SPMI, it is important to remember to keep the content simple and tailor it to individual clients' levels of functioning and understanding. As in the previous session, the focus once again is on a few key ideas that provide a biological reason for the unique risks experienced by SPMI clients who use drugs. The key concepts of this session include: (1) substance use affects brain chemicals; (2) when people with SPMI use street drugs they get a "double whammy"—brain chemicals that are already not functioning normally are further disrupted, causing even more changes in feelings and behaviors and perceptions that are the core of mental illnesses. Again, remember to keep language simple, and tailor the language and content to particular group members.

UNIT ON HIV AND HEPATITIS C

There are four sessions that focus on the prevention of HIV and hepatitis and how drug use relates to elevated risk of contracting these diseases: (1) HIV definitions, transmission, risky behaviors; (2) reducing HIV risk and explaining condom use; (3) practice requesting safe sex; (4) hepatitis prevention. Overall, the sessions focus on the connection between substance use and elevated risk, with the goals of providing clients with another set of reasons to reduce or stop their drug use, as well as to help them learn to be as safe as possible when they do use. In addition, high-risk sexual situations (i.e., clients are at high risk for having unsafe sex) are often connected to drug use, with many clients using drugs before and during sex or having sex with drug-using partners. By providing education about HIV and hepatitis and connecting it to substance use, our goal is to help clients learn ways in which their present-day use can have longer term consequences.

An important issue for these sessions involves clients and their connection to HIV or hepatitis. Many dual diagnosis clients will knowingly have one or both of these diseases, others may be infected but not yet know, and others will, after learning about these diseases, want to receive HIV or hepatitis testing. These can be difficult topics to discuss for clients who are infected or who fear that they are. There are several strategies to keep in mind. First, some clients will disclose that they have HIV or hepatitis in the group and want to talk about it. Such a client may have some knowledge about these disorders, and if he or she freely talks about it, then the client can be used as an "expert" to tell about symptoms, testing, medication, and so on. This client can also provide valuable information concerning how drug use has impacted his or her health, given the client's HIV/hepatitis status. Second, others may have HIV or hepatitis but do not want to discuss it within the group. Do not ask a client to talk about his or her HIV status unless the person has volunteered the information during the group and has been talking about it already. It is important for the client to feel comfortable in the group, and disclosing disease status must be up to the client. Third, make sure you have information on locations and costs of HIV or hepatitis testing in your area. If these sessions inspire a client to get tested, we help the client to arrange this, along with informing the client's primary psychiatric treatment provider.

There are optional components included in these sessions that have been added over the years as clients asked important questions about risk and health. For example, there is some information included in the definitions session on sexually transmitted diseases because some clients ask for this information. In the session on condom use, information about and instructions for using female condoms is provided, based on our experience with women who knew they would not be successful in getting male partners to use protection.

HIV DEFINITIONS, TRANSMISSION, RISKY BEHAVIORS

This session is devoted to definitions and statistics. First AIDS and HIV are defined and modes of transmission are reviewed. While some of this content is difficult to discuss, most clients know at least something, and others a great deal, about HIV transmission. This provides a good opportunity for clients to answer questions and be reinforced for participation and interest in the topic. Next, the discussion of risky behaviors often has a serious tone. For example, most clients are serious, and some may get somewhat upset when reviewing behaviors that most clients engage in (unprotected sex, sex with multiple partners). It is important to provide this information in a serious way, but also be able to help clients see that their efforts to reduce or stop using drugs are going to help keep them healthy and lower their risk of infection. The approach here should be one of reminding clients that HIV risk is something that they can impact by learning to control their behaviors—the emphasis is on problem solving and helping clients feel competent to be able to make good behavioral choices.

The other important goal of this session is to identify drug use as a risky behavior, one that can lead to unsafe sex. The link here is as follows: drug use makes you think less clearly, when you think less clearly you make bad decisions, one bad decision is to have unsafe sex. Therefore drug use can lead to a bad decision to engage in unsafe sex. This is a link that needs to be taught and repeated throughout the session.

REDUCING HIV RISK AND TEACHING CONDOM USE

Many SPMI clients will have little or no experience using condoms. The goal of this session is to link condom use with safe sex, which reduces the risk of HIV. Be prepared to show clients how to use condoms, and as the demonstration is proceeding, to talk about how condom use reduces the risk of contracting HIV. This session has a much lighter tone to it, owing largely to the fact that most of the session involves practicing condom use on wooden penis models. Most clients find this funny and have fun with it. This is a good tone to perpetuate in this group—the goal here is to get everyone to practice using condoms, and a humorous and fun atmosphere is more likely to draw in clients who may initially be embarrassed or uncomfortable. Modeling by the therapist is very important in this regard. A therapist who feels uncomfortable talking about topics related to sex and condoms use is going to have a difficult time making SPMI clients feel at ease. Be sure to practice this session before you do it for the first time so that the subject matter flows smoothly.

This session also includes discussion of alternatives to having sexual intercourse, including other ways to be intimate with someone, and substituting nonintimate activities for spending time together. Again, these are options that many clients with SPMI, who often have drug-related sexual encounters or are taken advantage of within their sexual relationships, have never even considered. Clients often criticize these alternatives to sexual intercourse. The therapist, rather than try to convince clients that cuddling is better than sex, must offer these as options to clients along with sex, and have clients think about times when they might not want to have sexual intercourse (when drugs are involved, when sex would be unsafe).

PRACTICE REQUESTING SAFE SEX

This session involves role-playing situations in which clients tell partners that they do not want to have sex or they want to only have safe sex. This will likely be a new skill for most if not all clients in the group, and many clients have a difficult time with these steps. This makes it important for clients to do multiple role-plays, in order to figure out the words that are right for them and to get comfortable saying them. Again, it is important to present to clients the idea that there are alternatives to sexual intercourse and that if sexual intercourse is preferred, there are ways to have sex that are safer than others. Role-plays need to be tailored to each client's situation and what they want to say to a partner. For example, one client may want to have intercourse and so needs to practice talking about safe sex with her partner. Another client may want to try alternatives to intercourse and so needs a role-play to practice this. Remember, the goal is to get clients to practice the steps and to apply them to some situation that would be useful to them with the goal of reducing their risk of contracting HIV. That is, if a client cannot come up with a situation that applies to their present world, have them do the role-play that you want them to do in order to practice the steps. For those who feel uncomfortable or who insist that they would never do this in the "real world," the following rationale can be useful:

Client: When I want to have sex, that's what I want. I don't need a condom and I won't use one if she asks me to. Condoms are bad.

Therapist: OK, so it seems sort of fake to you to ask your partner to have safe sex or to do something other than have sex.

Client: Yeah.

Therapist: Well, our goal here is to figure out a way for you to reduce your risk of contracting HIV. One way is to have safe sex by using a condom when you have sex. While using a condom right now seems like something you don't want to do, there may come a time when you want to have safe sex—for instance, if you know your partner has HIV, or if you are with a new partner and you don't know too much about her, and you want to make sure you don't contract HIV. So there might be times in the future when you want to suggest using a condom to your partner. So, for this role-play, let's say that you are with someone you don't know well and you want to reduce your risk of getting HIV so you are going to suggest that you use a condom. Let's set up the role-play now.

HEPATITIS PREVENTION

The session on hepatitis prevention includes information on all forms of hepatitis. Because of this, the session is dense and can take a long time. The Skills Sheet includes a thorough review of the types of hepatitis, how they are contracted, and ways to reduce risk of infection. This information must be tailored to the needs and level of the group members. That is, not all of the information needs to be presented. The session must include the information that clients in a particular group need to learn, and the level of presentation needs to be matched to the level of understanding among group members. For example, if clients are engaging in behaviors that put them at risk for hepatitis C and not for A or B, then information on C should be the focus of the session, especially since C is the most dangerous of the three.

COPING SKILLS SESSIONS

The coping skills training component of BTSAS involves helping clients learn how to identify triggers for substance use and the high-risk situations in which these triggers present themselves. We then teach clients how to escape or avoid these situations, and assist clients in problem solving so that escape and/or avoidance skills can be applied to different situations.

General Instructions to Therapists

In keeping with our overall approach, we use modeling and rehearsal to teach a few elemental cognitive and interpersonal techniques: (1) defining and identifying habits, cravings, and triggers; (2) defining and identifying high-risk situations; (3) defining and using avoidance to cope with drinking-related high-risk situations; and (4) defining and using escape to cope with drinking-related high-risk situations. The problems people are having with their goals will help the therapist know how to tailor the coping skills information to each individual client. For example, if a client has been having difficultly meeting a goal of staying clean between sessions due to social pressures to use, this can inform the selection of potentially effective coping strategies: the client can practice avoiding situations in which there will be social pressure to use, or can be taught how to escape situations when social pressure becomes evident.

It is important for the therapists to *generalize individual high-risk situations* to commonly experienced categories of high-risk situations. For example:

Client: I didn't meet my goal of not using for three days.

Therapist: What made it difficult for you?

Client: Danny came by and offered me a blast and I was really bored.

Therapist: So being bored is a high-risk situation for you. That can be a risky situation for lots of people. Has anyone else ever used drugs when they were bored?

Despite the fact that the client described a personal high-risk situation, the content of the situation can be framed as a general high-risk category: being bored. This generalization of individual high-risk situations is important for three reasons. First, it keeps information relevant for all group members and thus will help keep everyone engaged. Second, the limited cognitive ability of people with schizophrenia makes it essential to keep information to a limited number of key themes and problems that are repeated over and over again to increase learning. Third, the fact that this is a group intervention combined with the cognitive handicap make it impossible to cover every idiosyncratic problem faced by group members.

Habits, Cravings, Triggers, and High-Risk Situations

This session includes too much information for one 1.5 hour meeting. It is important to remember to tailor the information to the level of the group members, and not to present too much information at one time. It is better to present less information but to have good discussion about it, and to postpone some information for another group.

Tailoring the content of this session can take other forms as well. While the Skills Sheet for this session provides language on how to present these concepts, a particular set of clients might benefit from other language or different examples of the concepts. For example, the session plan talks about triggers, but many clients will have attended AA/NA meetings and might be more familiar and comfortable with the concept of "people, places, and things." Functionally these are two ways of saying the same thing, and the therapist should say things in a way that clients will relate to and understand. Some clients will have their own understanding of cravings. The signs and symptoms of cravings can differ, and clients may explain their experience of craving in different ways, or not fully be able to understand the concept. For example, some clients report that they do not experience cravings; they just use because they "feel like it". It is important to use the client's language when describing these concepts, and emphasize the concepts that are most applicable to each client.

Avoidance Coping

This session introduces the concept of avoidance, or not going into high-risk situations. This is a new concept for most SPMI clients, who often keep doing the same thing in spite of negative consequences, and often are not cognitively sophisticated enough to come up with a new way to do something if they are unsuccessful. Often simple suggestions can be very useful— using a different bus stop that can be reached without walking by a drug dealer; not answering the door when a drug using friend is knocking; not going to a family gathering if relatives will be drinking or using drugs. SPMI clients frequently do not realize that they have such options, that they can do things differently or decide to stay away from high-risk situations. In such cases, it is important when making a plan to avoid a high-risk situation to help a client figure out how to explain their avoidance to others if needed (e.g., tell family members why you are not coming to a family gathering). Clients also may not know that in some cases they do not need to provide an explanation to anyone (such as not answering the door when a drug using friend is knocking). In these sorts of cases, it is important to help the client find some alternative activity so that the avoidance can be successful (e.g., go in the bedroom and watch TV while the drug using friend is knocking on the door, go to an AA/NA meeting instead of the family gathering where drugs will be present).

Escape Coping

Escape, or quickly leaving a situation, is also often a new idea to SPMI clients. Again, these clients often don't realize that they can make a choice to leave a situation, and they may have difficulty providing an explanation for leaving when one is needed. This is another skill that needs review and practice in order for it to be useful to clients. It also lends itself to role-playing, so each client should be encouraged to come up with a situation in which escape would be useful and practice the steps during the group. As you will see on the Skill Sheet, the therapist is directed to review drug refusal skills with escape (leave the situation) as step 4.

It is important to review with clients why escaping a situation is difficult. This is likely to be different for each client. Some may not know what to say in order to get out of a situation. Others will not want to leave a situation when they are somewhere unfamiliar or do not have a way to get home. Many will find it difficult to leave a situation in which drugs are present because they will want to use drugs. It is important to solicit this sort of information from clients, acknowledge the difficult nature of leaving a high-risk situation, and then plan with a client how to address whatever difficulty is identified. The following is an example of how this might work:

Therapist: Now let's practice escaping a situation by setting up a role-play. Bob, can you tell me a high-risk situation that you think you would need to escape from quickly.

Client: When I run into my friend Ed on the street.

Therapist: Why would you need to escape this situation?

Client: Ed always wants to use with me. He likes to come over to my apartment to use. He likes to use in my apartment.

Therapist: So Ed has drugs on him when he sees you and he likes to go to your apartment to use. What makes it hard to escape this situation?

Client: Ed talks a lot and I don't know what to say. He always has drugs and wants to use them with me.

Therapist: OK, so it's hard to escape when you see Ed because he talks a lot and it's hard to know what to say. It's also tough because he has drugs and he offers drugs to you and that's pretty tempting.

Client: Yeah.

Therapist: Let's set up a role-play now. That will help us get down what exactly you can say to Ed. That means that even if he's talking a lot, you will already know what to say. If you already know what to say, you will be able to say it quickly and get out of there—that is going to help when you are tempted because you know Ed has drugs on him.

SUMMARY

In the education and coping skills training component of BTSAS, education is provided about the particular problems that clients with SPMI face when they use drugs. In addition, clients learn the meaning of and how to identify triggers for craving and drug use and high-risk situations. Coping skills such as avoidance and escape are taught and practiced so that clients learn strategies for not entering high-risk situations and getting out quickly and without using should they find themselves in one.

SKILLS SHEET: POSITIVE AND NEGATIVE ASPECTS OF USING

Goals

Group members will identify positive aspects of using alcohol and illicit drugs. Group members will identify negative aspects of using alcohol and illicit drugs.

Instructions to Therapists

1. **Conduct urinalysis before group and follow procedures in Urinalysis Contingency section.**
2. **Review goals and complete goal setting.**
3. **Brief review of last session**. In our last session we practiced using drug refusal skills and everyone did some really tough role plays. Let's review the steps in drug refusal skills, just to make sure we all have them memorized.
4. **Today's session: Introduce education and coping section**. *Today, we are going to start a new section of group. So far, you have been learning skills to help you make new friends, avoid conflict, and say "No" when you don't want to use drugs or alcohol. In this section of group, we want to help you learn other ways to either prevent yourself from using when you don't want to or to prevent a relapse after you have been clean for a while. During these group sessions, we will identify good and bad aspects of using drugs or alcohol, and how this leads to a habit; talk about the effects of alcohol and drugs on your brain; learn how alcohol and drugs can affect your medications and your illness; talk about cravings, and help you identify triggers and high-risk situations that lead to cravings; and help you each develop plans for how to deal with triggers and difficult situations. Today we'll start by focusing on helping you identify what you like about using alcohol and drugs and then some things you did not like.*
5. **What is positive about using?** *People usually use drugs and alcohol because they make them feel good—they like the high. Some people like it because it helps them be friendlier. It might be pretty unusual for you to be asked to think about why you liked to use drugs and alcohol. It's important to figure out what you thought was good about using because it helps us figure out strategies to help you cope with those situations without using. If you know why you like it, you will have a better idea of the situations in which you tend to use, and the situations in which you will be at risk to use. For example, if you liked using because it helped you feel confident around other people, then we know that situations in which you are around other people might be a time when you are at risk to use. Also, we can help you to find other ways to achieve these feelings without using. Using the same example, if you use drugs and alcohol to feel confident around other people, then we need to help you find other ways to feel confident that don't involve using. As another example, some people use drugs to help them feel calm when they are nervous. We can help you find other things to do to feel calm instead of using. So, why did you like using drugs and alcohol?*

Note to Therapist: List on board what participants like about using (draw from group members and information generated in MI sessions). If someone says, "It makes me feel better," then ask specific questions like "Better than what?" If someone says, "It makes my illness better," respond with "What symptoms of your illness does it make better?" (Therapist should keep this list for review in next session.)

6. **What is negative about using?** *There are lots of negative consequences of drug and alcohol use as well. You have all met in individual motivational interviewing sessions and talked about these—what are some of them?*

Note to Therapist: Probe for specifics regarding what exactly has happened to the group member where he or she experienced the particular negative consequence mentioned during group. For example, ask,

"What happened that you didn't like?" The therapist should be empathic here, "You had nasty hangovers. That must have been terrible." Therapist should keep a list generated by participants for review in the next session.

Some negative consequences are

You can get kicked out of treatment program	Could OD or die
Can get kicked out of housing	Makes it hard to sleep
Upsets friends and family	Increase Sx of mental illness
May cause you to lose children	Makes you anxious
You want to use more	Keeps you broke
Messes up the positive effects of medication	Makes you feel sick
Makes you depressed	Makes you shake
Causes you to throw up	Makes you tired
Gives you diarrhea	Once you start, can't stop
May go boosting or prostituting to pay for alcohol/drugs	
May get yourself in a dangerous situation and get hurt	

Note to Therapists: In the event that the group member mentions the concept of self-medication as a positive reason to use drugs and alcohol, various additions should be made to the content of the next few group sessions, including the following:

1. Distinguish whether the person is telling you that they are self-medicating to decrease symptoms of their illness or to decrease *side effects* of a medication taken for their illness.
2. If a group member is self-medicating for either of these reasons, it may be beneficial to help them through a role-play in which they speak with their physician/psychiatrist about how they need their medications changed either to decrease side effects or symptoms.
3. Then, in the following section effort should be made to describe the concept of medication side effects and the difference between using correct medication versus alcohol and drugs to decrease them.

If a member *does* communicate that he or she uses drugs or alcohol to reduce side effects resulting from medication, the therapist should explain briefly why side effects occur. The objective here is to teach members that there are *options* to self-medicating. The therapist should say the following, for example:

Bob, you said that you use cocaine to make you feel better when your medication gives you side effects. You're right. Cocaine can take away your side effects because of the way it affects your nerve cells. We will talk more about this later in this session. What happens is that when you take medicine for schizophrenia, it affects a chemical in your brain called dopamine. Dopamine acts in different parts of your brain to help control thinking and movement. Sometimes, medicine that helps you think more clearly also interferes with the part of your brain that controls movements. That's what causes side effects like feeling jittery, restless, shaky, or stiff. Your doctor can give you medication to help lessen these symptoms and that works more effectively and reliably than cocaine does. Sometimes the doctor will give you medicine like Cogentin or Benadryl.

Note to Therapist: Generally, however, this information on side effects will not be covered at this point unless the group members refer to decreasing their side effects as a major positive of using drugs and alcohol—this said with the intention of not wanting to run the risk of reinforcing that drugs and alcohol will be better than taking medications because the side effects aren't so bad as those from medications.

SKILLS SHEET: BIOLOGICAL BASES OF MENTAL ILLNESS

Goals

Group members will learn what neurotransmitters are and understand that they are related to symptoms of mental illness. Schizophrenia and major depression will be used as examples. Group members will understand that medications like neuroleptics and antidepressants help decrease symptoms of schizophrenia and major depression by decreasing levels of neurotransmitters. Group members will role-play explaining to family members or friends what causes their mental illness in order to reinforce learning.

Instructions to Therapists

1. **Conduct urinalysis before group and follow procedures in Urinalysis Contingency section.**
2. **Review goals and complete goal setting.**
3. **Brief review of last session.** *Last session we discussed how there are a lot of negative things that can happen to each of you when you use drugs and alcohol. For example, Mary, you said that your voices got worse when you used cocaine. What are some important reasons for you personally not to use street drugs or alcohol?*

Note to Therapist: Review each member's most important reasons and write on the board. Prompt for specific descriptions and provide empathic responses as appropriate. For example, "Joe, you said that you heard voices when you smoked crack. What did the voices say to you? How did the voices sound? Your voices told you that you're terrible? That must have been scary for you."

Clients may feel more comfortable with or better understand the term *brain chemicals* rather than *neurotransmitters*. After introducing the term *neurotransmitters* to group members, you can use either term, depending on which term you think the clients are better able to understand and use themselves.

4. **Today's session.**

Note to Therapist: The goal of this session is to increase awareness that the use of street drugs and alcohol can worsen the condition of people who have mental illness (i.e., to increase awareness regarding the negative consequences of substance use that are personally relevant to clients). Throughout this session, information should be supported by concrete examples and illustrations drawn on the board and distributed as handouts. Therapists should individualize material by asking questions that relate to group members' experiences and by using concrete examples that refer back to members' previously mentioned experiences with drugs and alcohol as they relate to topics discussed. In an effort to increase the perceived value of reducing their substance use, participants are prompted to relate their personal negative experiences with substances and are taught that substance use can have a particularly negative impact on their illness.

5. **Schizophrenia/mental illness, your brain, and drugs and alcohol.** *As we discussed in the last session, there are lots of reasons to use alcohol and drugs. We also have heard when we talk to you individually (pregroup assessments, ASI/Timeline Followback, MI) that there are a lot of negative effects from using drugs and alcohol. (Briefly refer back to members' personal experiences. For example, "Jane, you get paranoid; and Jack, you said you have symptoms such as—.")*

Have you ever thought about how drugs and alcohol affect your brain? Drugs affect the way your brain works. That is why people continue to use drugs even when negative things happen as a direct result of their use, because drugs affect the way the brain works. Drugs are chemicals that affect the way your brain works. We want to explain here some of the negative things that drugs and alcohol can do to your brain. Drugs can make your illness worse. To understand this, we will first need to review some basic information about your brain, how it works and how drugs and alcohol affect your brain.

Note to Therapist: From here on it is very important to make very frequent reference to handouts/flip chart.

6. What is the biological basis of schizophrenia/mental illness?

Note to Therapist: Pass out handout of neural network and refer to it while explaining the following:

Your brain is made up of thousands and thousands of tiny nerve cells; it's like a big jumble of electrical wires. Everything we do (thinking, moving, remembering) is controlled by all of these tiny nerve cells. For example, try moving your fingers. That's right. Now that seemed easy, but it was really very complicated. A number of things had to happen: You had to hear what I said *(move your fingers), the sounds had to be changed to electrical signals and sent to the part of your brain that controls hearing, that part of the brain connected to another part that tells you what those words move your fingers mean, and then a signal was sent to the part of the brain that controls movement in your fingers to tell it what to do. What is another thing you can show me now that your brain can tell your body to do?*

Now the interesting part of all of this for us is that the way the signals get sent from one nerve cell to another is by chemicals. It's kind of like when you turn on a light switch or turn on the TV: an electrical signal gets sent to make something happen. In our brain the signal is sent by chemicals. Let's look at this picture (refer to illustration of a nerve cell at the synapse): This shows two nerve cells next to each other. You see that while they are very close to each other, they don't touch. There has to be some way to carry a message over that gap from one nerve cell to the next. This is done by chemicals. There are many different chemicals in our brains that help send messages from one nerve cell to another. These chemicals are called neurotransmitters. The thing about neurotransmitters is that while they are involved in sending messages to nerve cells, they are also involved in our experience of moods and feelings such as sadness and anger and fear and anxiety, as well as how we perceive the world around us. So the same neurotransmitters/brain chemicals that are involved in sending messages from one nerve cell to another are also involved in mental illnesses that involve negative feelings and perceptions such as sadness, depression, fear, hallucinations, delusions, and anxiety.

For example, one of the most important of these brain chemicals is called dopamine. Have any of you ever heard of dopamine? Can you tell me what it is? Dopamine is a very important brain chemical because it is related to the mental illness of schizophrenia. Another important chemical in your brain is serotonin. Has anyone here ever heard of serotonin? Serotonin is a very important brain chemical that is related to depression. (Another class of brain chemicals is called catecholamines, which have been found to be related to anxiety disorders such as PTSD). *In order to get a better understanding of how these brain chemicals work, as well as how they are related to mental illness, let's use dopamine as an example.*

Note to Therapist: Regularly point at and follow along with illustration while presenting this section: it is very important to emphasize words with reference to the graphic representations.

In our brains dopamine is released from this nerve cell into this space (refer to synapse). Dopamine sends information/messages to the next cell by fitting into tiny spaces on that cell, like a key fitting into a lock (refer to dopamine/key and receptor cell sites/locks). *In most people, there are just the right amount of spaces. But when you have schizophrenia, there are more spaces, so more dopamine goes into the next cell through these extra spaces. The dopamine then sends more information than normal. This information tells the brain that something is happening when it is not because too much dopamine is being sent through the cell. This is what causes the voices that you hear, or the hallucinations that you see as a part of your mental illness.*

7. Compare a schizophrenia nerve cell to a normal cell illustrating more receptor sites.

Note to Therapist: As another example, the therapist can talk about serotonin and its relationship to depression. Too little serotonin is linked to depression. So:

In our brains serotonin is released from this nerve cell into this space (refer to synapse). *Like dopamine, serotonin also sends information/messages to the next cell by fitting into tiny spaces on that cell, like a key fitting into a lock* (refer to dopamine/key and receptor cell sites/locks). *In most people, just the right amount of serotonin is available to fit into the spaces on the next nerve cell. However, in depression, there is not enough serotonin to fit into the spaces. So there is not enough serotonin to carry the message to the next nerve cell. This means that the serotonin sends less information than normal. This is what causes the depressed mood, hopelessness, problems eating and sleeping, and suicidal thoughts when a person is depressed, too little serotonin.*

8. What is the biological basis of neuroleptics/medication for schizophrenia/mental illness?
   The next important thing to understand is that the medicines you take to reduce your symptoms of schizophrenia or other mental illness work by impacting neurotransmitters/brain chemicals and the spaces that they fit into on the nerve cells. For example, in schizophrenia, medications work by closing off or filling in these extra spaces in the cells (or "lock" of the lock and key model—again, continue to refer to the illustration) *so that not all of the spaces can be filled with the dopamine that is sitting between the cells. This way, less information is being sent through the cell. When you get the right amount of information being sent through your cells by the dopamine, your symptoms (like hearing voices, having unusual thoughts and paranoia) decrease.*

In the case of depression, medications work to increase the amount of serotonin available to get the message to the next nerve cell. This way, the right amount of information is being sent through the cell. When you get the right amount of information being sent through your cells by the serotonin, your symptoms (like feeling depressed and being suicidal) *decrease. This is true for other mental illnesses as well. Medications work to fix problems in neurotransmitters/brain chemicals and nerve cells such that messages are being sent from one nerve cell to the next in the appropriate way. For some mental illnesses, medications work by increasing the amount of a neurotransmitter/brain chemical. For others, medications work to fill up receptor sites or decrease the amount of a neurotransmitter/brain chemical that is available. Whatever the case:*

   (a) Neurotransmitters/brain chemicals are important for the proper functioning of your brain.
   (b) In mental illness, there is some disruption or imbalance in the normal flow and work of neurotranmitters/brain chemicals, leading to symptoms of mental illness.
   (c) Medications for mental illness work to correct this disruption or imbalance, leading to a decrease in symptoms of mental illness.

   What are the medicines that each of you takes for your mental illness?

Note to Therapist: Write a list on the board of the medicines commonly taken for schizophrenia: Thorazine, Mellaril, Navane, Stelazine, Haldol, Prolixin, Clozaril, Olanzapine, and Risperdal. Ask clients: "How do your medicines reduce *your* symptoms?"

   9. Role-Plays.

Note to Therapist: Lead participants through role-play activities involving conversations with friends or family members about the biological cause of their schizophrenia to keep group members engaged and to reinforce learning the material.

   10. Summarize the information presented so far.

SKILLS SHEET: INTERACTION OF DRUGS/ALCOHOL AND SPMI

Goal

Group members will understand that substance use alters neurotransmitter levels in the brain and can initiate/exacerbate symptoms of mental illness.

Instructions to Therapists

1. **Conduct urinalysis before group and follow procedures in Urinalysis Contingency section**
2. **Review goals and complete goal setting.**
3. **Brief review of last session.** *Last session we reviewed information about mental illness, your brain, and how your medicines help to reduce symptoms of mental illness like schizophrenia and depression. Who can tell me what the brain chemical important to schizophrenia is? That's right! Dopamine. How about the neurotransmitter/brain chemical that is important in depression? That's right–serotonin. We also talked about how medicines work to help symptoms of mental illness. How do your medicines help to reduce your symptoms?*

Note to Therapist: Continue to review session II material by asking specific questions. Reinforce all effort. Continue to use the lkey/lock analogy and the dopamine hypothesis of schizophrenia to further illustrate how drugs and alcohol additionally affect brain function. Remember to pull for feedback and examples from group members, thereby breaking up the didactic nature of the session.

Clients may feel more comfortable with or better understand the term *brain chemicals* rather than *neurotransmitters*. After introducing the term *neurotransmitters* to group members, you can use either term, depending on what you think the clients are better able to understand and use themselves.

4. **Today's session: What is the interaction between drugs, alcohol, and the brain?** *Street drugs and alcohol also affect dopamine, serotonin, and other neurotransmitters/brain chemicals and how your brain functions and sends information. Some street drugs cause too much of a neurotransmitter/brain chemical to be at work in the brain, while others cause less of some neurotransmitters/brain chemicals to be at work in the brain. The thing for you to remember is that drugs alter how neurotransmitters/brain chemicals work, which results in your brain not sending messages the way it is supposed to.*

Let's use cocaine as an example. (Distribute illustration of cocaine being inhaled). *Whenever cocaine is injected, smoked, or snorted, it is carried through the blood into the brain. Cocaine causes dopamine to sit in this space and send more information than normal to cells* (refer to diagram of neuron when cocaine is present and compare with the picture of a normal neuron).

Note to Therapist: Note that cocaine does not *increase* dopamine. It inhibits reuptake. However, therapists should not attempt to explain reuptake. The goal is to convey the basic concept of excess amounts of dopamine at the receptor site.)

This can make you feel good when you first use it (ask group members what the cocaine high/rush feels like). *You may feel more alert, excited, confident, or powerful.*

Cocaine can also make you paranoid, cause hallucinations (hearing voices or seeing things), *or cause you to have strange or unusual thoughts because there is too much dopamine being sent to the nerve cells. Have any of you had an experience like this when using cocaine? "—, tell me about a time when you used coke and your voices got worse?"* (Probe for feedback and shared experiences from group members here.)

This same process is at work with other types of drugs and other neurotransmitters/brain chemicals. When you use street drugs, they go through the blood to your brain. All street drugs alter neurotransmitters/brain chemicals in your brain. What happens is that street drugs and alcohol mess up how the neurotransmitters/brain chemicals work in your brain. All neurotransmitters are involved in how people feel, behave, and perceive the world around them. So whatever the street drug, it affects neurotransmitters in the brain, which alters how we feel, behave, and think about things.

5. **What is the interaction between drugs, alcohol, and mental illness?** *So what is the connection between drugs, alcohol, and mental illness? Remember that street drugs affect how neurotransmitters work in the brain and they mess up neurotransmitter functioning. This in turn alters how you feel and behave and think about things. Now remember that people with mental illness already have altered neurotransmitter functioning, such that they are already experiencing disruption in thoughts and feelings and behaviors because of the mental illness. So when a person with mental illness uses street drugs it's like a double whammy: neurotransmitters that are already not functioning normally are further disrupted, causing even more changes in feelings and behaviors and perceptions that are the core of mental illnesses.*

Let's continue with our example of dopamine and schizophrenia. Remember how we said that the person with schizophrenia has too many spaces on their brain cells and too much information gets sent? Cocaine also affects people with schizophrenia by upsetting the amount of information that gets sent through brain cells (show illustration). In addition to having those extra spaces on your cells for dopamine to fit into, the cocaine makes it so that even more dopamine can fit into those spaces. So if you have schizophrenia and you're using cocaine, you could relapse or make your symptoms worse even when you only use a little bit of it. Other drugs such as alcohol can also make your symptoms worse and possibly put you in the hospital. So, when you have schizophrenia, why shouldn't you use drugs and alcohol? Because you get too much dopamine which increases your symptoms.

Cocaine can also make symptoms of depression worse. After the rush of using cocaine, certain neurotransmitters are used up—this leads to people feeling very down, tired, lethargic, and depressed when they are coming down from cocaine. These feelings of depression can last for days after a person has used cocaine. Has this ever happened to anyone here? Has anyone ever gotten depressed after using cocaine? What was that like? How long did that last?

This same process is at work with other types of mental illness. What happens is that street drugs and alcohol mess up how your neurotransmitters work in your brain. This leads your brain to not function normally—your nerve cells wind up sending the wrong messages to other nerve cells. But remember that people with mental illness already have altered neurotransmitter functioning that causes symptoms of mental illness. So a person with mental illness who uses street drugs or alcohol gets a double whammy: neurotransmitters aren't functioning correctly due to the mental illness, and street drugs and alcohol only make this whole process a whole lot worse. That's why using street drugs and alcohol can make symptoms of mental illness worse. So whatever the case in terms of the type of mental illness you have:

(a) *Neurotransmitters are integral to the proper functioning of your brain.*

(b) *In mental illness, there is some disruption or imbalance in the normal flow and work of neurotransmitters, leading to symptoms of mental illness.*

(c) *Medications for mental illness work to correct this disruption or imbalance, leading to a decrease in symptoms of mental illness.*

(d) *Street drugs and alcohol further disrupt neurotransmitter functioning, and this messes up how your nerve cells send messages to one another.*

(e) *People with mental illness who use street drugs or alcohol get a double whammy: neurotransmitters are altered from both the mental illness and the drug use. This makes symptoms of mental illness even worse.*

6. **Summarize the information presented so far.**
7. **Role-plays.**

Note to Therapist: Lead members through role-play activities involving conversations with friends/family members about the interaction between drugs, alcohol, and schizophrenia to keep members engaged and to reinforce learning.

8. **Review the negative aspects of using again.** Tie this review in with discussion about substance use and symptoms of SPMI.

We have now talked about another way in which using drugs can be negative, particularly for people with SPMI—symptoms can be caused or get worse from drug use. Remember that we have talked about lots of other negative consequences of drug and alcohol use as well. Let's review some of the consequences we had on our list.

Note to Therapist: Probe for specifics regarding what exactly has happened to the group members where they experienced the particular negative consequence mentioned during group.

Some negative consequences are:

You can get kicked out of treatment program	*Could OD or die*
Can get kicked out of housing	*Makes it hard to sleep*
Upsets friends and family	*Increase Sx of mental illness*
May cause you to lose children	*Makes you anxious*
May go boosting or prostituting to pay for alcohol/drugs	*You want to use more*
May get yourself in a dangerous situation and get hurt	*Keeps you broke*
Messes up the positive effects of medication	*Makes you feel sick*
Makes you depressed	*Makes you shake*
Causes you to throw up	*Makes you tired*
Gives you diarrhea	*Once you start, can't stop*

SKILLS SHEET: HABITS, CRAVINGS, TRIGGERS, AND HIGH-RISK SITUATIONS

Goals

Define and give examples of habits, cravings, triggers, and high-risk situations. Explain how high-risk situations (HRS) make it hard to say "No" to drugs and alcohol. Group members will describe how they experience cravings, identify some of their own triggers, and identify their own HRS.

Note to Therapist: This section can be split into two sessions if needed. A logical place to break would be at high-risk situations.

Instructions to Therapists

1. **Conduct urinalysis before group and follow procedures in Urinalysis Contingency section.**
2. **Review goals and complete goal setting.**
3. **Brief review of last session.** *Last session we reviewed information about SPMI, your brain, and about how alcohol and drugs affect your brain and your mental illness. We also discussed important reasons for you not to use drugs and alcohol* (mention one of each member's reasons), *and what symptoms of your mental illness could get worse if you used—what was one symptom you experience that gets worse when you use?* (Review with each member.)
4. **Today's session: Discussion of habits.** *We know about the negative consequences of drug and alcohol use and how these consequences cause problems for you; and we talked about how cutting down could help make life easier for you. It seems hard then to understand why people keep using, doesn't it? So, why do you think people still use even though bad things can happen to them?*

Note to Therapist: If people answer by listing the good reasons to use (e.g., because the high feels good), then state:

> *You're right, one reason people continue to use even though bad things can happen to them is because using makes them feel good. A person uses despite all of the negative consequences because he or she has developed a habit of using that drug/alcohol. That is, they have gotten used to doing the drug/alcohol over and over again, like a routine, without thinking about it—like sitting in the same place every day during group. Habits are things we do without automatically thinking. Some habits are useful, like saying "Thank you" when someone holds an elevator door open for us. Other habits are not useful, like biting your fingernails or scratching a sore. Using drugs can be a bad habit like that: you can do a drug without thinking about whether you really want to or not because you are used to doing it at a certain time or in a certain place, or when someone asks you to. Has anyone used a drug without thinking about it? Like a habit? That makes it hard to cut down or stop using even when you don't want to use. We are going to teach you some ways to break that bad habit.*

5. **Discussion of craving.** *Another reason people use drugs is because they have cravings to use. Cravings are very strong physical urges or needs to use the drug; sometimes they can be so strong they hurt, and we can't think of anything else until we take the drug to reduce the bad feelings.*

Note to Therapist: Engage the members in a discussion about their own experiences with cravings. Use prompt questions such as the following: "Has anyone had cravings? What are they like for you? What happens when you get cravings?" The purpose of this discussion, as with the discussion of habits, above, is to get members to understand the concept by relating it to their personal experiences and to gather material to be used in developing intervention strategies. The discussion should be kept brief, and should not evolve into an extensive discussion of each member's personal reasons for using and problems in quitting.

Does anyone know why we have cravings to use drugs/alcohol? Cravings are the body's way of telling us that it really needs something, like hunger pangs. In the case of hunger, the body has a natural need for food, and when it needs more, it sends out signals that are hard to ignore, kind of like an alarm going off that says, "Feed me." Cravings for a drug are a little different, because it is not a natural part of life. Drug cravings occur because drugs gradually make changes to the brain. When you first start using drugs the brain doesn't expect it: so it just reacts to the sudden change caused by the chemicals. Gradually, the brain starts to adapt. Remember when we talked about how the brain adapts to dopamine and to medication to help control your illness? The chemicals caused the nerve cells to function differently. Well when you keep taking drugs the nerve cells adapt and after a while they need the drug to function properly: they sort of get used to having so much drug every so often. They are dependent on the drug. When the supply runs short, like when your body needs food, the cells start sending out signals. Instead of saying "feed me" they say "give me cocaine" or heroin or whatever they have become dependent on. Unlike your stomach, brain cells don't mess around by sending out gentle little reminders to eat: they hit you with a sledge hammer: "I want drugs now and I'm going to make you feel miserable until I get some."

Note to Therapist: This dialog should be related to individual group members by referring to symptoms of craving identified earlier. *"OK, so what do you do now that you know what cravings are? The most important point is that a craving doesn't last forever."* Draw diagram of sine curve (a series of bell curves) on a flip chart to explain craving hitting a peak and recurring periodically.

When a craving begins, it will continue to increase for several minutes, hit its peak (the point where it feels the worse), and then begin to fade away. Depending on what drug you use and how much you use, this process may take as little as about 7 to 10 minutes. One reason that people become dependent on drugs is that the drug immediately removes the craving and any uncomfortable feelings that come with it. But, remember, the craving will go away on its own without you having to use the drink or drug to make it go away! You just have to wait it out for that 7 minutes or so. Later, we will talk about ways to cope with those times when cravings seem really overwhelming. One of the things we can do is teach you how to relax and distract yourself.

The longer that you go without using drugs or alcohol, the number of cravings you experience will decrease. So, if at first, you have five cravings every hour, once you've been clean for a while, you may only have one or two. Also, the longer you are clean, the amount of time between cravings increases. So, when you first stop using, you may have one craving after another. But after you have been clean for a couple months, you may have a craving and then not have another one for an hour or more! Later, you're going to learn some skills to help you avoid situations that produce cravings and make it easier to wait it out until the craving goes away.

6. **Discussion of triggers: Physical versus trigger causes of cravings.** *As we were just saying, the longer you are clean, the fewer cravings you will have. But cravings can still occur even after you have been clean for a while. That's because cravings can be physical like we just talked about, and cravings can be caused by people, places, or things that you connect to using. These things, people, and places can trigger, or cause a craving. You will remember the pleasurable feeling you used to get from using drugs or alcohol when you are around those people, places, or things. This causes a craving.*

Note to Therapist: Put the flowchart on the board:

Triggers or Causes	⇒	People, Places, Things, etc. Physical Symptoms	⇒	Remember pleasurable feelings	⇒	Cravings Urge to Use/ Physical Symptoms

Note to Therapist: Therapist should use information gathered during motivational interview to assist group members in identifying their triggers.

Let's go over what some different types of triggers are now.

People: *Sometimes being with a person that you have used with in the past or that you use with now, is all it takes for you feel like you want a hit or a drink.*

Places: *Just being somewhere that you used, or even being in the area where you use or used can cause you to crave.*

Things/Times of Day: *Sometimes different things or certain times of the day can be a trigger for some people to want to use drugs or alcohol. For example, seeing the drug, or maybe seeing a pipe may trigger you to want to use. Also, you may want to use more when you have just gotten paid, just eaten a meal, or when you get up in the morning, or before you go to bed at night.*

Smells/Sounds/Sensations: *For some people, the smell of the drug/alcohol, or even the smell of cigarettes can be triggers to use. Also, the sound of traffic or certain kinds of music can be a trigger. Some other triggers may include seeing someone having a drink or taking a hit.*

Feelings: *Sometimes people use when they feel a certain way. Some people use when they are feeling good, and other people tend to use more often when they are feeling bad.*

Bob, what are some of your triggers?

Note to Therapist: Get feedback from different group members for each category and put on the board under the trigger category with different color markers for each group member. Continue to probe each group member for at least one or two triggers that they come up with on their own.

Combinations of triggers: *As you can see, several triggers will often occur together (illustrate this point by using one of the member's examples). This can make it really difficult to say "no" to drugs or alcohol, when you don't want to use. There are many different things telling you to use. For example, you may be with your good friend near your favorite bar when you just got paid, and you are really craving a drink. All of these things, these triggers, are telling you to use. That's why it is really important for you to learn how to deal with those situations.*

7. High-risk situations. *We said that triggers are the people, places, or things that you connect to using drugs or alcohol. Because triggers are associated with the pleasurable feelings you had when you were using, they can cause you to crave drugs or alcohol. So, when you are in a situation where your triggers are present, you are in a high-risk situation. These situations are called high-risk situations or HRS because there is a high risk that you will use when you are in them. Where there is a trigger there is a high risk for you to use.*

High-risk situations occur where there might be more than one trigger. High-risk situations can occur when more than one trigger acts at the same time. For example, Alex, can you tell us about a time when you didn't want to use, but some or all of the triggers you just told me about were there, and you ended up using?

Note to Therapist: Insert an example given by a member using the list of triggers he or she previously identified.

In that situation, there were several triggers acting at the same time that increased the chance that you would use the drug/alcohol automatically. What negative consequences happened as a result of using drugs in that situation? So in this situation, you faced lots of triggers and it led to a craving for the drug which made it really hard for you to say "No" to it, even though you knew that negative consequences would happen if you used.

One trigger that is really strong. *Another example of an HRS could be when there is one trigger that is so strong, you will use almost automatically. For example, if there is one person who you use with each time you see him, that may be enough to cause you to use automatically. Or, it could be one trigger that is very hard for you to avoid. For example, the person you live with is a strong trigger for you if you use with that person every day because it would be really hard for you to avoid that person. So for you, this would be a high-risk situation. What negative consequences might happen if you used with that roommate who is a trigger for you?*

Let's go through an example so that we all have a clear understanding of what high-risk situations are. Bob, what is a situation when you find yourself almost always using?

Note to Therapist: Go through the triggers that make up a client's HRS. Refer to the type of HRS that their example represents and further describe the multiple/single trigger HRSs.

8. **Have all group members identify their own high-risk situations.** *What we want to do now is to help you identify some of these situations in your own lives so that we can help you to cope with them and avoid using at these times when you don't want to use. Everyone who has a problem with drugs and alcohol has at least a few high-risk situations.*

When people try to use less or quit, they usually can do it in easy situations. When you run out of money to buy drugs, you can't use because you can't buy. Or if you go into the hospital for a while, it can be easier to not use because you can't get out to buy drugs. Being on conditional release can also make it easier to stay clean because you know that if you use, you will go back to jail. Has anyone here been on conditional release? What was it like keeping clean when you knew you would go back to jail if you used/drank?

Note to Therapist: Probe for information from participants who were able to stay clean for a certain amount of time when they were in jail, on conditional release, on probation or parole, in the hospital, or broke.

It's really hard to stay clean when you are in a high-risk situation. You may automatically drink or use drugs at certain times or in certain places or with certain people. We have learned that if you know what your triggers are ahead of time, then you can plan ahead and make a plan to avoid them. A plan will give you something you can do to prevent yourself from getting into a situation where you would automatically use. Bob, for you that plan might be staying away from your brother when you know he wants to use or has drugs on him.

Let's find out what some HRSs are for each of you. Fred, think of a time when you didn't want to use, but you did. Tell us about it.

Note to Therapist: Help members identify HRSs by asking leading questions similar to those from the trigger session regarding person, place, feeling, sensation (smell, sight). Try to concretize a time period for the person by asking them to think about a period of time when they were not using; for example:

"Think of a time in the last week/between now and this past Christmas/between now and your last birthday, etc." Then ask: "So, why is that a high-risk situation for you? And what were the negative consequences that you could face if you did end up using?" If no group member is able to think of a time, the facilitator should make use of information gathered from the motivational interviews at this point.

List on the board each HRS and trigger components of that HRS, followed by the possible negative consequences for each group member. If a client has difficulty answering, ask other members to help. It is important to help participants focus on what they were feeling, doing, where they were *before* they actually used, as they may have trouble distinguishing between what they were doing or feeling before when they were actually using.

SKILL SHEET: AVOIDANCE

Goal

Define avoidance as a strategy for coping with triggers and high-risk situations. Group members will identify avoidance strategies for coping with triggers and high-risk situations. Group members will role-play avoidance strategies *as appropriate*.

Instructions to Therapists

1. **Conduct urinalysis before group and follow procedures in Urinalysis Contingency section.**
2. **Review goals and complete goal setting.**
3. **Brief review of last session.** *Last session we talked about cravings, triggers, high-risk situations (HRS), and how they can lead to you using drugs/alcohol automatically, even when you don't want to. Can anyone explain what a craving is? (It's when your body tells you it needs the drug by giving you physical symptoms) Good, can you give me an example? (You feel nervous, anxious, or may smell the drug). Excellent! Who can tell me what a trigger is? That's right, a trigger is something that makes you really want to use. A trigger automatically makes you want to use drugs because when you did use drugs before, the trigger was always there, like a certain person or a certain place. Bob, what is one of your triggers? Now, who can tell me what an HRS is? Good, that's right. An HRS is one where you are likely to use drugs/alcohol almost automatically. This type of situation can happen when (a) several triggers act at once* (use a participant's example); *(b) when there is one trigger that is very strong* (example); *or (c) when there is a strong trigger that is very hard for you to avoid* (example). *For homework, we asked you to write down situations that are high risk for you.*

Note to Therapist: Ask each member what his or her situations are and what some of the negative consequences of use are. Go over general goals with group members, tying these substance use reduction goals to the strategies to be learned in sessions 5 and 6.

Today we are going to help you learn how to develop a plan to meet your goal even when you're in an HRS.

4. **Today's session: Avoidance coping strategies.** *We've found that when you know what your HRSs are, you can be on the lookout for them. It's always easier to deal with an HRS when you know that it is coming. Then you can be prepared and have a plan ready to help you deal with it. There can be more than one way to cope with an HRS. The plans we work on today will help you avoid this type of situation. Then, in the next few groups we will work on other ways you can deal with an HRS (escape or refusal).*

Defining avoidance. *Like we just said, one of the ways that you can cope with your triggers and HRSs is by avoiding, or staying away from them. For example, instead of going to a bar and trying to say no or trying to keep yourself from drinking that cold beer that you see on the counter, you just don't go to the bar. That way, you don't see the beer, you avoid the trigger, and don't put yourself in that HRS. Some ways you can avoid your triggers or HRSs include: distracting yourself with a movie, the television, or other activities, doing relaxation training, going somewhere like an NA/AA meeting, or getting together with or calling your sponsor if you have one. You can do all of these things instead of going to the places or hanging around with the people who are triggers for you.*

For example, one of Mary's HRSs is to use crack with her friend Josephine when she is in Josephine's apartment. She has been clean now for a few weeks and does not want to use today. Mary's goal in this situation is not to use today. One thing Mary can do to avoid this HRS is to call Josephine instead of going over to her apartment. What else can she do to avoid putting herself in this HRS? (Probe and elicit possible avoidance coping strategies from group members.) Other solutions could be: don't go to Josephine's apartment, meet Josephine in the park instead of in her apartment, go to a movie with Josephine, talk with Josephine on the telephone instead.

5. **Generating avoidance coping strategies for triggers and HRSs.** *So, in the past few groups we talked about your triggers and HRSs. Now let's have you come up with some plans of how you can avoid them. Who would like to start?*

Note to Therapist: At this point the facilitator will draw from one group member's previously discussed goal and high-risk situation, and go through devising an avoidance strategy with them using the following format:

(a) Review individual goal.
(b) Discuss individual HRSs.
(c) Identify the problem and the negative consequences that could result from using.
(d) Help member identify what could be done to avoid his or her HRS.
(e) As members come up with avoidance strategies, ask, "Why might it be hard to use that strategy?" or "What might go wrong with that?" and "What could you do instead if that didn't work?"
(f) Role-play the situation (when appropriate to the individual's situation)

Following is an example:

Bob, your goal has been to cut down to smoking weed only on weekends, right? And you told us here in group that one of your HRSs is when you are at your friend Johnny's house, because he always seems to have weed and usually keeps it sitting around where you can see it. Right? So, let's say that Johnny calls you up on a Friday afternoon, the two of you have not seen each other in a while, and he wants to get together to catch up on things. What is the problem that you could have in making a plan to do something with Johnny and trying to stay with your goal of decreasing how much weed you smoke on the weekend? Right, you know that you most often end up using with Johnny when you're in his house. If you agree to go there, you may as well be smoking that joint already and you will have blown your goal for the weekend. How can you use avoidance to stay out of a HRS with Johnny and the weed?

Note to Therapist: Keep in mind the participants' goals and that these goals do not *have* to be abstinence oriented.

Good, you can make a plan in that phone call to meet Johnny at the restaurant, or down at the Inner Harbor. OK, if you were to meet Johnny at the restaurant, why might it still be hard to not use or why might that not work? What could you do instead? Good. You could meet him at his sister's house where he doesn't get high. That's another way to meet your goal. Let's role-play that and see how it goes.

Note to Therapist: Have group members continue to generate avoidance-related solutions until each individual has been able to use their own particular trigger or HRS to come up with a solution.

Depending on the makeup of the group, therapists may want to have each member define the situation which puts them at most risk, identify one coping strategy, and then go around to each member again to identify another HRS. Another option would be to generate several solutions for one key situation per member. As appropriate, therapists or other members should role-play solutions with members to try them out and see if they would work. Therapists should be specific and ask members if they have different triggers for different substances.

SKILL SHEET: ESCAPE AND REFUSAL

Goal

Define escape and refusal as strategies for coping with triggers and HRSs, group members will identify escape and refusal strategies to cope with triggers and HRSs. Group members will role-play their escape and refusal strategies as appropriate.

Instructions to Therapists

1. **Conduct urinalysis before group and follow procedures in Urinalysis Contingency section.**
2. **Review goals and complete goal setting.**
3. **Brief review of last session.** *Last session we talked about one way to deal with your HRS situations. Can anyone tell me what that coping skill is? Good. Avoiding your triggers and high-risk situations is one way to keep yourself from "automatically" using when you don't want to. For homework, we asked you to write down examples of ways in which you could avoid your HRSs.*

Note to Therapist: Probe for individuals who actually have been able to avoid their HRSs, then use an example of someone whose avoidance coping strategy did *not* work as a bridge to the escape and avoidance skills. If clients all say that avoidance has worked, the facilitator can encourage use of the additional strategies with this comment:

Well, even though you were successful, sometimes you can't always avoid an HRS. In those cases, you will need other ways to deal with your triggers or HRSs. Today we are going to help you develop a plan to say "No" to drugs/alcohol when you don't want to use, but may be in an HRS. We will help you do this by using escape and refusal coping strategies.

4. **Today's session: Defining escape and refusal coping strategies.** *Sometimes you may not be able to avoid an HRS because you find that you are already in that situation. One thing that you can do if you find yourself in a HRS is escape, or leave the situation. Another thing you can do is to refuse the drug or alcohol that is being offered to you. Has anyone ever been in an HRS where he or she either escaped or refused and were able to keep themselves from drinking/drugging?*

You probably remember all of the time we spent a few weeks back working on drug refusal skills. Remember how we practiced step 4, leave the situation? This is exactly what escape is—leaving the situation. Who can tell me some situations in which you would want to leave the situation immediately? That's right, when the person has drugs on them you want to get out of there as fast as you can. Let's review the steps in drug refusal skills with "Leave the Situation" as our Step 4:

Step 1: Make eye contact
Step 2: Say no
Step 3: Give a reason
Step 4: Leave the situation—escape

Note to Therapist: Therapist should discuss the steps in the same way that was done during the drug refusal skills sessions.

5. **Generating escape and refusal strategies.** *Okay, now let's have you come up with some plans of how to escape or refuse drugs and alcohol when you find yourselves in your HRS. Bob, one of your HRSs was being with your brother when he wants to use drugs, right? So the problem here is that you are with your brother and he wants to use drugs and you don't. So what would be your goal in this situation?*

Note to Therapist: Keep in mind the participants' goals and remember that these goals *do not* have to be abstinence oriented.

So, your goal here is to—. OK, what can you do to achieve your goal of—? (Have client generate a solution. If member has trouble coming up with a solution, ask other group members for assistance). *OK. If you were to do—, why might it still be hard for you to say no to using —? OK. So what might you do instead of —? Good, that's another way to deal with that HRS and meet your goal of—. So then for this HRS, one solution would be to—, and if that didn't work, then you could try—. That's excellent!* (Repeat this process with each member).

Note to Therapist: Have group members continue to generate escape or refusal-related solutions until each individual has been able to use his or her own particular trigger or HRS to come up with a solution.

6. **Role-playing escape and refusal coping strategies.**

Note to Therapist: Have each group member role-play his or her own self-generated escape/refusal coping strategies.

SKILLS SHEET: HIV PREVENTION I—DEFINITIONS, TRANSMISSION, RISKY BEHAVIORS

Goal

Define HIV and AIDS, review the routes of transmission, and identify risky behaviors.

Instructions to Therapists

1. **Conduct urinalysis before group and follow procedures in Urinalysis Contingency section.**
2. **Review goals and complete goal setting.**
3. **Brief review of last session.** *Last time, we talked about ways for you to deal with your HRSs. Can anyone tell me what skills we used to help you cope when you may be in a HRS and don't want to use? That's right, we used escape or refusal skills. Escaping or refusing is one way that you can keep yourself from using when you don't want to use.*

Over the next few groups we will be talking about a deadly, incurable disease called AIDS and how people like you and me can get it or give it to other people. I'm sure you have all heard of HIV and AIDS. What do you know about it? Do you know anybody with HIV/AIDS?

Note to Therapist. This gives clients a place to say that they are HIV positive or have AIDS, if they want to share this with the group.

Today we want to give you information about HIV/AIDS. You might have heard some of it before, but other information you will be able to take with you into other contexts. Our focus over the next few sessions will be talking about HIV/AIDS and how drug use makes a greatly increased risk of contracting it. What's important is that there are ways to keep from getting it and that's what we are going to focus on here. We will talk about what is safe behavior and what isn't safe behavior when having sex or just messing around. Also, people who use needles or other works can be at risk of getting HIV. If someone is using and can't seem to stop, there are ways they can still protect themselves from HIV.

Please remember our group guideline about confidentiality. We want this part of group to be helpful in some way to everyone here. Not talking to people outside of group about what we say to each other here in group will help us all to feel more comfortable.

Note to Therapist: If it is known that a member in the group is HIV+, the therapist should spend additional time talking about reinfection, why it is important to prevent reinfection, and how to prevent reinfection. Issues include reinfection making medications less effective, developing immunity to a medication: "You might contract a type of HIV that is immune to medication, you will then be less responsive to treatment because you can get a strain that is not responsive to medication."

Also, the therapist should discuss that once someone has been infected, with current medications and medical treatments, the length of time between being diagnosed with HIV, and developing AIDS continues to grow.

4. **Today's session: Education about HIV and AIDS**

What is HIV/AIDS? *Now let's spend a little bit of time discussing the facts about HIV and AIDS so that everyone knows what it is* (distribute handouts with simple definition). *Can anyone tell me what HIV stands for? What about AIDS?* (Write both terms on the board.)

HIV(human immunodeficiency virus): This is a kind of virus (show picture) *that gets spread from one person to another. Can someone tell me what a virus is? That's right, a virus is like what people have when they have a cold—it is important to understand that it is much harder to spread the HIV virus than it is to spread a cold. But, once a person has the HIV virus in their body, it does not go away as a cold does. Once this happens, the person is called HIV positive and from this point the HIV positive person can give the virus to someone else and make him or her sick with HIV. Also, if a person who already has the virus gets more of it into their body from someone else, they may get sicker more quickly. This is called reinfection.*

AIDS (acquired immune deficiency syndrome). People can have the HIV virus in them for a long time—over 10 years—before they actually get the sickness or "syndrome" that we call AIDS. This is when a person gets certain diseases that happen because the part of the body that fights viruses and infections is weakened by having to fight off illnesses like pneumonia, certain cancers, and other infections. A lot of people get certain kinds of pneumonia that they end up dying from. But just because you have one of these diseases does not mean that you have HIV (list other diseases if group members seem interested).

How do people get HIV/AIDS? (Give group members handouts with most frequent transmission routes and draw on board). *There are lots of ways that people can get the human immunodeficiency virus—we'll call it HIV from now on. What is one way? Right, Bob, a person, man or woman, can get it by having sex with someone without using some sort of protection* (or whatever other way someone comes up with, be reinforcing). *What's another way?* (Keep probing until ideas are exhausted and list on board in columns by route of transmission). *Okay, so these are some, and there are some other ways that I'll add now. The way that the virus is spread is through one of three types of body fluid: What are they? Blood, semen, or vaginal fluid, and a mother's breast milk* (refer to handout of routes). *When these fluids go from someone who is already infected into someone who is not infected, that is how the virus* (show picture of the virus) *goes into another person.*

Statistics in Maryland. *Maybe some of you know people who have HIV or AIDS. Maybe you have even been tested for it before. What I do here in group and what educators do all over the world is talk about how to keep from getting it—why is that so important? Right, because there is no cure once someone has it. We already know that a lot of people—people right here in Maryland and in Baltimore—are HIV positive and have AIDS. Because there is no cure for the disease, people who have it will eventually die.*

Does anyone here know how many people in Maryland may be HIV positive? Well, the Department of Health says that enough people to fill two thirds of Camden Yards stadium have had the HIV virus (as of March 2001, 23,158 people in Maryland were living with HIV/AIDS; 55% were HIV cases and 45% were AIDS cases)! Some of them have gotten sick and died and some are still alive and don't even look sick yet—maybe they don't even know they have it yet! (Show colored handout of Camden Yards). *Every single one of those people could give it to someone else, too.*

Note to Therapist: You should collect statistics for your own city, county, etc. and tailor material accordingly.

Risky behaviors. *What is a behavior? Right, it is something that a person does, an action. For example, thinking about going to the beach is not a behavior—getting up and walking to the beach is a behavior. Or, dreaming about having sex with a hot guy or woman is not a behavior, but actually having sex with them is. What's another example, Bob? What do you do when you get up in the morning? That is a behavior* (list group members' responses on the board). *People get HIV because of their behavior. So, it's not that a certain kind of person—such as a gay person, or prostitute, or African American—gets HIV, but people who behave in certain ways are at risk of contracting the HIV virus. And that can be anyone!*

The thing to remember here is that there are different behaviors that you can do that can put you at greatly increased risk for contracting HIV. For example, remember that HIV can be spread through body fluids including blood and semen or vaginal fluid or mother's milk. Different behaviors are more or less risky for spreading these fluids and getting HIV.

Note to Therapist: Go over the body fluids and then relate them to the risk behaviors by following categories or use green/yellow/red dots next to behaviors to show level of risk.

> *Risky sexual behavior:* "What kind of things do people do when they are messing around that are risky behaviors?" (List responses on board)
>
> *Oral sex:* Sores make it more risky, don't do it without protection like a cut condom, dental dam, saran wrap. *Anal sex:* This is considered the highest risk behavior when unprotected, use two condoms to keep from breakage.
>
> *Intercourse:* Unprotected, pulling out, sores make it more risky.
>
> *Touching:* When sores are present and blood is exchanged.
>
> *Hooking/prostituting:* Either paying for sex or getting paid to have sex, prostitution is more dangerous because of having sex with someone who has had a lot of partners, being with more partners, violence, or drug use.
>
> *Risky drug use behavior:* "What kind of things do people do when they are using drugs and alcohol that are risky behaviors?" (List responses on board)
>
> **Shooting up**
>
> **Sharing needles**
>
> **Smoking rock/crack**
>
> **Getting high/drunk makes it more likely to make bad decisions**

It's easy to plan to have safe sex when you're sober but you won't always keep your goals when you are high. A lot of unsafe sex occurs when people are high. People put themselves at much greater risk when they use drugs—they lose the ability to use good judgment.

Note to Therapist: Some clients will have HIV. If they disclose this in the group and want to talk about it, they can be used as "experts" to tell about symptoms, testing, or medication. Do not ask a client to talk unless he or she has volunteered the information during the group and has been talking about it already.

Information on Other STDS, Add If Needed

These risky sexual behaviors and risky drug use behaviors can put you at risk for other diseases in addition to HIV. Sexually transmitted diseases such as syphilis, herpes, chlamydia, and gonorrhea are all contracted through the risky sexual behaviors we have been discussing today. Research has shown that people with these sorts of STDs are much more likely to contract HIV if they are exposed to it. That is because some of these STDs involve sores or tears that can let HIV into the body. So understanding these risky sexual behaviors is important in terms of reducing risk for HIV as well as other sexually transmitted diseases.

> **Bacterial STDs:** treated with antibiotics
>
> **Viral STDs:** can't be cured but can be managed with medications (e.g., herpes)

Other STDs

> **Bacterial vaginosis**
>
> **Chlamydia:** often no symptoms
>
> **Gonorrhea**
>
> **Herpes:** *most people with it don't know they have it. It can be spread even when symptoms are not visible (i.e., it is not true that it can only be spread during an outbreak)*
>
> **HPV (human papillomavirus):** *commonly associated with genital and anal warts, often leads to cervical cancer*
>
> **Syphilis**
>
> **Trichomoniasis:** *can lie dormant for months or years*

SKILL SHEET: REDUCING RISK AND DEMONSTRATING CONDOM USE

Goals

Identify ways to reduce risk of HIV infection and set goals to reduce members' risky behaviors. Demonstrate appropriate condom use.

Instructions to Therapists

1. **Conduct urinalysis before group and follow procedures in Urinalysis Contingency section.**
2. **Review goals and complete goal setting.**
3. **Brief review of last session.** *Last time we covered a lot of stuff. Let's review a little bit now. What is the name of the virus that we talked about? Good, what are some of the ways that people can get HIV?* (List on board) *Great! What is the disease called when people get sick from having the HIV virus in their system? That's right, AIDS. We also talked about behavior—risk behavior for HIV. What is a behavior? Right, something that a person does. What is one risk behavior for HIV?* (Have members generate a list and write it on the board.) *Good, these are all behaviors that will increase your risk of contracting the HIV virus. For your homework, I asked each of you to write down two things that you may be doing or that you have done in the past that put you at risk for getting HIV. Remember I said that we all have things—habits, behaviors—that we can change.* (Refer to therapist master list copy and review each person's healthy behaviors and add behaviors to be changed.) *Bob, what did you put down or think of between last group and today* (go through practice with all group members). *So, what could you do differently to change that behavior so that you are not at risk?*
4. **Today's session: Protecting yourself from HIV.** *So, these are some of the behaviors that can lead to getting HIV and AIDS. What are some things you can do to protect yourselves from HIV?*

Instead of Having Intercourse

Note to Therapist: Generate list of other things that people can do besides having sex to show that they care about each other or to make each other feel good. The list can include masturbation, other sexual activity that does not result an exchange of body fluids but is pleasurable, being together but not having sex, cuddling, kissing, going out and doing something fun. Give each member a condom in a wrapper to hold.

What About When People Do Drugs?

Note to Therapist: Generate list and hand out bleach bottle pamphlets if appropriate. Take a harm reduction approach. Remember that drug use is a high-risk behavior in and of itself due to loss of judgment and risk of not staying with goal of having safe sex that goes along with being high. Message is don't use drugs. If you do use drugs, then have safe sex or no sex. If you are going to a place where there will be cocaine, take a condom with you. Don't inject drugs. If you inject, have clean needles and don't share needles. Discuss needle exchange and distribute handouts on programs in the city where the group is located if needed. Women—don't be vulnerable. How to reduce vulnerability—have group members generate ideas.

What Does Not Work to Protect You From HIV?

Note to Therapist: Generate list including pulling out, washing afterwards, having sex with someone who "looks" healthy. Also, many popular methods of female birth control (the pill, Norplant, Depo-Provera, sponge, diaphragm, IUD) cannot reliably prevent HIV infection or remove the risk of getting other STDs.

Everyone has different risk behaviors, but it's important to know all the ways of protecting yourself and then figure out for yourself which are the most important and effective ones for you to use.

5. **Using a male condom.** *For people who have had unprotected sex in the past and want to change that behavior, one thing you can do is to use a condom, or, if you are having sex with another man, get him to use a condom too. Using a condom is not as safe as not having sex at all, but it is a lot safer than not using anything.*

I am going to show you how to use a condom correctly and then I'll ask each of you to do the same thing with the condom you have. Some of you may have used a condom before, some may not have, and some of you may have never been taught how to use a condom correctly.

There are some important things to make sure of when you are using a condom. What kind of material should a condom be made from? Latex, that's right. And what about the lubricant, or wet stuff, that you can use if you want—what kind should it be to use safely with a condom? This is K-Y water-based jelly, one kind of lubrication that is okay to use. You need to make sure that you use a lubricant that is water based. Don't use Vaseline, or baby oil, or anything with oil in it because this can make the condom break. Here are the steps to putting on a condom the right way.

Note to Therapist: Put blown-up handout on board and distribute handout. Follow steps and demonstrate condom use. Demonstrate with coleader first, if present, or do it alone once and then ask for group member participation.

"Okay,—, you can follow along with me now." (Prompt each group member through the steps and ask why each part is important. Do this with all members).

There are a few other things to remember when using condoms. Make sure you use a new one each time you have sex, and handle them carefully so that you don't break them with you nails or teeth. Condoms can expire—that means that they can't be used after a certain date because they get old. Don't forget to check the expiration date on the condom wrapper to make sure that it's still good. Also, don't keep condoms in your wallet to carry them around with you. The problem is that either the condom can be in there so long before you use it that it will be expired by the time you use it, or it gets worn out from all that time in the wallet when you carry your wallet in your back pocket and sit on it all the time.

6. **Using a female condom (optional).** *There is also a female condom that women can use in order to protect themselves when having sex. Remember that using a female condom is not as safe as not having sex at all, but is a lot safer than not using any protection. Let's practice using a female condom. I am going to show you how to use a female condom correctly using this model, and then I'll ask each of you to try it with the female condom you have. Some of you may have seen or used a female condom before, some may not have, and some of you may have never been taught how to use a female condom correctly.*

Note to Therapist: Therapists can use Female Condom Chart or pamphlet on female condoms to show group members the basics of how to use the female condom.

A few things to remember about the female condom. First, you have to use a new for each time you have sex. Second, do not remove the inner ring in the female condom. The ring helps keep it in place during sex. Third, don't use the female condom and a male condom at the same time—pick one or the other or else neither condom will stay in place the right way. Fourth, be careful not to rip the female condom. When you put it in, make sure you don't rip it with your fingernail or with your jewelry. If it does rip, make sure to take it out and use a new one. Finally, if the female condom slips out during sex, put in a new one. Here is a handout with instructions for using the female condom. Let's try it out with the model now.

Note to Therapist: The handout has seven steps for using the female condom. Make sure you go through them all.

This is the *very short* version.

Open package. Make sure the condom is covered with lubricant.
Hold condom with open end down. Squeeze top (inner ring) and insert.
Push in with index finger. The inner ring should be just past the pubic bone.
The open end (outer ring) should be lying against the outer lips.
The outer ring may move during sex. If it begins to slide inside, stop and insert a new condom.

Note to Therapist: Add to this information if needed and tailor to group members' needs and interests:

Remember that risky sexual behaviors can also lead to other sexually transmitted diseases in addition to HIV. Doing things to protect yourself from HIV such as wearing condoms, having safe sex, not having sex, and doing other sorts of things that feel good can also protect you from getting other sexually transmitted diseases. Wearing condoms is really important. When used consistently and correctly, male condoms are effective in preventing the sexual transmission of HIV and can reduce the risk of getting other STDs. Female condoms also may reduce the risk for STDs and HIV when used consistently and correctly. **Important***: Condoms do not cover all exposed areas, but they are very good at preventing STDs that are transmitted through fluids (gonorrhea, chlamydia, HIV). For STDs that are transmitted by skin to skin contact (herpes, syphilis), the best form of prevention is trying some other activity that feels good but does not involve sexual contact.*

7. **Role-Plays.** *Today I am going to ask you to think about all of the risky behaviors we've talked about so far. I want you to think about the risky behavior you identified in your previous homework or during group. We would like you to work on a goal to stop participating in that behavior, to reduce your risk by participating in that behavior less, or to participate in a safer, less risky behavior like we talked about today. Bob, you mentioned that your risky behavior is—, your goal then would be to—. What steps must you take to reach that goal?*

Note to Therapist: Elicit suggestions from the subject. If he cannot come up with steps, probe the group. If there are no suggestions, establish some concrete steps the subject can take to reach that goal (e.g., get some condoms, always have a condom, always use a condom). These steps, along with the subject's goal are written on the goal sheet used for homework. Repeat this for each group member.

Between now and next group, I want each of you to come up with some positive consequences to reaching each of your individual goals. Write them on your goal sheets and bring them in to our next group.

Note to Therapist: Also, have clients continue to work on goals.

Information for therapists who are asked questions regarding safer sex for lesbian couples:

Wear latex, vinyl, or nitrile (contains no latex) gloves for penetrative sex and anal sex.
    Protects against contracting infection through cuts on hands.
    Make sure nails are filed smoothly.
    Put on fresh gloves when you switch activities.
    Use water based lubricant
Use condoms to cover vibrators and other tools; put on a fresh condom when switching activities.
Use dental dams or plastic wrap for oral sex.
Clean tools with warm water and antibacterial soap, clean before every use. (for more information see, Newman, 1999).

SKILL SHEET: HIV PREVENTION, PRACTICE

Goal

Role-play members' goal related situations.

Instructions to Therapists

1. Conduct urinalysis before group and follow procedures in Urinalysis Contingency section.
2. Review goals and complete goal setting.
3. Brief review of lastsession.

Note to Therapist: Review each individual's goal to reduce risky behavior. Discuss positive consequences of achieving goal.

Last session we talked about how to use a condom. What is one important step in putting a condom on? Right, there has to be space in the end for the semen (or slang word if it fits with the tone of the group). What else? Right, you have to make sure that you, or the person you are having sex with, if it's another man, pull out before getting soft so the semen doesn't leak out the sides of the condom. Good! What else is important to remember about asking someone to use a condom? Did anyone get a chance to practice using the condom? —, why don't you help me review for the rest of the group how to put one on correctly.

4. **Today's session: Role-play goal related situation.** *There will be times when you find yourself with someone who you want to have sex with and who wants to have sex with you. It will be important for you to be able to remember your goal, and to do what you need to do to reach your goal and reduce your risk of HIV. These situations may come up without warning and you must know what to do. If you practice skills to reduce your risk behavior beforehand, you will be more capable of thinking about what to do when the situation actually happens. The following are the steps you can take to reach your goal. (List on board and give handouts).*

Step 1: *Clearly state your position or request (lets your partner know that you mean no)*

No, I can't have sex with you	*I want to use a condom*
No, I don't want to fool around	*I want to only have safe sex*

Step 2: *Give a reason why (helps your partner to understand your position)*

I don't have sex if it's not safe	*I don't have sex*
I don't know you that well	*I'm not in the mood*
I don't want to get pregnant	*I don't want to do anything risky*
I just don't feel right about it	*I'm staying celibate/don't have sex*

Step 3: *Suggest a safe alternative OR number 4*

Let's just hug and watch TV.	*Why don't we go out for pizza instead?*
Let's wait and talk about this more.	*Why don't you let me put a condom on first?*

Step 4: *Leave the situation (if the person trying to persuade you becomes violent or you think they may get violent)*

I have to leave now.
You have to leave now.

Note to Therapist: After modeling a role-play situation for group members, set up role-play with each group member. Make sure to use a scenario that reflects the individual's goal and be very specific with each individual about what would really happen and whom it would be with. Probe to check for any sign that a situation could become threatening to the member's health or safety. In this case, advocate for *leaving the situation or avoiding* the person entirely.

If role-playing with male participants, they may not need to convince their female partner to use a condom. If this is the case, set up a role-play scenario in which the participant explains to his "little brother"/son/nephew, etc., the reasons he should use a condom (e.g., his brother is about to have sex for the first time with his girl friend and doesn't want to use a condom).

SKILL SHEET: HEPATITIS PREVENTION

Goals

Group members will learn how the liver works and why it is an important organ. Group members will learn the definitions of the three types of hepatitis, what causes them, behaviors that put a person at risk for them, what the symptoms are, and how to get tested. Group members will identify behaviors that can put them at risk for contracting hepatitis and understand how to prevent getting hepatitis or giving it to others. Group members will learn about the medical treatments for hepatitis and understand how and why hepatitis C and HIV/AIDS are important to think about together.

Instructions to Therapists

1. **Collect urines before group and complete Urinalysis Contingency section.**
2. **Review goals and complete goal setting.**
3. **Brief review of last session.** *For the last several sessions we have been talking about behaviors that put people at risk for contracting the HIV virus. Last session we did role-plays to practice what to do when you find yourself with someone who you want to have sex with and who wants to have sex with you, and how to talk to them about having safe sex so that you can reduce your risk of contracting HIV. In the role-plays we practiced four steps. The first was to clearly state your position or request. Can anyone remember why it is important to clearly state that either you don't want to have sex or that you want to use a condom? Right, it lets your partner know that you really mean no. Next you practiced giving a reason why, and this is important because it helps your partner to understand your position. The next step was to suggest a safe alternative, such as using a condom or just being together without having sex. Finally, we talked about how if the person doesn't want to do an alternative you have suggested, you need to leave the situation, especially if the person keeps trying to persuade you or he or she becomes violent or you think the person may get violent.*
4. **Today's session.** *Today we are going to learn about another disease that affects many people, called hepatitis. There are actually several kinds of hepatitis and all can be contracted through the sorts of risky behaviors that we have talked about in our sessions on HIV/AIDS. The three most common types of hepatitis are A, B, and C. They are all caused by viruses that get into your body and then damage your liver. Some of them (especially hepatitis C) can cause really bad liver damage, leading to cirrhosis (or scarring), liver failure, and cancer. In today's group we are first going to talk about your liver and why it's an important organ. Then we will talk about the types of hepatitis, what causes them, and what their symptoms are. We will also tell you about ways to get tested in case you are ever interested, either now or in the future.*

What is the liver and why is it important? *Let's start out by talking about what the liver does and why it's important. Your liver works like a filter and cleans toxic stuff out of your blood. It also makes proteins that help your blood clot (so you stop bleeding when you have a cut), helps you digest food, and stores sugar and vitamins that provide your body with energy. Bottom line, you cannot live without your liver. So it's best to take care of your liver since you only have one and you need it to live. When it goes, so do you.*

There are many ways to take care of your liver. One of the most important is to avoid drinking a lot of alcohol, as well as not mixing alcohol with drugs. Both drinking and using drugs makes your liver do a lot of extra work, and for many people it gets to the point where their liver is tired and unhealthy from all that extra work. Has anyone here ever had problems with their liver? Can you tell us about it? In addition, to keep your liver healthy it is important to make sure that you don't take more medicine than is prescribed by the doctor or recommended on the bottle.

There are also lots of unsafe behaviors that put people at risk for getting hepatitis. To keep the liver healthy, it is important to know what these risky behaviors are and avoid them! We will be talking more about these behaviors as we talk about what exactly hepatitis is.

What is hepatitis? There are several types of hepatitis. Hepatitis A is the most common form of hepatitis and the easiest type to get. Hepatitis A is usually spread when people don't wash their hands after making a bowel movement. Food can spread the virus when people who prepare the food don't wash their hands after using the bathroom. The virus can also be transmitted during sex by rimming (sticking your tongue in someone's anus). Because touching poop can spread the virus, changing diapers and not washing afterwards is another risk. Hepatitis A can also spread through contaminated water in countries where the water supply is not kept clean.

Hepatitis B is usually spread through sexual intercourse (both vaginal and anal). If you have unprotected sex (intercourse without a condom) you are at risk for getting hepatitis B. Because it is also spread through blood contact, it can be spread by sharing needles, toothbrushes, and shaving razors (unlike hepatitis A, hepatitis B is not spread through food or water).

Hepatitis C is the most serious kind of hepatitis. It is also the most common among people who shoot drugs. It is spread primarily through blood when people share needles to use heroin and other drugs. Sharing straws to snort drugs also spreads hepatitis C, as does sharing toothbrushes and shaving razors, because these things all have blood on them. Also, the hepatitis C virus can live outside of the body for up to two weeks. So if it gets on a toothbrush or razor, for example, it can live for a long time and infect someone else if they use it. Unprotected intercourse (again, both vaginal and anal) can also spread the virus, although this hasn't been proven for sure yet.

Symptoms of hepatitis. The different types of hepatitis have different symptoms. If you get infected with hepatitis A, you will get quite ill: yellowy skin, fatigue, nausea, vomiting, abdominal pain, dark urine, light poop, and fever. However, the infection and all symptoms usually clear up on their own in a few weeks or months with no serious aftereffects or long-term liver problems. There is a vaccine for hepatitis A. You should check with doctor to see if he or she thinks you should get it.

In terms of hepatitis B symptoms, you may not get any, but if you do symptoms include flulike symptoms, dark urine, light stools, yellow skin and eyes, fatigue, and fever. As with hepatitis A, most people pass the virus without any long-term damage to the liver. In some people, however, hepatitis B can continue a silent attack on your liver and cause scarring or cancer. There is a vaccine (actually a series of three shoots) against hepatitis B. You should check with your doctor to see if he or she thinks you should get the shots.

Hepatitis C is the most serious of the three and the one most likely to cause long-term liver problems, including cirrhosis and cancer. First of all, what are the symptoms? Actually, most people who get hepatitis C don't even know they have it until their liver stops working and they get really sick. If you do get symptoms they might include getting jaundice (yellow skin); fatigue or tiredness; abdominal pain; loss of appetite; intermittent nausea and vomiting. Unlike the other kinds of hepatitis, which usually go away or end without causing any liver damage, the vast majority of people with hepatitis C become chronically infected. The disease can be long and drawn out, but people who are chronically infected with hepatitis C are likely to develop cirrhosis, liver failure, and cancer. Many people with hepatitis C end up needed a liver transplant. Also unlike hepatitis A and B there is no vaccine. Also even if you've had A and B you can still get C. Because most people don't get any symptoms it is important to get tested so you can start doing something about it before it destroys your liver.

The reason hepatitis C is so serious is because there is no simple and effective treatment or cure. A liver transplant may help, but the virus could come back and destroy the new liver. There are treatments (like interferon and ribavarin) that have helped some people. However, these treatments can also make you very sick and they are not good for everyone. For example, if you have HIV/AIDS you may not be able to take them at all.

Hepatitis C testing. *While there is no vaccine for the virus, there is now a blood test to see if you have been exposed to hepatitis C. If you think you might have hepatitis C, you should ask about hepatitis testing. There is a test that can tell you if you have antibodies to hepatitis C. You can ask your doctor about getting tested, or if you are interested we can work with you to find out how to get tested. If the test is positive, you will need to take other tests to see if you have the virus and to see if it has damaged your liver.*

Risky behaviors and hepatitis. *Now we are going to talk about the kinds of behaviors that put you at risk for getting hepatitis and what you can do to prevent getting it or spreading it. Remember that several sessions ago when we were talking about HIV/AIDS we talked about risky behaviors: things that people do that increase their risk of contracting HIV. We talked about risky sexual behaviors and risky drug use behaviors. Can anyone remember some of the risky sexual behaviors we talked about? That's right: any sort of sexual activity including oral sex, anal sex, and intercourse can be high risk, especially when sores are present and you are not using protection. Hooking/prostituting is also a very high-risk sexual behavior because of having sex with someone who has had a lot of partners, being with more partners, violence, or drug use. And can anyone remember any of the risky drug use behaviors we talked about? Yes, shooting up, sharing needles are two extremely high-risk behaviors. We also talked about how simply getting high/drunk is a risky behavior because it makes you think less clearly and so it makes it more likely that you will make bad decisions, such as having unprotected sex.*

Some of these same behaviors are also risky when it comes to contracting hepatitis. Since there are different types of hepatitis, there are different risky behaviors associated with each one. Let's start with hepatitis A, which is spread through fecal/oral contact. Hepatitis A is usually spread when people don't wash their hands after making a bowel movement. Food can spread the virus when people who prepare the food don't wash their hands after using the bathroom or changing a diaper. Hepatitis A can also be spread during sex by rimming (that's using your tongue to lick someone's butt). So for hepatitis A, not washing your hands after you go to the bathroom is a risky behavior. It is one that is easily addressed by making sure that you wash your hands every time after you go to the bathroom. In addition, as we have talked about before, having safe and protected sex is a good way to make sexual transmission less of a problem.

Now let's talk about hepatitis B. Remember that the hepatitis B virus is found in blood, semen, and vaginal secretions. It can be spread by unsafe sexual contact and contact with blood through sharing needles or tattoo/body piercing instruments. Any unsafe sexual practice that involves a direct exchange of infected bodily fluids like blood, semen, or vaginal secretions will put you at risk. The same sexual behaviors that put you at risk for HIV/AIDS also put you at risk for hepatitis B. (Review again the list of high-risk sexual behaviors, write it on the board, have clients look at handouts if they need to.)

OK now let's talk about hepatitis C, the most dangerous of the three because it is the one most likely to cause longer-term damage to your liver. The hepatitis C virus is found in blood and spread through sharing needles. It is also a really strong virus and can live outside of the body for a long time (in some cases up to several days). This means that it can also be spread through sharing razors, toothbrushes, nail files, barber's scissors or clippers, tattooing equipment, body piercing or acupuncture needles if contaminated by the blood of an infected person. It can also be spread by sharing straws to snort drugs.

Finally you should know that hepatitis C was only discovered a little while back. Because of this, anyone who has had a blood transfusion before 1992 or received any clotting factors made before 1987 is at risk for hepatitis C because there was no way to screen for it. Remember that you can't tell if a person has hepatitis C just by the way they look. Most people who get infected with hepatitis C don't have any symptoms. Unlike the other kinds, which usually go away or end without causing any liver damage, the vast majority of people with hepatitis C become chronically infected. The disease can be long and drawn out, and people who are chronically infected with hepatitis C are likely to develop cirrhosis, liver failure, and cancer. Many people with hepatitis C end up needing a liver transplant. Also, unlike hepatitis A and B there is no vaccine. Also even if you've had A and B you can still get C.

How to decrease your risk of contracting hepatitis C. Let's talk now about what you can do to keep from getting and spreading hepatitis C. Remember it is found in blood. Can anyone name one thing that you can do to keep from getting/spreading hepatitis C? Right, not sharing stuff like razors or needles, and being really careful in handling anything that may have blood on it. What's something else? That's right—not using needles to do drugs and not sharing needles. Remember that it's extremely easy to spread hepatitis C (and HIV) by using and sharing needles. Of course it's better if you don't shoot drugs at all. If you do, there's always going to be blood around, even if you can't see it. The blood will be on the needle, inside the needle, and it will be around your skin where you inject. When you touch the needle or your skin, the blood gets on your hand. Then everything you touch **with that hand gets blood on it.**

So, if you're going to use needles to shoot drugs, the best thing to do is to have your own clean area for fixing. Don't touch or use anyone else's stuff. Have your own needle, water, cooker, matches, lighter, tie, filter, etc. And don't let anyone use any of your things. To keep all your stuff clean, use a newspaper or magazine to spread everything out on. That area and everything on it is your clean space. If you use with other people make sure they have their own space and their own equipment. If you have to help someone get off, just help them get a vein and let them do everything else.

Another way to reduce the spread of hepatitis C, HIV, and other infections is to wash your hands with soap and water. Washing your hands and injection sites before and after you fix will keep you much healthier. It doesn't matter what kind of soap you use, just use a lot, rub your hands together, get all parts soapy and scrubbed, and then rinse real good. In addition, while getting hepatitis C through sex is less common, you should still be sure to practice safe sex each and every time you engage in sex. What does it mean to have safe sex? That's right—use a condom.

What to do if you have hepatitis C. If you do find out that you have hepatitis C there are some important things you can do. You should stop drinking alcohol altogether because alcohol can speed up the liver damage associated with the hepatitis. Also if you haven't already gotten them you should talk to your doctor about getting vaccinated against hepatitis A and hepatitis B. This is really important because if you have hepatitis C and then get hepatitis A as well, it can actually cause a very serious liver condition that could kill you pretty quickly.

Summary of Units on HIV/AIDS and Hepatitis

As we have talked about before, there are lots of similarities in the behaviors that put you at risk for hepatitis C and HIV/AIDS. Both are caused by viruses and can be spread by sharing needles and other things that might have blood on them or by having unsafe sex. While they may cause different illnesses, you can take the same basic steps to prevent both HIV/AIDS and hepatitis. Let's review again the types of risky sexual and drug use behaviors that put people at risk for both of these diseases and what you can do to keep from getting/spreading them.

Note to Therapist: Review again prevention and risk reduction tips with special emphasis on those that are relevant to both HIV/AIDS and hepatitis. Make sure clients have handouts, and use handouts and charts to review this information. Get participants to generate as much information as possible.

Chapter **10**

RELAPSE PREVENTION AND PROBLEM SOLVING

INTRODUCTION

Achieving abstinence from drugs is a process that unfolds over time. Motivation waxes and wanes as a function of a host of neurobiological, psychological, and environmental factors. Success may breed complacency that increases exposure to high-risk situations. Stress and life events produce negative emotional states that rekindle memories of drug use, increase urges, and decrease willpower to resist drug use. Cues that were associated with drug use in the past may be encountered unexpectedly and awaken urges to use. Lapses are common, and present a risk of becoming full-blown relapses. These various risks are of concern for anyone attempting to stop drug use, but they are particularly problematic for people with SPMI given the deficits many of them experience in the ability to exert self-control, to conduct effective problem solving, and to see the continuity of events over time. In addition, the prevalence of poly-drug abuse is common in this population, and different substances must be targeted sequentially for most clients. In that regard, skills and motivational factors relevant for one substance will not automatically generalize to abstinence from other substances. Consequently, treatment must be extended over time so that training in skills and coping strategies can be applied across substances, to high-risk events that occur intermittently, and in periods of decreased motivation. To do this, treatment must include sessions on relapse prevention and problem solving, in which clients identify high-risk situations that are likely to occur in the future and apply the skills that they have learned to coping with these situations without drug use. Relapse prevention and problem solving (RP/PS) is the unit of BTSAS in which these issues are addressed.

The structure of the RP/PS sessions is identical to the skills training sessions. Each session in the RP/PS unit begins with urinalysis, reinforcement, and goal setting. The RP/PS sessions then involve introducing clients to a range of high-risk situations, and having them identify the best skills to use to cope with the situation without using drugs. Clients then practice coping in these situations both by using the skills that have already been taught (refusal, escape, avoidance) or others that are discussed in the course of the group (e.g., calling someone for help/support). Many sessions will include problem solving in high-risk situations that clients have encountered or will encounter in the near future, as well as others that clients may not have previously considered. Other sessions will vary according to the needs of individual group members.

The basic training strategies (e.g., rehearsal, extensive use of prompts, having participants repeat information in their own words) employed in earlier training sessions continue to be used throughout the RP/PS unit. In addition, material covered in earlier sessions is systematically reviewed and related to current experience when the core curriculum is completed (typically by the end of the fourth month). Entire units (e.g., refusal skills training, education about dopamine and schizophrenia) are repeated as needed for new members. We have created Skills Sheets with guidelines to correspond to all RP/PS sessions. It is important to remember that these sessions are guidelines that need to be tailored to the specific needs of the clients in the groups.

MAKING RP APPLICABLE TO SPMI CLIENTS

In designing the RP/PS module, it was important to select situations that are relevant to SPMI clients and have a high likelihood of leading to relapse. In addition to providing relevant content, BTSAS therapists must make the RP/PS relevant to clients in other ways. This is important because clients with SPMI, due to their cognitive deficits, have difficulty imagining the future and applying things learned in the present to what might happen at a later time. The therapist must always make RP/PS relevant in the here and now and encourage the client to think about how to use these skills as they work to reduce or stop drug use. That is, RP in the primary substance abuse literature is geared toward substance abusers who have achieved some reduction or abstinence in their use, and who now need to work on coping with situations that can lead to relapse (hence the name *relapse prevention*). In BTSAS groups, some clients may have reduced or stopped using, but others will be current users. In order for this content to apply to everyone, it must be presented as relevant to getting clean as well as staying clean. This can be done in several ways. First, the sessions must be presented in the here and now, with therapists soliciting and using current information on clients to illustrate the topics of the RP/PS sessions. For example, if the topic of the session is coping with stress, the therapist can ask for current examples of stress: "Bob, in our last group you talked about being really stressed out about your housing situation. Since that kind of stress can lead you to use cocaine, let's talk about how you can handle that stress without using drugs."

Second, it is important to incorporate RP/PS topics into goal setting. For example, a client who is struggling with low motivation and has completed the RP/PS session on coping with low motivation, can be directed during goal setting to try out some of the coping strategies learned in the RP/PS session. A client who is currently struggling with medication side effects can discuss during goal setting having a talk with his doctor about this and have as his goal to talk to the doctor before the next BTSAS session.

CONTENT OF THE RP/PS UNIT

The RP/PS unit is aimed at teaching clients to address the dysphoria, depression, anxiety, and boredom that play a significant role in substance use for SPMI clients. The intervention uses behavioral techniques (e.g., modeling, role-play, imaginal rehearsal), and is tailored to the preferences and needs of each individual client. The group format of BTSAS facilitates the training, as clients can suggest strategies to one another, share concerns and successes, provide mutual support, and learn from observation of their peers. The emphasis is on distraction, avoiding social isolation, and checking the validity of dysfunctional thoughts by checking assumptions with others.

Most clients have a number of high-risk situations in which they have much more difficulty coping without substance use. In the RP/PS unit, each client is helped to identify the three to four most risky situations for him or her through group discussion. It might also be useful to identify these situations via a self-report questionnaire such as the Inventory of Drug-Taking Situations (Turner, Annis, & Sklar,

1997), a paper and pencil inventory that surveys usage patterns. We then use a limited problem solving strategy to teach clients how to anticipate these situations and help them identify specific ways to avoid them. The goal here is to identify specific risks and solutions, rather than teach a generic strategy that clients can use to deal with any new situation they might encounter. Once again, our premise is that SPMI clients are not likely to initiate or effectively implement a multistep problem solving routine in the face of real life pressures, but they can benefit from a circumscribed strategy that involves few choices and makes modest demands on executive functions. The aim is to teach clients about the persistence of high-risk situations and to help them identify situations that will be risky in the near future and devise coping strategies for each.

The content of the RP/PS unit will vary somewhat according to the needs of individual clients. Several topics are considered integral to the unit and should be covered in all groups. Other modules have been developed for use with certain groups depending on the clients in the group and the issues being presented. The standard modules include: Introduction and review of drug refusal and coping skills (avoidance and escape); introduction to relapse prevention and review of high risk situations; coping with lapses; addressing other substances of abuse; coping with boredom; coping with depression or stress; coping with symptoms of schizophrenia and mental illness I: Talking to your doctor about symptoms and side effects; coping with symptoms of schizophrenia and mental illness II: Other ways to cope; coping with low motivation; and money management.

The optional modules, done selectively depending on the needs of group members, include: violence and victimization and substance abuse; dealing with partners that use drugs; creating a drug free social support network; general assertiveness training; anger management; employment skills (connecting with job training, how to prepare for a job interview, etc.); and relaxation training.

These sessions reflect general issues that need to be addressed, but all are not conducive to one-session discussions only. That is, these are topics that require ongoing monitoring, discussion, and intervention. These modules are designed to give therapists a starting point for addressing these topics, but these topics are not ones that can be covered in a single sessions. Each topic needs to be repeatedly discussed and client progress toward goals needs to be continuously monitored. For example, addressing other substances of abuse is an important part of the RP/PS unit. This is a topic that cannot be adequately addressed in one session. The session can serve as the mechanism for approaching the topic both generally in the group and more specifically for individual clients. However, other substance use and abuse must be continually monitored, and client progress toward reducing or abstaining from a secondary substance must be repeatedly addressed. This might take the form of a client who has successfully abstained from a goal drug then changing his or her designated goal drug to a secondary substance (e.g., from cocaine to marijuana). For many clients, the secondary drug of abuse will be alcohol. Efforts to reduce or abstain from alcohol need to be reinforced and addressed following the RP/PS session that deals with seconday substances. Other RP/PS sessions involve helping clients create plans for coping with some high-risk situation. These topics and the plans that were generated need to be frequently revisited; plans might need to be updated or completely changed in the event that a client has found a plan unworkable. For example, the RP/PS session on money management involves therapists helping clients develop plans for managing their money. This is not a one-session type of topic—therapists need to determine if the client has designated a payee, opened a bank account, gotten direct deposit, or otherwise followed through on plans that were established during the session.

STANDARD MODULES

The aim of the RP/PS sessions is to teach clients to identify high-risk situations that they are likely to encounter in the future and to devise coping strategies for each.

Relapse Prevention (RP)

The general framework of RP is presented, and subsequent sessions involve identifying high-risk situations (either ones that clients come up with or ones that therapists come up with), and applying the principles of RP to each (i.e., planning for each high-risk situation).

Coping with Lapses

Lapses (isolated occasions of use) can easily become relapses (full-blown return to use). Thus a lapse is a high-risk situation. The primary focus is to make clients aware of the distinction between lapses and relapses and the danger of moving from the former to the latter. Given that most people with SPMI have difficulty with abstraction, the focus must be concrete and specific. Ask clients when they last had a lapse, and then refer to that situation throughout the session so that the client can continually pair the content of the session with a specific recent event. Also, do not belabor the point if a client does not fully understand the lapse/relapse distinction. This will likely be a very new concept for clients, most of whom will have been told repeatedly that any use in any amount or for any length of time is a relapse. Clients have had similarly harsh negative consequences for lapses and relapses (any use can get a client kicked out of his or her housing or treatment), and many will adamantly disagree with the notion that a lapse can be contained. Rather than try to convince a client that you are right and he or she is wrong, the following explanation can be used:

Client: I don't agree with that. Any use is bad, even one time or one joint or one sip or anything.

Therapist: So to you even a very little bit of use seems just as bad as a lot of drug use. I'm glad you told me that. As we talk today about how to keep a little bit of use from becoming a full-blown relapse, it will be really important for us to figure out how to apply what we talk about to you and how you see all of this.

Addressing Other Substances of Abuse

Data show that if you use one drug you are at substantially increased risk to relapse for another. Thus continued use of a secondary substance is a high-risk situation for relapse. Clients who have addressed a primary drug (e.g., cocaine) but are still using a secondary drug (e.g., alcohol) are at higher risk for relapsing to cocaine as long as they are drinking. There are several issues that often arise here. Some clients for whom this is an issue will not want to admit to other drug use. Clients have many reasons for keeping substance use secret, and just because they have disclosed use of one drug does not mean that they will feel comfortable being honest about any other use. For example, consider a client who is working in the BTSAS group on reducing her crack use, taking methadone for her heroin use, and drinking frequently with some consequences (missing appointments, drinking throughout the day), although she has not discussed her drinking with anyone on her treatment team. She may not want to disclose the extent of her drinking due to the potential consequences of this disclosure (getting terminated from treatment or housing, implications for child custody). Relatedly, clients may not want to change their use of other drugs and may not consider use of other substances a problem. This is particularly true for clients who smoke marijuana or drink. Clients will sometimes voice the opinion that drinking is the only fun that they have left, that their drinking is not a problem for them. In addition, clients might abuse substances that they do not consider to be drugs of abuse, such as medications that they are prescribed for anxiety or sleep but that they are using to get high. It is important to remember that the goal of BTSAS is not to make clients admit that they have a problem, accept ideas that they are not willing to accept, or make them believe the things that we believe. Rather, the goal is to provide information that clients can understand and absorb, with the approach that clients will gain skills that they did not have before, and will have information to use in the future. In addition, the focus should be on how use of other drugs is a high-risk situation that can lead to use of the client's goal drug. The following example illustrates how a therapist might handle this sort of situation:

Client: I don't have a problem with other drugs. I do crack and that's it. I drink on the weekends with my friends, and that's not going to change.

Therapist: It sounds like you see your crack use as the problem that you need to work on —that's great! Your drinking doesn't seem to concern you and it's something you do with your friends and it's fun. Tell me, have you ever gotten into any trouble when you are drinking with your friends on the weekend—maybe some trouble with the police or something?

Client: A couple of times I got warned by a cop when we were out and drank and were yelling at people. At a bar once I almost beat up a guy and got thrown out of the bar.

Therapist: What about the day after you drink? How do you feel?

Client: Not too good. Tired. It's hard to get up and go to work. But that's what happens when you are out with your friends and have a good time.

Therapist: So you see your drinking as a way to have a good time with friends. There have been times though when it's not all good—like when you got into a bar fight and when you got warned by the police officer or when you wake up the next day and feel pretty bad. My point here is not to tell you or convince you that you have a problem with drinking—you just told me that there are times when you drink and things that are not great happen to you, so you seem pretty clear about some of the ways that drinking can get a person into trouble. What I want to do is help you figure out how to make sure your drinking doesn't lead you to use crack. You have been working really hard here in group on stopping your crack use. Your hard work has really paid off and you have a lot to be very proud of—you're doing a great job! For lots of people, drinking makes them do things they wouldn't ordinarily do if they weren't drinking. You just gave me a good example—you got into a fight in a bar, which probably wouldn't have happened if you weren't drinking. What we want to do today is talk about how drinking or using other drugs can be a high-risk situation for using crack, because you will not be thinking as clearly and you might do something that you wouldn't ordinarily do, in this case, use crack.

In addition, the BTSAS therapist has a powerful tool at his or her disposal—other group members. By generating discussion among group members in this session, it is often the other clients who point out to each other the impact other drug use is having on someone's life. It is important for the therapist to keep this discussion among clients positive and reinforcing, rather than confrontational and accusatory. The following exchange continues the one from above to illustrate this strategy:

Client (Bob): That wouldn't happen. When I drink I just drink.

Therapist: It sounds like, for you, drinking is seen as a separate thing from crack use. One thing that we know from working with other people with both mental illness and drug use is that things that aren't planned can happen at any time. Has anyone here ever had a time when they went out drinking and they wound up using drugs at some point that night?

Client 2: That happened to me. I don't even like crack—I do heroin. But when I drink I can get really out of it. This one night I was drinking and someone pulled out some crack and I was messed up and just did it. I felt really bad about that.

Client 3: Me too. One time I drank and woke up the next morning and I didn't know where I was or what had happened. Then I had to get a drug test at the clinic and it was positive. You should watch it Bob. That could happen to you.

Therapist: Those are great examples of how drinking can sometimes lead you to do things, in this case use drugs, and you don't even know it. So drinking or using other drugs, even if those are not your drug of choice, can get you out of it enough so that if your drug of choice is around, you might use it. That's exactly what we call a high-risk situation. Bob, what do you think about that? Has there ever been a time when you drank too much and wanted to use crack?

Client: I want to use crack all the time, when I'm drinking and when I'm not drinking.

Therapist: Well the important thing here is to think about how when you drink, it could put you at risk to use crack. There may come a time when this is an issue for you, so learning this stuff now may be a help to you if you ever are in this situation in the future.

Coping with Negative Affect

Data show that negative affective states are the most common reasons for relapse. Also, studies on reasons for substance use among clients with schizophrenia find that one of the most common stated reasons for use is coping with negative affect, especially boredom. Thus negative affect is a high-risk situation. The goal here is to help clients plan for negative affect and to discuss other coping strategies other than substance use.

Boredom

Coping with boredom is a very important and challenging topic to address with SPMI clients. It is important because these clients list boredom as one of the main reasons they use, and it is challenging because it is difficult both for clients and therapists to come up with things to do to decrease boredom. Clients with SPMI often have few social contacts or relatives to visit, lack jobs, lack skills to secure and succeed in jobs, and often live in impoverished circumstances where they lack access to interesting activities or money to engage in them. These factors make it extremely important for the BTSAS therapist to be creative and resourceful when helping clients learn to cope with boredom. First, learn what resources and activities your clinic, hospital, or treatment center has to offer its clients. Often treatment centers have open groups that clients can attend, drop in support groups, or center-related activities that clients might enjoy. In addition, many clinics offer self-help meetings or client seminars that can be informative as well as offer something to do with other people that doesn't involve substance use. Second, we suggest researching free activities in your town or city. These might include going to a local library, volunteering at some local organization, or going to free lectures or other free city events. Third, research free "recovery-themed" activities in your city. Self-help meetings and organizations and churches are excellent places to find free activities that are oriented toward wellness. It is important to talk with a client about what sorts of things he or she would enjoy and would be willing to do (many clients have had past experiences with self-help groups and will not return, some clients may not be interested in church-related activities, clients who can't read may not enjoy spending time in a library). Then, in goal setting, clients can be directed to try out some of these activities. Part of goal setting might need to include how a client would get to and from an activity, how the client would pay for the activity if payment is required.

Depression and Stress

Clients with SPMI and substance use disorders generally use drugs to help them feel better when they are depressed, stressed, or experiencing some other form of negative affect. Helping clients learn and try out alternatives to drug use in such situations is a key feature of BTSAS. As you will see on the Skills Sheet, we offer a range of options for coping with these negative emotions without using drugs: (1) increase pleasant activities; (2) talk to someone; (3) get help/solve the problem that is causing you to feel depressed/stressed; and (4) talk to your psychiatrist about medication. You will see these solutions are offered in many RP/PS sessions. Remember, our goal is to provide clients with a limited range of options, and have them learn and implement these options in high-risk situations. That is, rather than presenting a long list of options that clients would forget, or change potential solutions to fit specific situations, we stress providing a few simple options, things that these clients could do and do correctly with little effort, which are likely to be useful in many different situations. Over the course of the different RP/SP sessions, therapists should remind clients of these potential solutions, while also asking clients for other options. In this way, the group can be tailored to individual clients.

Coping with Symptoms and Side Effects

Another one of the big reasons clients with SPMI give for their drug use is to cope with SPMI symptoms and medication side effects. In the education module, we review how drug use most often makes symptoms and side effects worse. In RP/PS, the goal is to give clients other drug-free options for improving symptoms and side effects. We have broken this down into two sessions. The first focuses on teaching clients how to talk to their doctors about symptoms and side effects. The second involves other strategies for coping with symptoms and side effects, including distraction and talking to someone about them.

Overview and Talking to Your Doctor

Clients with SPMI are often not good at describing how they are feeling, and they often report feeling nervous when talking to their doctors. In this session, we teach clients how to talk to their doctors about their symptoms and side effects, and then role-play with them so they can practice how to do this. As is our custom, we break this skill down into steps: (1) Make eye contact and be firm; (2) tell your doctor that you are having more symptoms or medication side effects; (3) tell your doctor what the symptoms or side effects are; and (4) ask your doctor if he or she can change your medication or give you something that will help these symptoms/side effects. It is important to talk with each client about how he or she talks with the doctor, if this makes the client nervous or anxious, and give the client additional coping strategies for these feelings if needed. For example, if a client gets anxious when talking to his doctor because he fears that he will forget the important things he needs to tell the doctor, the therapist can help the client make a list of issues to talk about in the appointment with the doctor. If a client does not like her doctor, helping her to remain calm, to understand the need for her to work with the doctor despite her not liking him, and to stick to the issue (the increase in symptoms or medication side effects) is going to be critically important. Again, these examples illustrate the great importance BTSAS places on tailoring content to individuals within the group.

Distraction, Alternative Ways to Cope, and Talking to Someone

The second session in this series is on other ways to cope with increased symptoms or medication side effects. We suggest several strategies: (1) distraction; (2) increase activity levels; (3) initiate social interaction; (4) modify physiological state—breathing and relaxing; (5) talk to someone. This is another situation in which we present a limited set of suggestions and then help clients figure out how to implement them. This session is a particularly good opportunity for general discussion among clients regarding what works for them and how they have implemented these strategies in their own lives.

Other High-Risk Situations

Both low motivation and money management are high-risk issues for clients.

Low Motivation

Motivation to maintain abstinence waxes and wanes over time. Periods of low motivation are high-risk situations for drug use. Clients often say that they never want to use drugs again, with little understanding that there will be temptations and periods of time when they are less motivated to maintain abstinence.

Money Management

Money is a continuous source of risk for many clients. This unit covers practical strategies for controlling that risk by minimizing the person's access to money. Tactics include formally establishing representative payees, giving benefit checks to case managers or significant others for deposit rather than the client cashing them, establishing concrete goals for savings (e.g., to move to a better apartment, to buy kids Christmas presents), and not carrying money unless going directly to a store for a specific purchase.

Optional Modules

Once the group has completed the standard RP/PS modules, the BTSAS therapist must tailor the remaining RP/PS group sessions to the specific needs of the clients in the group. There are several options for therapists:

1. Repeat standard RP modules as needed. If clients need more practice with specific RP/PS skills, review and practice those skills. High-risk situations such as coping with boredom, coping with lapses, coping with depression or stress, coping with low motivation, coping with symptoms and side effects, and money management are all important enough to be reviewed and practiced again. This can be introduced to clients in the following manner (coping with symptoms and side effects is used as an example because this is something that clients often have a lot to say about):

Several weeks ago we talked about symptoms of mental illness and medication side effects as two high-risk situations that often lead people to use drugs. We had a great discussion on the symptoms that people have and how they have tried to use drugs or alcohol to cope with these symptoms or side effects. We thought that this was such an important topic, and one that was relevant to so many of you, that we would spend today's group reviewing what we learned and practicing how to cope with symptoms and side effects without using drugs or alcohol.

2. Therapists can consider covering the optional RP/PS modules if the topics are relevant to any group members. Specific optional modules (again, all related to coping with high-risk situations) include: dealing with a partner who uses drugs; creating a drug free social support network (how to meet people who don't use drugs); general assertiveness training; and employment skills (connecting with job training, how to prepare for a job interview, etc.). These optional sessions follow the same pattern as the standard sessions: urinalysis, goal setting, review of the last week's topic, explanation of the new topic with input from group members, discussion of coping strategies, and practice/role-plays as needed.

It is important to remember that these sessions are guidelines that need to be tailored to the specific needs of the clients in the groups. These sessions reflect general issues that need to be addressed, but all are not conducive to one-session discussions only. That is, these are topics that will need to be repeatedly addressed and discussed throughout the course of the PS/RP unit.

We present here some brief information on these optional sessions. The sessions are grouped here according to general topic areas. Remember that you can pick and choose which optional sessions to present based on the needs and interests of group members.

Optional Sessions that Focus on Social Situations that Impact Drug Use

The optional sessions that focus on social situations that impact drug use include: (1) violence and victimization and substance abuse; (2) dealing with a partner who uses drugs; and (3) creating a drug-free social support network. These are probably the most important optional sessions for many clients, especially those who live with drug using partners or roommates. The sessions devoted to violence and talking with a drug using partner are designed to give clients safe ways to talk to the people in their lives who may cause them harm. It is common for clients with SPMI to be in dangerous relationships that are maintained for a range of reasons (financial support, housing, children, no other options). Telling clients simply to leave the partner is often not accepted by the client as a good solution, and depending on the situation, may really not be a good solution. These sessions offer a way to talk with clients about these issues, get clients thinking about the sorts of changes in their relationships they might need to make in order to maintain abstinence, and tell clients where they can go if they need help. As part of these sessions, lists of agencies and groups that help people in violent relationships should be provided, as well as names and contact information for shelters and other forms of temporary housing. In addition, clients might disclose to you information that they have not told their primary treatment team. In such cases, it is important to help the client discuss these issues with her treatment team, as those professionals who know the client best are in the best position to secure any needed services.

The session on creating a drug-free social network is also important, as many clients leave BTSAS groups and return to environments where everyone they know uses drugs. Given the social skills deficits of SPMI clients, making new nonusing friends and finding activities that are not connected to drug use is a clear challenge. This session gives ideas and is a good place to solicit ideas from group members about how to meet people, things to do with other people, and how to keep from using when others in one's environment continue to do so. It is important to remember the settings that most SPMI clients live in; make sure strategies for meeting others are relevant to these settings. Also, be sure to review the first two BTSAS on making small talk and making plans with a friend—both are relevant to building a social network that is not based on drug use.

Optional Sessions that Focus on General Social Skills

The optional sessions that focus on general social skills include general assertiveness training and anger management. We included these sessions because being able to tell other people what you are feeling, refuse requests, and communicate effectively with others are important skills needed to stay drug-free. In the session on general assertiveness training, we stress that letting people know how you feel is better than leaving feelings bottled up inside, and we review three skills: (1) expressing negative feelings; (2) expressing positive feelings; and (3) review of refusing a request and offering an alternative (from BTSAS session 3). It is not necessary to review all of these skills in this session—you can select the one or two that are most relevant, or spread the content across two or three sessions if you want to review and practice all of these skills. Alternatively, you can introduce all three skills, and have the client select which one he or she needs to practice the most. If you choose this latter option, be careful not to confuse clients with too many steps. Rather, you can discuss generally why talking about things is important, review in general the three skills, have the client select which one he or she wants to practice, and review the steps for that skill while setting up the role-play. The anger management session focuses on teaching clients the benefits to them of handling anger appropriately and the steps for doing so: (1) keep calm; (2) say how you are feeling and why; (3) say why this situation or behavior has made you angry; and (4) make a suggestion to keep this from happening in the future.

Optional Sessions that Focus on Continued Skills Building

The optional sessions focus on continued skills building, include employment skills and relaxation training. In these sessions, we try to teach clients some skills that can help them as they progress into more long-term abstinence from drug use. The session on employment skills is designed to help clients prepare for post-drug-use life. Many clients have never had a job or tried to get one, often because their drug use kept them from working. Once abstinent, many clients will express interest in working, and this session is designed to help them with this process. It can also be relevant to clients who are not ready to work yet but who might be interested in employment some time in the future. We stress in this session the idea that these are good skills for anyone to know who might want to work at some point, and we get everyone involved in the discussion by providing examples and discussing past experiences (clients who are not currently working may have worked in the past). Finally, the relaxation training session is useful for several reasons: it teaches a useful skill that clients can use easily in their real lives, and it can be used throughout the BTSAS program if many clients come to group anxious or distressed. That is, once the skill is taught, the therapist can incorporate some brief relaxation into a session periodically if clients show up angry or otherwise distressed. It is also a good skill to use to cope with cravings, and as such can be introduced during that session and used periodically in group if clients experience cravings during the BTSAS session.

SUMMARY

The RP/PS component of BTSAS focuses on helping clients learn to cope with the high-risk situations they are likely to encounter as they work to achieve reductions in drug use. The focus is on developing a plan of action so that clients are prepared when such risks are encountered. The goal is to prepare clients for difficult situations so that they are ready to cope effectively and without drug use.

SKILLS SHEET: INTRODUCTION TO RP/PS/REVIEW OF DRUG REFUSAL AND COPING SKILLS

Goals

Group members will review and practice drug refusal skills. Group members will review and practice coping skills, including escape and avoidance.

Instructions to Therapists

1. **Conduct urinalysis and and follow procedures in Urinalysis Contingency section.**
2. **Review goals and complete goal setting.**
3. **Brief review of last session.** In our last meeting we talked about Hepatitis – the different types of hepatitis and the different risky behaviors that can lead to someone getting Hepatitis. Can anyone tell me some of the things that we talked about and learned about Hepatitis?
4. **Today's session: Introduce the problem solving and relapse prevention section:** *We have now completed several months of this skills group and we have talked about many things that will help you stay clean. Today we will begin a new section of the group called "Problem Solving and Relapse Prevention." The goal of this section of the group is to think about things that could happen in the future that could tempt you to use drugs, and develop a plan for dealing with them now. If you have a plan, then when you find yourself in a high-risk situation, you will be prepared to deal with it without using drugs. We will continue to talk about high-risk situations and how to cope with them, and we will talk about different high-risk situations, some that you may not even have thought about before. We will develop plans for dealing with these situations, and then practice our plans in the role-plays so that they become easy to do and automatic. The plans that we come up with will involve skills that you have already learned and practiced, including drug refusal skills, escape, and avoidance. We will also talk about other things that you can do in high-risk situations if things like refusal, escape, and avoidance are not enough.*

(a) Drug refusal skills (put these on the board and give a handout). *In today's group, we are going to review the skills that we have learned so far during group. We will then be able to apply these skills to different high-risk situations. We have learned three sets of skills so far for dealing with high-risk situations. The first is drug refusal skills. Can anyone tell us what drug refusal skills are? That's right: Drug refusal skills involve telling someone that you don't want to use drugs, as well as telling them that you don't want them to ask you again about using drugs. You might remember that we learned and practiced steps for drug refusal skills. Let's review these now. Can anyone tell me what the first step in drug refusal skills is? Yes, the first step is making eye contact. Why is it important to make eye contact? This gets the person's attention. The second step is telling the person in a firm voice that you don't want to use drugs or alcohol. Why is it important to use a firm voice? That's right: this helps make it clear that you do not want to use/drink with the person. When you are firm with someone they will know that you mean what you are saying. What's the next step? Give a reason why you don't want to use. Why is this important? It helps the person understand why you don't want to use drugs or alcohol. The last step is requesting that the person not ask you to use/drink. Why is it important to tell someone that you don't want them pressuring you to use alcohol or drugs? That's right: You want them to know that you don't want to have to keep saying no to them, that you want them to leave you alone. We have also talked about what you could do once you have told someone not to ask you to use drugs or alcohol, including suggesting an alternative or leaving the situation. When do you think it would be a good idea to suggest an alternative to someone? That's right—when you and that person have other things that you like to do together, you can suggest that instead of using drugs, you could do something else, like get some coffee, talk, or take a walk. When do you think it's a good idea* to just leave the situation? When you and the person have nothing else that you like to do together other than use drugs, or when the person has the drugs right there and doesn't want to do anything else except use (also, when the person is a drug dealer).

(b) Escape. *Drug refusal skills are really important when you are in a high-risk situation and someone is offering you drugs and you don't want to use. We also learned another coping strategy to use to cope in high-risk situations called escape. Does anyone remember what escape involves? That's right: escape means that you leave the situation. Has anyone ever been in a high-risk situation and coped by escaping or leaving the situation and was able to keep him- or herself from drinking/drugging?*

(c) Avoidance. *OK, so we use drug refusal skills when we are in a high-risk situation and someone is offering drugs and we don't want to use. Another strategy to use in a high-risk situation is escape—just get out of the situation—leave as quickly as possible. There is also another thing that you have learned to do to cope with high-risk situations. Remember that when you know what your high-risk situations are, you can always be on the lookout for them and not even get into the situation at all. That is, you can use avoidance and avoid the high-risk situation all together. Can anyone tell me what avoidance is? That's right: Avoidance is when you cope with a high-risk situation by staying away from that situation and never getting into the situation at all. For example, instead of going over to the place where you always used drugs (e.g., instead of going into the high-risk situation), you could avoid going to that place. Instead, you could go somewhere else, call a friend, go to an AA/NA meeting—something that is not at the place where you used. If you do that, you are not faced with the really strong temptation to use drugs. That way, you don't see the place where you used to use, so you avoid the trigger, and you don't put yourself in the high-risk situation.*

Let's use an example (use an example from a group member, the following is an example): One of Mary's high-risk situations is to use crack with her friend Josephine when she is in Josephine's apartment. She has been clean now for a few weeks and does not want to use today. Mary's goal in this situation is not to use today. One thing Mary can do to avoid this HRS is to call Josephine instead of going over to her apartment. What else can she do to avoid putting herself in this high-risk situation?

(d) Role-playing drug refusal skills, escape, and avoidance. *Now let's do some role-plays to practice how to use all of these coping skills to stay clean and not use drugs. When we set up the role-play you can decide which strategy you would like to practice: refusal skills, escape, or avoidance. First, we (i.e., the therapists) will do a role-play to show you how it will go. How about if we do a role-play and practice drug refusal skills? In our role-play, let's pretend that Tara (coleader) asks me to use alcohol and drugs with her. She has drugs with her and she is pressuring me to use and asking me several times to go and use with her. I want to say no because I am not using drugs and I want to stay clean. I also want to tell her to stop asking me to use and to stop pressuring me. I am not going to suggest an alternative since Tara has the drugs with her. Instead, I'm just going to leave the situation. As we do the role-play, you watch and see if we do all four steps.*

How did we do? What did you like about that role-play? Did you watch for the steps? How was my eye contact? How did I do giving a reason that I didn't want to use?

OK, now let's do some more role-plays. Bob, how about if you go first. Can you think of a high-risk situation that you had to deal with recently or one that you are going to have to deal with in the next few days that we can practice? That's a good one—your friend is coming over this weekend and you think he is going to want you to go out and get drugs with him and use. OK, now which coping strategy do you want to use? Can you use avoidance and avoid the situation? That would mean you telling your friend not to come over. If you are not going to tell your friend not to come over, then how about we practice refusal skills so that when he asks you to use, you can tell him no.

Note to Therapist: Let clients describe the situation, and then come up with which strategy they should use or might want to use to cope in that high-risk situation. Make suggestions but come up with a plan that the client feels that he or she could actually do. For example, if Bob's friend is coming over, avoidance (i.e., Bob telling the friend not to come over) would be a good strategy, but if Bob is not going to do that, then set it up for him to practice refusal skills).

Avoidance is harder to role-play if the client is deciding by himself to go somewhere. For example, if the client says that when he goes to a particular bar, say, it's a high-risk situation, work with the client to come up with a plan that includes what time he is likely to want to go to the bar, where else he can go instead of going to the bar, how he can get to that place. Be very concrete. This will be the client's practice for how to avoid a high-risk situation.

Another avoidance scenario is one in which the client is approached by someone else, and that person wants to go into a high-risk situation. For example, the client is asked by a friend to go to the bar in question, which is a high-risk situation for the client. In this situation, *you can use the refusal skills steps:*

> *Make eye contact*
> *Say no*—state that you do not want to there (e.g., go to the bar)
> *Give a reason*—"I used to use drugs there and I don't want to be around there anymore."
> *Suggest an alternative/leave*—"Let's go to the cafeteria instead/you will have to go there without me."

No matter what skill they are practicing, write the steps on the board for each skill:

> *Refusal skills: Eye contact, state no, give reason, suggest alternative/leave.*
> *Escape: Eye contact, state no, give reason, escape/leave immediately.*
> *Avoidance: Eye contact, state no, give reason, suggest alternative/leave.*

SKILLS SHEET: INTRODUCTION TO RP/REVIEW OF HIGH-RISK SITUATIONS

Goals

Group members will learn the basic principles of relapse prevention. Group members will review high-risk situations and practice coping with upcoming HRSs through role-plays.

Instructions to Therapists

1. **Conduct urinalysis before group and complete Urinalysis Contingency section.**
2. **Review goals and complete goal setting.**
3. **Brief review of last session.** *In our last group, we reviewed skills to use to deal with high-risk situations. There were three skills that we reviewed. Does anyone remember any of the skills? Right, one was drug refusal skills. What are drug refusal skills? That's right: telling someone that you don't want to use drugs and that you don't want them to ask you to use drugs again. We did role-plays and practiced the steps involved in drug refusal skills—making eye contact, saying no, giving a reason, and suggesting an alternative, or telling the person to stop asking you to use. Did anyone use drug refusal skills in the last week? We also reviewed two other skills to use to deal with drug use situations. Does anyone remember the other two skills we reviewed? That's right, one was escape—leaving a high-risk situation. Has anyone been in a high-risk situation and coped by escaping or leaving the situation this week? The last skill we talked about in the last group was avoidance. Can anyone tell me what avoidance is? That's right—avoidance is when you cope with a high-risk situation by staying away from that situation and never getting into the situation at all. Bob, give me an example of avoidance. That's right. Instead of going over to the bar where you always used to use drugs (i.e., instead of going into the high-risk situation), you could avoid going to the bar. Instead, you could go somewhere else, call a friend, or go to an AA/NA meeting. That way, you don't see the place where you used to use, so you avoid the trigger, and you don't put yourself in the high-risk situation. Did anyone avoid a high-risk situation this week and just not go into the situation at all? Tell us about it.*
4. **Today's session: Introduction to relapse prevention.** *Now that you have been in group for a while, many of you (or all of you if everyone in the group has been clean for a while) have had some clean time and have been working hard to not use drugs or alcohol. That's great and it's our goal here to help you keep this good work going so that you don't use drugs/alcohol. In our next several groups we are going to talk about different high-risk situations that could come up that might be tough to handle and we are going to plan for them so that you will know what to do if you find yourself in that situation. This is called relapse prevention—talking about the high-risk situations that could happen and figuring out how to deal with them now. Our goal is for you to have a plan so that you can keep clean from drugs/alcohol. Bob, why do you think it's good to have a plan for dealing with a high-risk situation? That's right, a plan will help you know what to do in a tough situation, so that you will be able to not use drugs or alcohol. A good example of why we talk so much about having a plan is that of a fire drill.*

Has anyone here been in a fire drill recently? In a fire drill, we practice what we would do in the event of a fire so that if a fire were to happen we would have a plan and we would know what to do—listen for the alarm, use the stairs instead of the elevator, know where the exits are so that you can get out of the building quickly. At places like the VA we have fire drills regularly so that clients and staff know what to do and where to go if there is a fire. So we have a plan just in case there is a fire.

We take the same approach here in this group when we talk about drug/alcohol use—it's good to have a plan just in case you find yourself in a high-risk situation so that you will know what to do to stay clean. We have talked before about learning new behaviors, and how that takes a lot of practice. So we will make plans and then practice them a lot by doing role-plays. In the next several groups we will talk about many different high-risk situations, ones that we have talked about before and others that haven't yet come up. We will talk about what to do when you are feeling stressed or depressed or bored so that you won't use drugs in those situations. We will talk about ways to cope with symptoms of mental illness instead of using drugs or alcohol to do that. We will also talk about situations that people in the group find tough to deal with and practice over and over what to do when those situations occur.

5. **Review of group members' high-risk situations.** *We have talked a lot in here about high-risk situations in which there are lots of drug-use triggers present that might cause you to crave drugs or alcohol or just make you want to use. Remember that these situations are called high-risk situations (HRSs) because there is a high risk that you will use when you are in them. Where there is a trigger there is a high risk for you to use. What we have talked a lot about in group is how to identify your own high-risk situations that happen in your own lives so that you can figure out what to do in these situations so that you won't use drugs. When you have problems with drugs or alcohol it's very hard to stay clean when you are in a high-risk situation. You may automatically drink or drug at certain times or in certain places or with certain people. Bob, you said that when you get together with your friend Fred, you guys always just do cocaine. That is an example of a high-risk situation—one in which you have always used in the past and it's really hard to be in that situation without using drugs. Over the next several groups we are going to spend time talking about different high-risk situations and figuring out what to do in those situations so that you won't use drugs. We will make a plan for dealing with different high-risk situations. A plan will give you something you can do to either not get into a high-risk situation, or give you something you can do if you get into the situation so that you don't use drugs. Bob, for you that might be using avoidance, staying away from your friend Fred, or using drug refusal skills to tell Fred that you don't want to use drugs with him anymore and that he should stop asking you to use. Right now, let's talk about some of the high-risk situations that people have been in lately and see what they have done or could do to cope in those situations without using drugs. Bob, have you been in a high-risk situation in the last week—one in which you found it really hard to be in without using drugs? (Also find out whether clients have successfulyl avoided a high risk situation).*

Note to Therapist: Review high-risk situations with each group member. The high-risk situation can be one that the client has been in recently or one that the client is likely to face in the near future. Make a plan for the high-risk situation using coping and refusal skills, then role-play the plan. If the plan is to use drug refusal skills, write the skills on the board and what the client will say for each one. If the plan is to use escape (i.e., the client is in an HRS and plans to leave immediately), write the steps on the board (eye contact, say no, give a reason, leave the situation) and what the client will say for each one.

If the client plans to use avoidance to cope with an HRS, work with the client to come up with a plan including what time he is likely to want to go to the bar or wherever the place may be, where else he can go instead of going to that high-risk place, how he can get to that low-risk place. Be very concrete. This will be the client's practice for how to avoid a high-risk situation. Another avoidance scenario is one in which the client is approached by someone else, and that person wants to get into a high-risk situation. For example, the client is asked by a friend to go to a particular bar. In this situation, you can use the refusal skills steps: (1) Make eye contact; (2) say no—state that you do not want to go there (e.g., go to the bar); (3) give a reason—"I used to use drugs there and I don't want to be around there anymore"; (4) suggest an alternative/leave—"Let's go to the cafeteria instead"/you will have to go to there without me.

No matter what skill the clients are practicing, write the steps on the board for each skill:

Refusal skills: Eye contact, state no, give reason, suggest alternative/leave.
Escape: Eye contact, state no, give reason, escape/leave immediately.
Avoidance: Eye contact, state no, give reason, suggest alternative/leave.

SKILLS SHEET: COPING WITH LAPSES

Goals

Group members will learn the meaning of relapse and lapse. Group members will review having a lapse as a high-risk situation and practice skills for coping with lapses.

Instructions to Therapists

1. **Conduct urinalysis before group and follow procedures in Urinalysis Contingency section.**
2. **Review goals and complete goal setting.**
3. **Brief review of last session.** *In our last group we talked about relapse prevention. Does anyone remember what relapse prevention is? That's right, it's planning ahead for high-risk situations so that you will know what to do if you find yourself in that situation. Last group we talked about different high-risk situations that many of you either were facing or might be facing in the near future. We talked about these high-risk situations and made plans for how to deal with them now. Why is it good to plan ahead and to have a plan for dealing with high-risk situations? That's right, it's good to have a plan just in case you find yourself in a high-risk situation so that you will know what to do to stay clean. Did anyone find themselves in one of the high-risk situations that we had planned for in our last meeting? How did it go and what did you do? (Or, did anyone find themselves in a high-risk situation in the past week? Did you have a plan for that situation? What did you do? How did it go?)*
4. **Today's session: Relapses and lapses.** *One of the things we know about giving up drugs is most people have a bad day sooner or later. They may think they have it licked and decide they can do just a little. Or, maybe they are having a bad day and lose self-control. Lots of people who give up drugs talk about how hard it is not to do drugs when they are feeling stressed out or depressed, and that these bad feelings lead them to want to use. Sometimes they just have a weak moment and forget why it is so important for them to stay clean. Lots of people tell us that peer pressure sometimes gets so bad that they have trouble saying no. Whatever the case, most people who are giving up drugs make a slip at one time or another and use. We call these times slips or lapses.*

The big problem with lapses is that they can become full-blown relapses or return to drug use. Sometimes lapses make people feel they have failed so they just give up and start using again. Or sometimes they feel they can control drug/alcohol use and continue to do a little but they gradually get caught up again. So a lapse is a high-risk situation because a little bit of drug use can quickly turn into a full-blown relapse.

The most important thing for you to remember is that a lapse does not have to become a relapse. You need to just get back to your hard work the next day. We have found that it is easier to keep a lapse from becoming a full-blown relapse if we talk about it in group and figure out what to do if a lapse happens. Remember that it would be great if you never had a lapse at all, and that is something to really work toward. But, in this group we always plan ahead so that if you find yourself in a high-risk situation you will know what to do. So, it's important to talk about lapses—we don't want it to happen but if it does, you will be prepared. So it's better when there is a plan— some sort of idea of what you could do if you experience a lapse. Why do you think it's better to have a plan? That's right—if you have a plan, you will already know what to do, and you will be able to quickly get back on track again instead of the lapse turning into a full-blown relapse. Many people who don't have a plan don't know what to do if they have a lapse, so they just throw in the towel and go back to using. That is very common when people are trying to change a really tough behavior like drug use. A person will have a lapse, feel really bad about it, and just say "I screwed up, I'm no good and I can't do this. I'm just going to forget about being clean and go use." Has that ever happened to anyone here—you had stopped using for a while, then had a lapse, and then said "Just forget it" and you went back to using? What we do in here is talk about what else you could do if a lapse happens instead of going back to using, so that you have a plan to get back to after the lapse occurs.

5. **Planning for lapses.** *OK, so let's figure out what each of us can do if we have a lapse. Right after the lapse occurs is the most difficult time to know what to do and a time that you are at very high risk to have a lapse become a full-blown relapse. There are three steps for you to use right after a relapse:*

Step 1: Stop! Keep calm! *A lapse is a warning signal that says that you are in danger of going back to using, similar to the way a warning light goes on in your car to indicate mechanical trouble. When you see the warning light in your car, you pull over to the side of the road to assess the situation. You can do the same thing with a lapse—it's the warning signal that is telling you to stop, leave, or escape the high-risk situation in which the lapse occurred, and look at and listen to what is happening. Go to a quiet, safe place. Most people who have a lapse feel really bad afterward, guilty, like they have failed. This reaction is normal and will pass with a little bit of time. You might feel bad for a while, but the bad feelings will pass if you let them. Remind yourself that the lapse was a one-time thing, a mistake, and one that you will learn from and plan for so that you will be able to cope with it next time. It is not a sign of failure—everyone makes mistakes.*

Step 2: Remember your hard work. *Often after a lapse people say, "What's the use, I've blown it already" and they go back to using. There is something you can do instead. Review all the reasons that you wanted to be clean in the first place—to feel better, to look better, to get along with people better, to get out of the dangerous drug lifestyle, or whatever it was that made you want to be clean. Think about how far you have come already and how much hard work you have put into getting and staying clean. You could say to yourself, "I have been working really hard and I have done a really good job getting clean and staying clean. I have made one mistake, but that's not worth giving up all the hard work that I have done!"*

Step 3: Implement a plan. *The more quickly you can get back on track after a lapse the better off you will be and the more likely that a lapse won't turn into a full-blown relapse. First, get rid of all drugs or alcohol that is around as well as any other triggers that are present. Second, escape the high-risk situation. Third, go do something else that will take up your time and that will get you involved in something other than drug use. For example, you can go to an AA/NA meeting, go to a group, go meet a friend who doesn't use drugs, or go for a walk.*

Step 4: Ask for help. *Other people can help you cope with a lapse so that it doesn't turn into a full-blown relapse. Talk to your therapist, your counselor, or doctor, to other group members, to family members, or anyone else who is helpful to you. There are also treatment and crisis centers that you can call in times of need. We have some listed on the handout.*

Note to Therapist: Write steps on the board and give group members handouts and wallet cards before explaining each step. Get group members' thoughts on each step: have they done such a thing before, would they add anything to that step.

6. **Making a lapse plan for each group member.** *Now we want to talk about high-risk situations that could involve a lapse and then plan for what to do if a lapse occurs. Who would like to start? How about you John? What's a high-risk situation for you that could lead to a lapse if you don't plan ahead?*

Note to Therapist: Give the client time to come up with a high-risk situation. If they have trouble thinking of one, present a situation to the client based on what you know about the person and his or her use, such as the following:

I know it's tough to think of one. You know, you always used to use with your ex-wife right? Let's imagine you run into her this Saturday night at a party, and she persuades you to smoke a joint, just like old times. You say no, you don't do that anymore, but she talks and talks and you finally give in and decide to just do one. The next day you're feeling really rotten for giving in and feel like all your hard work is down the drain. That's an example of a lapse. OK, let's apply the lapse steps to this situation. The first step is stop. What would you do?

Note to Therapist: Go through each step with the group member and write his or her plan on the board under each step. Be as concrete as possible. Incorporate role-plays where appropriate. Role-plays might be particularly useful for steps 4 (escaping the situation) and step 5 (asking for help). For example, if the group member is in a situation with other people and needs to leave the situation, the role-play can center on the group member telling the other people that he or she is not going to use drugs any more and needs to leave the situation. Write the escape steps on the board and then do the role-play.

No matter what skill they are practicing, write the steps on the board for each skill:

Refusal skills: Eye contact, state no, give reason, suggest alternative/leave.
Escape: Eye contact, state no, give reason, escape/leave immediately.
Avoidance: Eye contact, state no, give reason, suggest alternative/tell person they will have to do that without you.

SKILLS SHEET: OTHER SUBSTANCE USE AS A HIGH-RISK SITUATION

Goals

Group members will identify and discuss their use of other/secondary substances of abuse. Group members will learn that use of other drugs/alcohol is a high-risk situation for relapse to their primary drug of abuse. Group members will set goals for reducing/stopping other substance use and practice refusal, escape, and avoidance skills related to other drug use situation.

Instructions to Therapists

1. **Conduct urinalysis before group and follow procedures in Urinalysis Contingency section.**
2. **Review goals and complete goal setting.**
3. **Brief review of last session.** *In our last group we talked about lapses and what to do to cope with lapses when they occur. Does anyone remember what a lapse is? That's right, it's a slip—using drugs once in a specific situation. What is the important thing to watch out for if you have a slip? Right, a lapse can turn into a full-blown relapse. But, the important thing to remember is that it doesn't have to. A lapse is a high-risk situation, but if you know what to do ahead of time (if you plan ahead) then you can get back to your hard work and not have a lapse turn into a full-blown relapse. We have found that it's better when there is a plan—some sort of idea of what you could do if you experience a lapse. Why do you think it's better to have a plan? That's right—if you have a plan, you will already know what to do, and you will be able to quickly get back on track again instead of the lapse turning into a full-blown relapse. We also talked about steps for coping with lapses. Can anyone remember any of the steps that we discussed? (**Step 1:** Keep calm; **Step 2:** Implement a plan; **Step 3:** Ask for help). Did anyone have the opportunity to use these steps or give any more thought to them?*
4. **Today's session: Other substance use as a high-risk situation.** *As we have talked about before, the goal of the relapse prevention section of the group is to think about high-risk situations and plan ahead so if you get into such a situation, you will know what to do to cope with that situation and not have a full-blown relapse. Over the past couple of groups we have talked about lots of different high-risk situations and how to cope with lapses. Another high-risk situation that we are going to talk about today is using alcohol or other drugs besides the one that you have been working on in this group.*

Note to Therapist: Review for the group each group members' primary drug, or the drug that they have been working to cut down/stop using since the beginning of the group.

So many of you have been working on getting clean from cocaine, and some of you have been working to stop using heroin. However, we haven't talked a lot about other drugs that you might have been using while you have been cutting down from the cocaine or the heroin. For example, how many group members drink alcohol? How many days in the week do you drink? How much do you drink when you do drink? As another example, sometimes people continue to smoke marijuana even when they are clean from cocaine or heroin.

We want to spend our time talking today about the other drugs or alcohol that you might use, and practice applying the refusal, escape, and avoidance skills to alcohol or other drugs. That way, if you have been thinking about cutting down or stopping drinking or other drug use, or if you want to do so in the future, we will have practiced applying the skills that you have learned and you will have a plan and know what to do. Remember, we think it's best for you to have a plan—to plan ahead— so that if you are ever in a high-risk situation like drinking or using other drugs, you will know what to do.

First, we need to start by talking about why drinking or using drugs other than your primary drug is a high-risk situation at all. Sometimes people think that as long as they are not using cocaine it doesn't matter if they drink or smoke pot. Why do you think that drinking alcohol or using another drug is a high-risk situation? Does anyone have an idea why drinking or using other drugs can put you at risk for relapsing to cocaine or heroin? There are a couple of ways that using alcohol or other drugs can be a high-risk situation for relapse to cocaine/heroin. Let's talk about the first way. Many of you have talked about how when you did cocaine you always drank too. So many times you did the two together—drinking and doing cocaine or drinking and doing heroin.

Interestingly, other people who use drugs say the same thing—lots of times they did several drugs or drugs and alcohol together. When you do two things together over and over again, they become linked together. Drinking or other drug use can be a trigger for cocaine use. Who remembers what a trigger is? That's right—a trigger is a person, place, thing, situation, or feeling that automatically makes you want to use. A trigger can be a person you used to use with, a street corner where you used to use, the smell of the drug being prepared to use, or anything that you associate with drug use. A trigger makes you crave drugs automatically—you don't even have to think about it for it to happen.

Drinking or using other drugs can be a trigger for cocaine/heroin use. That means that you have done the two together so many times that when you do one (for example drinking), you automatically want to do the other (for example, you will crave cocaine). We know that using anything can lead to a relapse to cocaine/heroin use.

There is a second way that alcohol or other drug use can be a high-risk situation. Can anyone think of another way that alcohol or other drug use can be a high-risk situation for relapse to cocaine/heroin? It has to do with how drinking and other drug use affects you and your brain. Alcohol and other drugs, like cocaine/heroin, affect your brain and your ability to think and make good decisions. Part of the reason that people like to drink is because it lowers their inhibitions, they have a good time, they do things that they wouldn't normally do when they were sober. In terms of relapse, this is a problem. When we drink or use other drugs, we don't think as clearly and we don't make as good decisions as we would if we were sober. What that means is that drinking or other drug use can lead to us not thinking clearly, and not making a good decision about using cocaine or heroin and so put us at risk for using cocaine/heroin. For example, suppose you have been drinking for a while and you feel drunk. Someone comes around and tells you they have some really good stuff and wants you to use with them. When you are drunk it's going to be much harder to use the refusal, escape, and avoidance skills you know and it's going to be much harder to tell people that you don't want to use cocaine/heroin.

Drinking and using other drugs is a high-risk situation in another way. Situations in which people are drinking and using some drugs are more likely to be situations in which cocaine or heroin is around and people are using. So just being around a lot of people who are drinking could potentially put you in a situation in which people are using cocaine/heroin too.

5. Set a goal to cut down or stop drinking or other drug use.

Note to Therapists: Repeat this information for all members who are drinking or using other drugs and have made progress in cutting down or stopping cocaine or heroin use.

Since drinking and other drug use can put you at high risk to use cocaine and heroin, we want you to think about cutting down or stopping any drinking or other drug use that you do. Remember that in this group we don't require that you do anything with regards to your drinking or other drug use, but we do think it's important for you to learn skills to use to reduce your drinking and other drug use. That way when the time is right for you and you are ready to cut down or stop drinking or other drug use, you will have had some practice using refusal, escape, and avoidance skills in drinking and other drug use situations. Would anyone like to set a goal to cut down drinking or other drug use this week? Bob, how about you? You have been clean from cocaine for a few months now, which is great, and you have been working very hard to stay clean from cocaine. You said that you have been drinking a few times per week and that when you drink you think about using cocaine. What kind of goal could you make with regards to your drinking that you think would help you to stay clean from cocaine over the next week? That's a good one—cutting out a day of drinking this week. How many days per week do you usually drink? OK, so if you usually drink five days per week, how about if this week you cut out one drinking day? Which day would you like to cut out? What else will you do? What will you do if you really feel like drinking?

Note to Therapists: Continue in this way for all group members who are drinking or using other drugs and who are willing to set some sort of goal with regards to those substances. The goal does not have to be that the group member totally stops using. If the group member is using a secondary drug quite frequently and he or she suggests stopping totally, consider whether the group member can do that successfully or if the goal should be scaled back to drinking/using on fewer days in the last week, or staying clean from everything for just the next week to try out being totally clean—a term for this can be sampling, being totally clean from all alcohol and drugs for one week to see how it would go.

6. **Practice skills to refuse, escape, and avoid drinking/other drug use.** *Now we want to practice applying the refusal, escape, and avoidance skills that you have learned and used in this group to drinking or other drug use situations. Who would like to start? OK Bob, the drug that you have been working on in here is cocaine. You have done a great job staying clean from cocaine for 10 weeks now. We have been talking today about how drinking or using drugs other than cocaine can be a high-risk situation for you to relapse to cocaine use. Can you think of a situation that you have been in recently in which other people were drinking or using other drugs? What happened in that situation? Did you drink or use other drugs? Was that a high-risk situation for cocaine use for you?*

Note to Therapists: Review a drinking/other drug use situation with each group member. The situation can be one that the client has been in recently or one that the client is likely to be in, in the near future. The situation should involve either the group member drinking or using other drugs or being in a situation in which he or she was offered or pressured to drink/use other drugs, or in which the person would have a hard time not drinking/using other drugs. Make a plan for the situation using refusal, escape, and avoidance skills, then do role-plays to practice. If the plan is to use drug refusal skills, write the skills on the board and what the client will say for each one. If the plan is to use escape (i.e., the client is offered alcohol and plans to leave immediately), write the steps on the board (eye contact, say no, give a reason, leave the situation) and what the client will say for each one.

If the client plans to use avoidance to cope with a drinking/other drug use situation, work with the client to come up with a plan including what time he is likely to want to drink/use other drugs, what he can do instead, where else he or she can go except to the bar, how he or she can get to that place. Be very concrete. This will be the client's practice for how to avoid drinking/other drug use situation. Another avoidance scenario is one in which the client is approached by someone else, and that person wants to go into a drinking/other drug use situation. For example, the client is asked by a friend to go to a bar/party. In this situation, you can use the refusal skills steps: (1) Make eye contact; (2) say no, state that you do not want to go there (e.g., go to the bar); (3) give a reason ("I'm trying to stay clean from cocaine and drinking makes me want to use cocaine, I don't do that any more"); (4) suggest an alternative/leave—"Let's go to the cafeteria instead"/"You will have to go to there without me."

No matter what skill they are practicing, write the steps on the board for each skill:

Refusal skills: Eye contact, state no, give reason, suggest alternative/leave.
Escape: Eye contact, state no, give reason, escape/leave immediately.
Avoidance: Eye contact, state no, give reason, suggest alternative/leave.

SKILLS SHEET: COPING WITH BOREDOM

Goals

Group members will understand why feeling bored is a high-risk situation. Group members will list activities to do when they feel bored and practice coping with boredom in role-plays.

Instructions to Therapist

1. **Conduct urinalysis before group and follow procedures in Urinalysis Contingency section.**
2. **Review goals and complete goal setting.**
3. **Brief review of last session.** *In our last group we talked about drinking or using other drugs as a high-risk situation for relapse to cocaine/heroin use. Does anyone remember the ways that drinking/other drug use is a high-risk situation? There are three ways: Drinking and other drug use can be a trigger for craving cocaine/heroin because the two things have been done together so many times in the past. Or, drinking/other drug use can be a high-risk situation because they cloud our judgment and cause us not to think clearly and to make bad decisions. Finally, drinking and other drug use can be a high-risk situation because if alcohol or other drugs are around, it's more likely that someone in that situation is using cocaine or heroin and they might offer you some. Did anyone have a situation this week in which they found drinking or other drug use, either by themselves or by someone else, to be a high-risk situation?*
4. **Today's session: Why boredom is a high-risk situation.** *We have talked a lot about the high-risk situations and triggers that lead people to use drugs. One important trigger that often is involved when people use drugs is feeling bored. Lots of times people use drugs just because they are bored and they can't think of anything else to do. Has this ever happened to anyone here—you used drugs because you were bored and couldn't think of anything else to do? Tell me about that.*

This is especially important for people who use drugs and alcohol and also have schizophrenia. Lots of times people with schizophrenia don't have things to do during the day and they find themselves at home with nothing to do. We know that sitting at home with nothing to do can get boring, and sometimes people with schizophrenia use drugs because they have nothing to do and are bored. However, when you are trying to stop using drugs, it's important to figure out what to do when you feel bored, instead of using drugs. Today we want to talk about what you can do when you are feeling bored so that you won't use drugs.

5. **When do you feel bored? What can you do when you are feeling bored?** *First we need to talk about when we are likely to get bored. Who would like to start? OK Bob, what is it like for you when you get bored? What time of day do you usually get bored? Why is that time of day boring for you?*

Note to Therapist: Have group members discuss when they are likely to get bored, where they are when it happens, what time of day, what they usually do, does it work, and so on. Have all group members participate in the discussion so that therapists get an idea of what being bored is like for each group member.

Now we need to figure out what we can do when we feel bored. We have to think of what we can do when we feel bored that will help us not feel bored any more. Let's think of things that we like to do with our time that don't involve using drugs or alcohol. Why is this important? It's important because if we don't want to use drugs or alcohol when we are bored, we have to come up with something else that we like to do. However, sometimes it's hard to think of things to do that don't involve drugs.

What do you like to do that doesn't involve using drugs or alcohol? We have created a list of things that lots of people like to do (Read over list). You see that some of these things you can do alone and some activities involve other people. What other things should we add to the list?

It's great that you all could come up with so many other things to do when you feel bored besides using drugs or alcohol. The next thing to do is to pick one of the activities on the list and try it out. Once you have thought of some things that you can do, you need to pick one and do it. It's important to make sure that it's something that you can do at that moment. For example, if you are feeling bored and you think of some things that you like to do and one of them involves going to your friend Bob's house but you know that Bob is not at home, that would not be a good activity to pick because you can't do it at that moment. If you like to walk in the park but it's a rainy day and not very nice for a walk, then you can't do that right at that moment. It's important to pick an activity that you can do right then while you are bored and not leave yourself any time to start using drugs or alcohol.

The last thing to do is to either keep doing the activity or pick another activity to do until you are no longer bored. Sometimes we pick something to do and we find that we are really enjoying it and that we are no longer bored. If that is the case, that's great! You have successfully coped with feeling bored, without using drugs or alcohol. However, it might happen that you pick an activity to do and you find that you are not really enjoying it and that you are still bored. In that case, you need to pick another activity to do that you will enjoy so that you won't feel bored and be at risk for using drugs and alcohol.

6. **Practice coping with boredom.** *Let's do some role-plays now to practice these steps in coping with boredom. Suppose we show you how by using a role-play first so you can see how the steps go* (coleaders role-play with each other then with each group member). *How about if we say that I am in my home with my friend and we are sitting around feeling bored* (therapists also might role-play a situation in which the client is at home alone and bored and needs to cope with boredom on his or her own).

Scenes to use in the role-play

- Sitting at home with a friend and not doing anything.
- Sitting at home alone feeling bored.
- At home alone and the plans that you had with a friend fell through.

SKILLS SHEET: COPING WITH DEPRESSION AND STRESS

Goals

Group members will understand that depression and stress are high-risk situations that can lead to relapse. Therapists will teach alternative strategies for coping with depression and stress. The group will include a discussion of depression and stress and what these experiences are like for group members. Group members will list strategies for coping with depression and stress and practice via role-plays.

Instructions to Therapists

1. **Conduct urinalysis before group and follow procedures in Urinalysis Contingency section.**
2. **Review goals and complete goal setting.**
3. **Brief review of last session.** *Last group we talked about being bored as a high-risk situation. Does anyone remember why being bored is a high-risk situation? Lots of times people use drugs just because they are bored and they can't think of anything else to do. When you are trying to stop using drugs, it's important to figure out what to do when you feel bored, instead of using drugs. Last group we talked about several things that you could do when you felt bored. Does anyone remember what some of those things were?*
4. **Today's session: Feeling depressed and stressed as high-risk situations.** *As we have discussed before, the goal of the relapse prevention section of the group is to think about high-risk situations and plan ahead so if you get into such a situation, you will know what to do to cope with the situation and not have a full-blown relapse. Over the past couple of groups we have talked about lots of different high-risk situations including coping with lapses and staying away from drinking or other drug use. Remember that lapses and drinking/other drug use are both high-risk situations for someone to have a full-blown relapse to cocaine/heroin. Today we want to talk to you about another high-risk situation that can lead to relapse—feeling depressed or stressed. How many of you here have ever felt really depressed or stressed or bad or upset? Has that ever led any of you to relapse to drug use? Bob, you have told us before that you get depressed? Do you find you use more or relapse when you are depressed?*

Note to Therapist: At this point, the therapist should engage group members in a discussion of how their use changes when they are depressed, stressed, or experiencing other negative affect, and whether they have experienced that they use more or relapse when they feel bad. Keep in mind that this is not meant to be verbal psychotherapy or an in-depth discussion of what depression or stress feels like for group members. Do not ask clients how they feel when they are depressed/stressed, what being depressed/stressed is like for them. What therapists should do is explore with group members the connection between negative affect and continued use/greater use/relapse to use so that they understand that depression/stress/negative affect is a high-risk situation: stay behavioral. Explore how depression/stress/negative affect is linked to greater use or relapse.

Examples

The client feels bad, stops going to treatment, uses cocaine to feel better and be able to get up and out of bed in the morning.

The client has a fight with a family member, feels stressed out, doesn't know what to do or say to the family members, so goes and gets high.

The client is having a problem of some sort that he or she doesn't know how to solve and feels upset by it so gets high.

Make notes on the board/flip chart as needed so that clients can see the pattern that feeling depressed/stressed/other negative affect is a high-risk situation that can lead to relapse.

We know that these sorts of experiences are common for lots of people who are trying to give up drug use. In surveys of people who have relapsed, the number one reason that people give for relapsing to drug and alcohol use is because they are depressed, stressed, angry, or upset. In other words, negative feelings very often lead people to relapse. So, feeling depressed or stressed or bad is a high-risk situation that we need to discuss and plan for. Remember that when we plan ahead, then we are better prepared for the high-risk situation—in this case negative feelings like depression or stress—when it happens.

5. **Coping with depression/stress/negative affect.** *Now you might be thinking: What else can I do when I'm depressed/stressed? I use drugs or drink because it helps when I feel bad. So what am I supposed to do to feel better? Let's talk now about what else you can do to feel better so that you don't use drugs or drink when you feel depressed or stressed. There are lots of things that people do to feel better that don't involve drug use. The hard part is finding what's right for you. What we want to do now is get a big list of things together that might help, and then you have to try them out and see what works for you.*

(a) Increasing pleasant activities. *One thing that we have found helps people when they feel bad is to do something pleasant or something that they like to do. Research shows that when people do things they feel better. They may not have all of their problems solved, but just doing something and getting up and out and active can improve your mood. Has anyone ever found that just doing something, anything, pleasant makes them feel better than doing nothing at all? Bob, tell me something about that.*

Now, doing something pleasant can be tough when you are feeling bad. For example, one thing that happens when people get really depressed is that they stay home in bed and stop doing things. What we have learned from working with other clients is that if you get involved in something pleasant, it may keep you from getting really depressed. The time to get up and do something pleasant is right when you notice you are feeling a little stressed or down—that way you don't wait until you are too upset/depressed to do anything at all.

So what can you do that's pleasant? Let's come up with a list. We need to name as many things as we can think of that are pleasant or can get your mind off feeling bad and might help you to feel better. Think of the things that you do when you are upset in order to feel better. Bob, can you start us off? What's one thing that you do that you find pleasant?

Note to Therapist: Generate a long list and get input from all group members. See handout to get started if clients are having trouble coming up with items for the list.

(b) Talk to someone. *Another thing that we have found that helps people when they are feeling depressed/ stressed/bad is to talk to someone about how they are feeling. Lots of times when we are upset we keep it to ourselves. Does anyone here do that—keep their feelings inside? Tell me a little about that. Does keeping things inside help you to feel better? What we have learned from other clients is that not talking about what's bothering you doesn't help you feel better. In fact, it usually makes you feel worse. Instead of keeping things all bottled up inside so that you feel worse, you can talk to someone about it and at least get it out there in the open. To do this, you have to think of someone who will listen to you. Sometimes that is a family member or a friend or a counselor or a therapist. Think now about who you could talk to when you feel bad? "Bob, who do you talk to when you feel bad?"*

Note to Therapist: Therapist should discuss this with all group members and figure out a person for each group member. Suggest counselor/therapist as often as possible, even for people who name a friend or a family member that they could talk to when they feel bad. Keep a list.

(c) Get help/Solve the problem. *Lots of times people get depressed/stressed/feel bad when they have a problem and they don't know what to do to solve it. Has that ever happened to anyone here? That's a good example Bob—you had a housing problem and you didn't know what to do and it made you really depressed. One thing that we know can help is to get help to solve the problem. That often will help people find a solution to a problem so that they don't have to feel really depressed/stressed/bad about it. Can anyone here tell us about a time that he or she had a problem and got some help to solve the problem and felt much better about it?*

Therapists should get examples from group members. Problems to ask about can be related to money (SSI checks, bills), housing, medication (running out of medication), family problems, and so on. Pull for examples of when group members got help with a problem and got it solved so that they didn't have to spend a lot of time feeling depressed/stressed/bad about it.

(d) Talk to your psychiatrist about medication. *These days there are lots of medications that help people with feelings of depression or when people feel stressed out. One thing that you can do when you are depressed/stressed out is to talk to your psychiatrist to see if any of these medications might be right for you. Only your psychiatrist can help you with this, so that's the person to talk to. Does everyone here have a psychiatrist that he or she sees for medication? Let's review how you might talk to your psychiatrist about this. First you would need to make the appointment. Second you would need to go to the appointment and tell the doctor that you are feeling depressed or stressed out. Third, you would need to ask the doctor if there are any medications that he or she thinks might help you feel less depressed or stressed out. Let's go around the room and practice.*

Note to Therapist: Therapists should go around the room and have clients discuss who their doctor is and how they would go about making an appointment. Then each client should do at least one role-play in which he or she uses the above steps to ask the doctor if there is a medication that would help the group member feel less depressed/stressed out.

(e) Plan ahead/Practice strategies (i.e., asking for help/problem solving). *Remember, we think it's best for you to have a plan, to plan ahead, so that if you are ever in a high-risk situation you will know what to do. So now we need to make a plan for each of you to follow when you are feeling depressed/stressed/bad. That way when you are in that situation, you will have a plan and know something that you can do so that you do not relapse. Who would like to start?*

Note to Therapist: If possible, find out what the high-risk negative affect is for a group member (i.e., what do they call it—being depressed, stressed out, upset, bad, etc.). You want to use their words. At this point in the group you might know from what a client has already said. If not, just use the term *feeling depressed or stressed*. We *do not* want a big discussion of what types of feelings the client has. Rather, we want to help the client make a plan for when he or she is feeling depressed/stressed/bad. Talk with each group member about what that person could do if he or she were feeling that way, using the three strategies discussed in group: doing a pleasant activity, talking to someone, getting help to solve the problem. Give examples for each category. For example, if Bob often feels stressed out, list some pleasant activities that he could do, a person that he could talk to, and how he could get help to solve a problem (who he would go to for help with different sorts of problems, or how to solve one specific problem that affects him repeatedly such as medication side effects, problems getting to treatment appointments, arguments with family members, etc.). Get input from other group members. For example:

Bob, you have said that you get stressed out and upset and lots of times it's because of arguments that you have with your sister. Let's make a plan for you for the next time you are stressed out or upset. First, you can do some pleasant activities. We made a list with input from everyone in group. Which things on the list do you think you could do when you are stressed out or upset that you think you would find pleasant? Great—taking a walk, going to a meeting, and listening to music are all really good ideas and things that you can do when you are feeling really stressed or upset that might help you to feel better. OK, what's the second thing we said people can do when they are stressed out or upset? Sue, can you remember? Right, they can talk to someone. Why is that a good thing to do Fred? Right, keeping negative feelings bottled up inside you doesn't help them go away and lots of times talking about them makes you feel better. So Bob, who could you talk to when you are feeling stressed out or upset when you have arguments with your sister? Can you think of anyone you could talk to? Can anyone think of someone that Bob could talk to in that situation? That's a great idea Fred—Bob could talk to his counselor. I also remember you saying you had an NA sponsor. Maybe you could talk to that person when you are stressed out or upset from an argument with your sister. What do you think? OK, can anyone remember the third part of the plan for dealing with being stressed out or upset? That's right Sue, get help to solve the problem that's making you upset in the first place. So Bob, you said that you get stressed out and upset most when you have arguments with your sister. Sounds like you need someone to help you talk to your sister sometimes. Who could help you with that? I think your counselor is a great idea. Maybe you could talk to your counselor and he or she could give you ideas for how to talk to your sister. Maybe you could even bring your sister to an appointment with your counselor so you could talk to her with your counselor there.

Note to Therapist: If the client reports getting depressed/stressed out due to someone asking them to use drugs or wanting them to do drugs with them, review refusal, escape, and avoidance skills and do a role-play of person using these skills in that situation. Write the steps on the board for each skill:

Refusal skills: Eye contact, state no, give reason, suggest alternative/leave
Escape: Eye contact, state no, give reason, escape/leave immediately
Avoidance: Eye contact, state no, give reason, suggest alternative/leave

SKILLS SHEET: COPING WITH SYMPTOMS OF SPMI/MEDICATION SIDE EFFECTS I—OVERVIEW AND TALKING TO YOUR DOCTOR

Goals

Group members will understand that having symptoms and side effects are high-risk situations that can lead to relapse. Therapists will teach alternative strategies for coping with symptoms and side effects. Discuss symptoms and side effects and what they are like for group members. **Group members will** list strategies for coping with symptoms and side effects and practice via role-plays when appropriate.

Instructions to Therapists

1. **Conduct urinalysis before group and follow procedures in Urinalysis Contingency section.**
2. **Review goals and complete goal setting.**
3. **Brief review of last session.** *Last group we talked about feeling depressed or stressed as a high-risk situation. Does anyone remember how feeling depressed/stressed out/bad can be a high-risk situation? That's right—people feel really bad or depressed and just wind up using to feel better or because they don't know what else to do. We know that these sorts of experiences are common for lots of people who are trying to give up drug use. We talked about planning ahead and made plans that involved doing pleasant activities, talking to someone, and getting help in solving the problem when you are feeling depressed/stressed out/bad. Did anyone use their plans this week to cope with feeling depressed/stressed out/bad?*
4. **Today's session: Symptoms of mental illness/schizophrenia and medication side effects as high-risk situations.** *As we have discussed before, the goal of the relapse prevention section of the group is to think about high-risk situations and plan ahead, so if you get into such a situation, you will know what to do to cope with the situation and not have a full-blown relapse. Over the past couple of groups we have talked about lots of different high-risk situations including coping with lapses, staying away from drinking or other drug use, and coping with feeling depressed/stressed out. Remember that these are all high-risk situations for someone to have a full-blown relapse to cocaine/heroin.*

Today we want to talk to you about two more high-risk situations that can lead to relapse: having symptoms of schizophrenia or other mental illness and medication side effects. Why do you think that symptoms of mental illness and medication side effects are high-risk situations for relapse to cocaine/heroin? What symptoms do you have that lead you to use drugs/alcohol? What side effects do you try to cope with by drinking or using drugs? How many of you here have ever had symptoms of your mental illness or medication side effects and used drugs or alcohol in order to try to make the symptoms/side effects go away or not be as bad? We have learned through our work with clients with severe mental illness that they will often use drugs or alcohol to cope with symptoms of mental illness, such as delusions, hearing voices, hallucinations, or feeling manic. Others tell us that they use drugs to cope with medication side effects such as fatigue and agitation. Can someone here tell us a bit about what's that's like for them?

Note to Therapist: Many clients will have heard of the concept of self-medication. Therapists should distinguish whether the person is telling you that they are self-medicating to decrease *symptoms* of their illness or to decrease *side effects* of a medication taken for their illness. The therapist needs to explain briefly why side effects occur. The objective here is to teach members that there are *options* other than self-medicating.

Drugs and alcohol can have some effect on symptoms and side effects. For example, Bob, you said that you use cocaine to make you feel better when your medication gives you side effects. You're right. Cocaine can take away your side effects because of the way it affects your nerve cells. Remember a few weeks ago we talked about your brain and a brain chemical called dopamine. What happens is that when you take medicine for schizophrenia, it affects a chemical in your brain called dopamine. Dopamine acts in different parts of your brain to help control thinking and movement. Sometimes, medicine that helps you think more clearly also interferes with the part of your brain that controls movements. That's what causes side effects like feeling jittery, restless, shaky, or stiff. Cocaine affects the dopamine in your brain and sometimes has an impact on these side effects.

However, there are many problems with using cocaine or other drugs to help cope with SMI symptoms and medication side effects. There is a difference between using drugs and alcohol to cope with symptoms and side effects and using the correct medication to help with those problems. Can anyone think of a problem with using drugs and alcohol to cope with symptoms and side effects? Well, one problem is that drugs and alcohol are not always effective in decreasing symptoms or medication side effects. Interestingly, clients also tell us that using drugs or alcohol is not always helpful when they are using it to cope with their symptoms of mental illness or with medication side effects. Lots of clients have told us that drug and alcohol use actually makes their symptoms and side effects worse—they have worse hallucinations or get more paranoid or more depressed when they use drugs or right after they use. Have any of you had that experience of using drugs or alcohol to cope with symptoms of mental illness or medication side effects and then finding that it's not really helpful after all?

Note to Therapist: Therapists should get client input throughout this discussion and ask clients for additional reasons why it is problematic using drugs or alcohol to cope with symptoms and side effects.

5. **Coping with symptoms of SPMI.** *The important point to keep in mind is that there are things that you can do to cope with symptoms of mental illness and medication side effects instead of using alcohol and drugs. There are things that you can do to cope with symptoms and side effects that will be a lot more effective than using drugs or alcohol.*

(a) Talk to your doctor. *When you have increased symptoms or side effects, the first person to talk to is your doctor. This is such an important thing for you to do that we are going to spend the rest of this group practicing ways to talk to your doctor about symptoms and side effects. The reason is that when you have symptoms or side effects, you might need your medication increased or changed. Such a change might help you feel better and relieve your symptoms. In addition, your doctor can give you medication to help lessen these symptoms and that work more effectively and reliably than cocaine does. Sometimes the doctor will give you medicine such as Cogentin or Benadryl.*

One thing that clients have told us is that it's hard to talk to their doctor and tell him or her about symptoms or side effects. Has anyone here ever found that to be hard? Why was it hard for you to talk to your doctor about symptoms and side effects? We have some steps here for talking to your doctor or counselor about symptoms and side effects. Let's go over these now:

Make eye contact and be firm. Why is this important? So the doctor/counselor knows that you are serious and that you have something important to discuss with him and her.

Tell your doctor that you are having more symptoms or medication side effects. Why is this important? Lots of times your doctor has a lot of questions for you when you come in to see him or her. By telling the doctor up front that you are having more symptoms or medication side effects, you make sure that the doctor knows that this is an issue that you need to discuss with him or her right away during that appointment, that it's not something that can wait.

Tell your doctor what the symptoms or side effects are. This is important so that the doctor knows what is happening with you. If you can't tell him or her what is going on, they will not be able to figure out how to help you. Sometimes it might be helpful to write a list of the symptoms or side effects that are bothering you so that you don't have to remember everything. That way you can just give the list right to the doctor and you won't have to worry about forgetting something important.

Ask your doctor if he or she can change your medication or give you something that will help these symptoms/side effects.

Note to Therapist: Therapists should role-play talking to the doctor about symptoms and side effects with all clients. In setting up the role-plays, therapists should ask group members for specific descriptions about the symptoms and side effects that bother them and build this information into the role-plays. The therapists should find out the name of the group member's doctor and use that name in the role-plays.

SKILLS SHEET: COPING WITH SYMPTOMS OF SPMI/MEDICATION SIDE EFFECTS II— DISTRACTION, ALTERNATIVE WAYS TO COPE, AND TALKING TO SOMEONE

Goals

Group members will understand that having symptoms and side effects are high-risk situations that can lead to relapse. Therapists will teach alternative strategies for coping with symptoms and side effects. **The group will r**eview symptoms and side effects and what they are like for group members. Group members will practice strategies for coping with symptoms and side effects via role-plays when appropriate.

Instructions to Therapists

1. **Conduct urinalysis before group and follow procedures in Urinalysis Contingency section.**
2. **Review goals and complete goal setting.**
3. **Brief review of last session.** *In our last group we talked about having symptoms of schizophrenia or other mental illness and medication side effects as possible high-risk situations. Can anyone remember why symptoms of mental illness and medication side effects are high-risk situations for relapse to cocaine/heroin? That's right: clients with severe mental illness will often use drugs or alcohol to cope with symptoms of mental illness, such as delusions, hearing voices, hallucinations, or feeling manic. Others tell us that they use drugs to cope with medication side effects such as fatigue and agitation. Can anyone remember the problem with using alcohol or drugs to cope with symptoms or side effects? Yes: drugs and alcohol are not always effective in decreasing symptoms or medication side effects. Lots of times drug and alcohol use actually makes symptoms and side effects worse—they make hallucinations worse or people get more paranoid or more depressed when they use drugs or right after they use. We then practiced talking to the doctor as an important way to cope with symptoms and side effects. Did anyone talk to their doctor in the past week in order to keep from using drugs or alcohol to cope with symptoms or side effects?*
4. **Today's session: Coping with symptoms of SPMI.** *Talking to your doctor is a very important thing to do when you are experiencing symptoms or side effects. There are also other things that you can do to cope with symptoms of mental illness and medication side effects instead of using alcohol and drugs. There are things that you can do to cope with symptoms and side effects that will be a lot more effective than using drugs or alcohol.*

(a) Distraction. *Distraction can be helpful when you are experiencing voices or hearing things that others can't hear. Sometimes voices are really strong or get worse and it's hard to know what to do. One thing that some clients find helpful is distraction—paying attention to something else rather than the voices. Research with clients with mental illness has found that when people pay attention to something else rather than the voices, sometimes the voices decrease a bit or don't make you feel as bad. There are several strategies that have been tried to help people distract themselves from voices: listening to music through headphones, reading out loud, listening to something on the radio, and listening to a book on tape. Can anyone here think of any other ways that someone could distract him- or herself when they are hearing voices? Has anyone here heard voices and found something helpful in terms of distracting them from the voices?*

Note to Therapist: Generate a list of ways to distract clients and get input from all group members. See handout to get started if clients are having trouble coming up with items for the list.

(b) Alternative ways to cope. *Sometimes people need something to do to cope with symptoms and side effects before they get to talk to their doctor. There is evidence that there are simple things that people can do to help themselves feel a bit better while they are waiting to see their doctor. I'll bet there are things that* *all of you have tried when you are experiencing symptoms or side effects that have helped you feel better at some point in your lives. Can anyone tell me something that he or she did to feel better when experiencing symptoms, which actually helped the person feel better? From our own and other people's work with clients with mental illness, we have found that several things can help when someone is experiencing symptoms or side effects:*

> ***Increase activity levels:*** *Do something, anything!*
> ***Initiate social interaction:*** *Call someone, don't isolate.*
> ***Modify physiological state:*** *Breathing and relaxing.*

(c) Talk to someone. *Another thing that we have found helps people when they are experiencing symptoms or side effects is to talk to someone about what's going on with them. Lots of times when something serious like symptoms/side effects is happening we don't tell anyone about it. Does anyone here do that—keep that stuff inside and not tell anyone? Does keeping things inside help you to feel better? What we have learned from other clients is that not talking about what's bothering you doesn't help you feel better. In fact, it usually makes you feel worse. Instead of keeping things all bottled up inside so that you feel worse, you can talk to someone about it and at least get it out there in the open. To do this, you have to think of someone who you think will listen. Sometimes that person is a family member or a friend or a counselor or a therapist. Think now about who you could talk to when you feel bad? Bob, who do you talk to when you feel bad?*

Note to Therapist: The therapist should discuss this with all group members and figure out a person that each group member could go to, when they are experiencing increased symptoms or side effects, who might be able to help them and would encourage them to talk to their doctor about the problem. Suggest a counselor/therapist as often as possible, even for people who name a friend or a family member that they could talk to. Keep a list of each group person's "go-to" contact.

6. **Plan ahead/practice strategies (e.g., asking for help/problem solving).** *Remember, we think it's best for you to have a plan, to plan ahead, so that if you are ever in a high-risk situation you will know what to do. So now we need to make a plan for each of you to follow when you are having symptoms or medication side effects. That way when you are in that situation, you will have a plan, and know something that you can do so that you do not relapse. Who would like to start?*

Note to Therapist: If possible, find out which is more common for each client—using to cope with symptoms or using to cope with side effects. At this point in the group you might know this from what a client has already explained his or her problem, but *get specific*—what specific symptoms and side effects do the group members experience? Talk with each group member about what the person could do if he or she were feeling that way, using the three strategies discussed in group: talking to the doctor, distraction, talking to a family member, or therapist/counselor. Give examples for each category. For example, if Bob often feels fatigue from his medication and he used cocaine to feel more up and awake, discuss how Bob could talk to his doctor about this side effect, alternative ways to cope, and talking to someone about it. Get input from other group members. **Important:** Put great emphasis on talking to the doctor and role-play talking to the doctor with each group member.

For example: *Bob, you have said that you hear voices and that sometimes they get worse. You have said that you used cocaine to deal with hearing the voices—when you used cocaine, the voices didn't bother you, probably because you were so distracted from using drugs that you didn't think about the voices anymore. Let's make a plan for you for the next time you hear voices so that you have something else to do instead of using cocaine. First, you can talk to your doctor. Let's role-play that right now.* (Give client a handout and set up and complete a role-play).

Note to Therapist: Do role-plays of talking to their doctor with all clients. Therapists can do a role-play first to model how the steps go. Then role-play with each client.

Those were great role-plays about talking to the doctor about symptoms and side effects. OK, what's another thing we said people can do when they experience symptoms or side effects. Sue, can you remember? Right, they can use distraction or get involved in an activity to get their attention focused on something else. Why is that a good thing to do Fred? Right: getting your attention focused on something else means you are paying less attention to your symptoms. People with mental illness have said that this is often helpful in making them feel a bit better when they are experiencing symptoms or side effects. So Bob, what could you do to get your mind on something else when you are experiencing symptoms or side effects?

We also discussed talking to someone as something that might help when a person is experiencing symptoms or side effects. Bob, who could you talk to in that situation? Can anyone think of someone that Bob could talk to in that situation? That's a great idea Fred: Bob could talk to his counselor. I also remember you saying you had an NA sponsor—maybe you could talk to that person when you are experiencing symptoms or side effects. Another good place to bring that up is in a treatment group like this one.

Note to Therapist: If the client reports experiencing symptoms due to someone asking them to use drugs or wanting them to do drugs, review refusal, escape, and avoidance skills and do a role-play with the person using these skills in that situation. Write the steps on the board for each skill:

Refusal skills: Eye contact, state no, give reason, suggest alternative/leave.
Escape: Eye contact, state no, give reason, escape/leave immediately.
Avoidance: Eye contact, state no, give reason, suggest alternative/leave.

SKILLS SHEET: COPING WITH LOW MOTIVATION

Goals

Group members will understand that motivation to reduce or stop drug use waxes and wanes over time and that low motivation is a high-risk situation that can lead to relapse. Therapists will teach strategies for coping with low motivation. The group will discuss motivation, how it waxes and wanes, and what this is like for group members. Group members will list strategies for coping with low motivation and practice via role-plays when appropriate.

Instructions to Therapists

1. **Conduct urinalysis before group and follow procedures in Urinalysis Contingency section.**
2. **Review goals and complete goal setting.**
3. **Brief review of last session.** *For the last few groups we have talked about having symptoms of schizophrenia or other mental illness and medication side effects as possible high-risk situations. Can anyone remember why symptoms of mental illness and medication side effects are high-risk situations for relapse to cocaine/heroin? That's right: Clients with severe mental illness will often use drugs or alcohol to cope with symptoms of mental illness, such as delusions, hearing voices, hallucinations, or feeling manic. Others tell us that they use drugs to cope with medication side effects such as fatigue and agitation. Can anyone remember the problem with using alcohol or drugs to cope with symptoms or side effects? Yes: drugs and alcohol are not always effective in decreasing symptoms or medication side effects. Lots of times drug and alcohol use actually makes symptoms and side effects worse—they make hallucinations worse or people get more paranoid or more depressed when they use drugs or right after they use. We have also talked about other ways to cope with symptoms and side effects, including talking to your doctor, distraction and getting involved in other activities, and talking to someone about it like your counselor. Did anyone use any of these skills this week to keep from using drugs or alcohol to cope with symptoms or side effects?*
4. **Today's session: The nature of motivation and low motivation as a high-risk situation.** *As we have talked about before, the goal of the relapse prevention section of the group is to think about high-risk situations and plan ahead so if you get into such a situation, you will know what to do to cope with the situation and not have a full-blown relapse. Over the past couple of groups we have talked about lots of different high-risk situations including coping with lapses, staying away from drinking or other drug use, coping with feeling depressed/stressed out, and coping with symptoms and side effects. Remember that these are all high-risk situations for someone to have a full-blown relapse to cocaine/heroin.*

Today we want to talk about another high-risk situation that we want to help you plan for —staying motivated to cut down or quit using drugs. Staying off drugs takes a lot of hard work. Lots of people tell us that sometimes they get tired of all of the hard work that it takes and sometimes they just want to throw in the towel and use, just because they are tired of doing all of the hard work all of the time. Quitting drugs can be like climbing a huge mountain—at the bottom you feel strong and have tons of energy and feel you can get to the top, but as you climb you get more and more tired, and your body feels really bad, and you just want to stop and give up. This is true with quitting drug use—sometimes you feel really great and motivated and glad to be doing the work, and other days you feel bad and just wanted to forget the whole thing.

Has that ever happened to anyone here? Lots of people who are trying to stop using drugs tell us that there are times when they have really low motivation to stop using drugs—they just don't feel like doing all the hard work anymore. Sometimes people just get tired and figure, "What's the use? I'm sick and tired of all of this hard work and this struggle. I should just forget the whole thing." Have any of you had times when you were really working hard to stop using and you really wanted to stop? Bob, you have told us that several years ago you stayed clean for six months straight. What was that like for you? Were you working really hard to stay clean? Has that happened to anyone else here?

Note to Therapist: Throughout the section you need to be soliciting input from group members and getting them to describe their experiences with low and high motivation.

We know that people who are trying to stop using drugs have both sorts of times. There are times when they are really motivated to stop and they feel great about working hard to stay away from drugs. At those times they go to all of their treatment appointments, go to lots of NA meetings, and feel really good about all the hard work they are doing to stay clean. However, everyone also has times of low motivation. At those times they find it hard to get to treatment appointments, don't want to go to NA or AA meetings, and generally feel like they are too tired to do what they need to do to stay clean. Has anyone here experienced either of these sorts of times? Can you tell us about them?

We have found that this low motivation and feeling tired is an important reason why people relapse. That's why we want to talk to you about what to do when your motivation is low and you are really tired and you think that staying away from drugs is just too much for you to do. By planning ahead for times when your motivation goes down, you will have some things that you can do so that you don't throw in the towel and relapse. Why would it be a problem to relapse when you are experiencing low motivation? For one thing, you have been doing a lot of hard work while you have been stopping your drug use, just like the mountain climber who gets in really good shape, gets all the best gear, and gets to Mt. Everest in top shape to climb. So you have done a lot of really hard work that you don't want to mess up by throwing in the towel. Why else is it important to cope with low motivation without using drugs or alcohol?

Note to Therapist: Therapists should get client input throughout this discussion and ask clients for additional reasons why it's problematic using drugs or alcohol to cope when they experience low motivation.

5. **Coping with low motivation.** *The important thing to keep in mind is that there are things that you can do to cope with low motivation instead of throwing in the towel and relapsing.*

(a) **Talk to someone.** *One thing that we have found helps people when they are experiencing low motivation is to talk to someone about what's going on with them. Lots of times when something serious like low motivation is happening we don't tell anyone about it. Does anyone here do that—keep that stuff inside and not tell anyone? Does keeping things inside help you to feel better? What we have learned from other clients is that not talking about what's bothering you doesn't help you feel better. In fact, it usually makes you feel worse. Instead of keeping things all bottled up inside so that you feel worse, you can talk to someone about it and at least get it out there in the open. To do this, you have to think of someone who you think will listen. Sometimes that is a family member or a friend or a counselor or a therapist. Think now about whom you could talk to when you feel bad? Bob, who do you talk to when you feel bad?*

Note to Therapist: Therapist should discuss this with all group members and figure out a person that each group member could go to when they are experiencing low motivation who might be able to help them and would encourage them to talk to their doctor about it. Suggest counselor/therapist as often as possible, even for people who name a friend or a family member that they could talk to when they feel bad. Keep a list.

(b) **Remember the "bad times."** *The fact that you are all in this group tells us that you have reasons for wanting to reduce or cut down on drug/alcohol use. You might remember that before you started group* *you met with Melanie for an interview and talked with her about some of the things that have happened to you because of your drug use. You might have talked about how using drugs has led you to do things that you didn't want to do, like steal or hurt someone or be mean when you are otherwise a very nice person. Has that happened to anyone here? Tell us about it. People have also said that using drugs gets them into trouble in other ways—they neglect themselves, spend all their money on drugs, and so can't pay their rent or pay for food. What problems have happened to you because of your drug use?*

Therapist Note: Probe for specifics regarding what exactly has happened to the group member where they experienced the particular negative consequence. For example, "What happened that you didn't like?" The therapist should be empathic here. "You had nasty hangovers. That must have been terrible." Therapist should keep a list generated by participants for review in the next session. If participants have difficulty coming up with consequences, give them an optional handout that lists negative consequences of drug use.

People who are trying to stop using drugs and alcohol tell us that one thing that helps them when they experience low motivation is to remember all the problems that they had when they were using.

One way to "remember the bad times" is to keep a list of some of the problems that drug use has caused you. That way when you experience low motivation to stop using and you are thinking of throwing in the towel, you can read over the list and remember the problems that drug use caused for you. We have a list here of some of the problems that you and other clients have told us about when they are using drugs. Where do you think you could keep the list so you could look at it when your motivation is low? (Find a place for each group member to keep the list.)

(c) Think about how things are better now that you are not using. *People tell us that remembering the "bad times" sometimes makes them see how well things are going now that they are not using. Another strategy for coping with low motivation is to acknowledge how things are better now that you are not using drugs. Lots of you talked in your motivational interviews about how your lives have changed since you cut down or stopped using drugs—you have a place to live, you're saving money, you're taking care of yourself and have nice clothes, you have enough money for food. Can anyone share how his or her life has changed since they cut down/stopped using?*

One way to remember how things have changed since you stopped using drugs is to keep a list of all of the good things that have happened since you cut down or stopped using. That way when you experience low motivation to stop using and you are thinking of throwing in the towel, you can read over the list and remember how all the hard work you are doing is paying off and how your life is much better since you have stopped using. We have a list here of some of the ways that you and other clients have told us their lives improved once they cut down or stopped using drugs. Where do you think you could keep the list so you can look at it when your motivation is low? (Find a place for each group member to keep the list.)

(d) Do something that feels good. *One thing that we have found helps people when they feel low motivation is to do something pleasant or something that they like to do. Research shows that when people do things they feel better. They may not have all of their problems solved, but just doing something and getting up and out and active can increase your motivation to stop using drugs. Has anyone ever found that just doing something, anything, pleasant makes him or her feel better than doing nothing at all? Bob, tell me something about that.*

Now, doing something pleasant can be tough when you are experiencing low motivation. For example, one thing that happens when a person has really low motivation is that they stay home in bed and stop doing things. They find it hard to get up the energy to get out and do things. What we have learned from working with other clients is that if you get involved in something pleasant, it may give you more energy so that your motivation to keep working hard goes up. The time to get up and do something pleasant is right when you notice you are feeling low motivation—that way you don't wait until you are totally unmotivated to do anything at all.

So what can you do that's pleasant? Let's come up with a list. We need to name as many things as we can think of that are pleasant or can get your mind off feeling bad and might help you to feel better. Think of the things that you do when you are upset in order to feel better. Bob, can you start us off? What's one thing that you do that you find pleasant?

Note to Therapist: Generate a long list and get input from all group members. See handout to get started if clients are having trouble coming up with items for the list.

6. **Plan ahead/practice strategies (i.e., asking for help/problem solving).** *Remember, we think it's best for you to have a plan, to plan ahead, so that if you are ever in a high-risk situation you will know what to do. So now we need to make a plan for each of you to follow when you are experiencing low motivation. That way when you are in that situation, you will have a plan and know something that you can do so that you do not relapse. Who would like to start?*

Note to Therapist: Get specific. When do clients find they experience low motivation? What has worked for them in the past? Talk with each group member about what they could do if they are feeling that way, using the strategies discussed in group—talking to someone, remember the "bad times," think about how life has improved since stopping drug use, doing something that feels good. Give examples for each category.

For example: Bob, you have said that you experience low motivation to keep working hard to stop using drugs on the weekends when all of your friends are out using. You have said that when everyone is using you just want to throw in the towel and join in. Let's make a plan for you for the next time you feel that way, so you have something else to do instead of using cocaine. First, you can talk to someone about it. Who could you talk to when you are feeling you have low motivation to keep working hard to stop using cocaine? Can anyone think of someone that Bob could talk to in that situation? That's a great idea Fred—Bob could talk to his counselor. I also remember you saying you had an NA sponsor—maybe you could talk to that person when you are experiencing symptoms or side effects. Another good place to bring that up is in a treatment group. OK, what's another thing we said people can do when they experience low motivation. Sue, can you remember? Right, they can remember the "bad times" and the problems they had when they were using drugs to remind themselves that using caused a lot of problems for them. Remember that we gave you a list of problems that happen when people use drugs. Are there any others that you would add to the list? Where could you keep the list so that you could look at it when your motivation to keep working is low? Some people tell us that they keep that list in their wallet so that it is with them all of the time. We have small lists made up that fit in a wallet so that no matter where you are you can remember the problems that drug use can cause.

OK, what's another thing we said people can do when they experience low motivation. Fred, can you remember? Right—think about all the good things that have happened in your life since you stopped using drugs. We put the good things that can happen on the other side of the wallet card so that you can see them wherever you are.

OK, what's another thing we said people can do when they experience low motivation. Sue, can you remember? Right, they can do something fun. Bob, what fun or pleasant things can you think of to do when you are experiencing low motivation?

If the client reports experiencing low motivation due to someone asking him or her to use drugs or wanting the client to do drugs with them, review refusal, escape, and avoidance skills, and do a role-play of a person using these skills in that situation. Write the steps on the board for each skill:

Refusal skills: *Eye contact, state no, give reason, suggest alternative/leave.*
Escape: *Eye contact, state no, give reason, escape/leave immediately.*
Avoidance: *Eye contact, state no, give reason, suggest alternative/leave.*

SKILLS SHEET: MONEY MANAGEMENT

Goals

Group members will understand that having money is a high-risk situation that can lead to relapse. Therapists will teach strategies for money management. The group will discuss how having money is a high-risk situation for group members. Group members will list strategies for money management and practice these strategies via role-plays when appropriate.

Note to Therapist: This can be done over two sessions if needed.

Instructions to Therapists

1. **Conduct urinalysis before group and follow procedures in Urinalysis Contingency section.**
2. **Review goals and complete goal setting.**
3. **Brief review of last session.** *Last group we talked about having low motivation as a high-risk situation for relapse. Remember that we talked about how sometimes people are really ready and motivated to cut down or stop using drugs and at other times they have a lot of trouble staying motivated. At those times they get tired of all of the hard work that it takes and sometimes they just want to throw in the towel and use, just because they are tired of doing all of the hard work all of the time. Lots of people who are trying to stop using drugs tell us that there are times when they have really low motivation to stop—they just don't feel like doing all the hard work anymore. Drug use is a really tough habit to break and sometimes people just get tired and figure, "What's the use? I'm sick and tired of all of this hard work and this struggle. I should just forget the whole thing." Remember that people who are trying to stop using drugs have both sorts of times. There are times when they are really motivated to stop and they feel great about working hard to stay away from drugs. At those times they go to all of their treatment appointments, go to lots of NA meetings, and feel really good about all the hard work they are doing to stay clean. However, everyone also has times of low motivation. At those times they find it hard to get to treatment appointments, don't want to go to AA meetings, and generally feel like they are too tired to do what they need to do to stay clean. We have found that this low motivation and feeling tired is an important reason that people relapse. We talked about things that you could do when you are feeling like you have low motivation to keep working to reduce/stop drug use. Does anyone remember some of the strategies we talked about last group? Right Bob, we talked about talking to someone, remembering the "bad times," thinking about how things are better now that you are not using, and doing something that feels good. Can anyone tell me why these things would help when you are feeling tired of working to stop using drugs?*
4. **Today's session: Why having money is a high-risk situation.** *As we have talked about before, the goal of the **relapse prevention** section of the group is to think about high-risk situations and **plan ahead** so if you get into such a situation, you will know what to do to cope with situation and not have a full-blown relapse. Over the past couple of groups we have talked about lots of different high-risk situations including coping with lapses, staying away from drinking or other drug use, coping with feeling depressed/stressed out, coping with symptoms and side effects, and coping with low motivation. Remember that these are all high-risk situations for someone to have a full-blown relapse to cocaine/heroin.*

Another important trigger for using drugs for many people is money. People who use drugs often find it really hard not to use when they have money or they know that they are going to get money sometime soon. For example, lots of times when people get a pay check or an SSI check, they get a big urge to use drugs because they have all of that money there and know that they can buy drugs or alcohol with it. So they go out and spend all the money on drugs or alcohol, but then they have no money left for anything else. Has that ever happened to anyone here—you use your monthly check and then use all of your money for drugs and then have no money left for anything else? Tell me about that.

The problem with using all of your money on drugs is that you don't have money left for the other things you might need or want. What are some other things that you need to spend your money on? That's right—you need to pay your rent, you need to buy food, you need to buy clothes. What else is there that you need to buy with your money? Yes, you need to pay for your transportation, and you might want some special things for yourself like a radio or a tape for your Walkman or a cup of coffee. What happens when you spend all of your monthly check on drugs—can you buy these things that you need like rent and food and clothes? Right, when you use all of your money on drugs, there is nothing left to use to pay your rent or buy food or buy clothes or pay for the bus, or anything else. Have any of you ever been there—used all your money for drugs so you have nothing left for anything else? What can happen if you have no money left for rent or food or clothes?

Today we want to talk about ways to manage your money so that you won't use all of it to buy drugs. This is called money management and it involves making sure that your money is safe and is not just sitting in your pocket waiting to be used to buy drugs. Why do you think that money management would be a good thing? That's right—if you manage your money, then you won't have a big amount to tempt you to use drugs and there will always be money for you to use to buy the things that you need like rent and food and clothes. Also, if you use money management, you might be able to save some money after you pay for all of your necessities so that you can save up for something special you might want.

> 5. **Strategies for money management.** *Talk to your social worker or counselor about banking services or getting a representative payee.*

Note to Therapist: You should find out something about having a representative payee before this group so that you are knowledgeable enough to answer client questions about it.

There are lots of services at the bank that can help you to save your money so that you don't have it on you and have to deal with it as a trigger for drug use. One thing that is very helpful is having a bank account. Does anyone here have a bank account? Bob, you have a bank account? Would you be able to tell everyone here a little bit about how it works? What kind of account do you have, when do you deposit money, when do you withdraw money, stuff like that?

Like Bob described, you can open a bank account and deposit your money in that account. That way you won't have it around all the time and have to deal with it as a trigger for drug use. Another service that you can use at the bank is direct deposit—your checks are automatically put into the account on the first day of the month or whenever you get the check. That way you don't have to pick up your check or get a big payment that might lead you to really crave drugs, and you might then go out and blow the money on drugs. Has that ever happened to anyone here—the day you get your check you go out and use it all on drugs? From our work with clients with drug problems and mental illness we have learned that it's a pretty common thing, that lots of times people will use the whole month's money on the day that they get their check. That's because they get their check, the check is a trigger that makes them really want to use, and they go cash the check, and spend all their money on drugs. Then they don't have any money left for food or rent or anything else. Has that happened to anyone here? Tell us about what that was like for you. With direct deposit, the good thing is that you never have to pick up the check because the money goes directly into your bank account. That way, the check will never be a trigger for drug use.

So opening a bank account and getting direct deposit of your check into your bank account are two ways to manage your money so that you don't find yourself with a lot of money on you all at once. Another one is having a representative payee or a rep payee—a person who manages your money for you and who makes sure your money goes into the bank. This person then gives you money for your needs each day, but keeps track of the money and makes sure that the rest of it stays in your bank account. Does anyone here have a rep payee? Can you tell the group how that works and what it's like for you?

Remember that for many people having money is a high-risk situation that leads them to use drugs. If you want to do either of these things, open a bank account or get a representative payee, you need to talk to your counselor/social worker about it. Your counselor/social worker will know all the things that you need to do to open a bank account and get direct deposit. Is anyone interested in talking to their counselor/social worker about opening a bank account or getting direct deposit? OK Fred, when do you think you can talk to your counselor/social worker about this? Let's write that down for you so you don't forget. I will also let your counselor know that you would like her help with this and to bring it up in your appointment tomorrow.

(a) Take someone with you who doesn't use drugs when you go to get your money. *Another thing that can help on the day you get your check is to take someone with you when you go to pick up your check, a person who can help you get the money without spending it on drugs. The person who goes with you should be someone who doesn't use drugs. Have that person come with you to the bank to make the deposit. Why would it be good to have a person who doesn't use drugs come with you to get your check and go with you to deposit it at the bank? That's right—that way when you have your check, that person can help you get to the bank and deposit your check without using the money to buy drugs. Does anyone do this when he or she picks up their check?*

(b) Write a budget. *Another thing that helps people manage their money is to write a budget and to figure out where all the money needs to go. Has anyone here ever written a budget? What did you do when you wrote a budget? Writing a budget involves writing down all the things that you need to have money for and the amount of money needed for each thing, and making sure that you have all the money that you need to pay all of your bills and take care of yourself. Why do you think that writing a budget would be a good thing to do to help you manage your money? We have found that when people see what they need to spend the money on and how much they need for things like food and rent and clothing, it helps them to keep motivated to deposit their check instead of using it on drugs. When someone really knows what needs to be paid for, and knows that if they don't have the money then they won't have a roof over their heads, sometimes it can help to remind them to go straight to the bank to deposit the check and not take a detour to buy drugs with the money. Has this ever happened to anyone here?*

(c) Select a nonusing friend, family member, or professional to help you manage your money. *Another thing that can be helpful is asking for help in managing your money. Asking for help involves selecting a nonusing friend, family member, or professional (such as your counselor or social worker) who can help you manage your money. Has anyone ever done this before? There are some housing programs that involve having a care provider or some other professional handle money and bills for a person, giving that person the money each week that they need for transportation to and from appointments, meals, and other activities. Has anyone ever done that before? Other people have a friend or family member who doesn't use drugs help them with managing their money, someone who will help them deposit their checks, pay their bills, and save money. Has anyone ever had a nonusing friend or family member help manage their money? Why do you think this is a useful thing to do in terms of money management? That's right—managing money is not easy and it's good to have help from someone who might know a bit more about it. Lots of people get help managing their money— it helps you get your bills paid, helps you save money for things that you want, and helps you to not spend your money on drugs.*

(d) Plan ahead/practice strategies (i.e., asking for help/problem solving). *Remember, we think it's best for you to have a plan, to plan ahead, so that if you are ever in a high-risk situation you will know what to* *do. So now we need to make a plan for each of you to follow when you have to deal with money. For most people the hardest time for them to deal with money and when they get cravings to use is when they have a large amount of money sitting in their pockets, like when they pick up their monthly check. So let's make a plan for each of you so that if you are ever in that situation, you will have a plan and know something that you can do so that you do not relapse. Who would like to start?*

Note to Therapist: Get specific. When do clients have money—many times in the month or just the first or 15th of the month? What do they do now when they have money? Do they have a bank account, direct deposit, a provider who deals with their money and gives them a allowance? What has worked for them in the past? Talk with individual group members about what they could do if they have money and want to use. For example, they could talk to their counselor or social worker about banking services, take a nonusing friend or relative with them to pick up and deposit the check, write a budget. Have them role-play where necessary, such as talking to their counselor about opening a bank account, or asking a nonusing friend or relative to come with them to pick up and deposit their check. Be specific and give examples.

For example: Bob, you have said that having money on you is a big trigger for you. When do you usually have money on you? Does that happen every day or just a few days in the month? OK, so you have money on you on the first of the month when you get your monthly check. What usually happens when you have that money on you? So, you pick up the check and go right across the street to the check-cashing place where you get cash and then you go buy crack. What do you do for money the rest of the month? It sounds like working out a plan for how to get that check and not use it for drugs would be a good thing for you. Let's make a plan for you for the next time you pick up your check so you have something else to do instead of using all the money to buy crack. First, you can talk to your counselor/social worker about banking services. Bob, do you have a bank account? So you don't have a bank account. That makes it hard for you to have a place to put your money once you pick up your check. If you had a bank account, you could take your check to the bank and deposit it. You could still take some money for the things you would need, but you wouldn't have a pocket full of cash—all that cash is hard to resist when it comes to crack, right? Another option after you have a bank account is to get your check automatically deposited into that account on the first of every month. That way you don't have to go to pick it up. Why don't we role-play you talking to your counselor/social worker about setting up a bank account.

> **Step 1:** *Make eye contact and speak firmly.*
> **Step 2:** *Tell your counselor that you would like to set up a bank account/direct deposit for your money.*
> **Step 3:** *Give her a reason why (so that I can deposit my money and have some place to put it so that I won't have it all in my pocket to spend on crack).*
> **Step 4:** *Ask what you need to do to set up a bank account/direct deposit and ask for his or her help in doing it (having help will make it easier for you and will help you to get the paperwork all filled out).*

OK, what's the other thing we said people can do when they have to deal with money? Sue, can you remember? Right, they can ask a friend or family member who doesn't use drugs to come with them to pick up their check and go to the bank with them. Remember that we said that having a nonusing person with you might help you to take the check to the bank instead of cashing it and using all the money on drugs. Bob, who do you know that might be able to help you? Do you have any friends or family members who don't use drugs? You had said that you have an NA sponsor, what about him? Good, you have your brother who helps you with lots of other things, and you think he would go with you and help you pick up and deposit your check. Great!

OK, what's another thing we said people can do to manage their money? Fred, can you remember? Right—write a budget. Bob, do you think you would be able to write a list of all the bills you need to pay each month and how much money you have available to pay each bill? Let's start you off now. Do you pay for rent? Oh, that's covered already. OK, what other bills do you have to pay?

Note to Therapist: Therapists should make a plan for each group member. Each plan does not have to include every strategy, and plans should be personalized for each group member. For example, if a group member's main problem is with getting his or her check on the first of the month, focus on that and write a plan just for that issue, which might include opening a bank account and having a nonusing person go with him or her to get and deposit the check. If a group member's main money problem involves using money on drugs throughout the month without first paying bills, then writing a budget and problem solving (i.e., figuring out how to get the bills paid, and which needs to be paid first) might be the appropriate focus.

If the client reports experiencing difficulty managing money due to being asked to buy drugs for someone else/use with that person, review refusal, escape, and avoidance skills and do a role-play of a person using these skills in that situation. Write the steps on the board for each skill:

Refusal skills: Eye contact, state no, give reason, suggest alternative/leave
Escape: Eye contact, state no, give reason, escape/leave immediately
Avoidance: Eye contact, state no, give reason, suggest alternative/leave

SKILL SHEET: VIOLENCE AND VICTIMIZATION AND SUBSTANCE ABUSE (OPTIONAL)

Goals

Group members will discuss the links between violence/victimization and substance abuse and discuss what can be done to escape or avoid violent situations.

Instructions to Therapists

1. **Conduct urinalysis before group and follow procedures in Urinalysis Contingency section.**
2. **Review goals and complete goal setting.**
3. **Brief review of last session:** Tailor this according to where in the schedule this session is completed.
4. **Today's session.** *When people use drugs, they often find themselves in risky or dangerous situations in which they could be harmed or become victimized, either physically or sexually. Many people don't realize it, but people who use drugs are at a much higher risk of being victims of many different kinds of violence. The reverse is also true—people who have been the victims of violence are at a much greater risk of using and abusing drugs and alcohol. In fact, experiencing violence is for many something that leads to relapse, but it doesn't have to be that way if you know other things that you can do to handle a violent or victimizing situation. Today we want to talk to you about some of the links between violence and substance abuse. In addition, we want to talk about what you can do if you find yourself a victim of violence and give you some strategies for dealing with the situation without using drugs or alcohol.*
5. **Links between violence/victimization and substance abuse.**

Note to Therapist: Try to have clients add to discussion. Be careful not to put group members on the spot to share experiences because they might not want to talk about personal experience of violence or victimization. However, try to elicit discussion whenever possible.

(a) Victimization causes stress which leads people to use drugs and alcohol. *Being the victim of violence is extremely stressful. That stress can make it very difficult to get through the day and take care of the things that you need to do. People will often say that one of the main reasons for a relapse is stress—they were stressed out and they didn't know how to handle it so they used drugs to help deal with the stress. In fact, lots of people who use drugs or alcohol say that one of the things that got them into using in the first place was being the victim of physical or sexual violence, and that after that they didn't know what to do to deal with the stress so they started using. So one way that victimization and substance abuse are linked is that victimization leads to stress, and stress can cause a person to relapse.*

(b) Victimization makes symptoms of mental illness worse, which leads people to use drugs and alcohol. *Another thing that we know about victimization and the stress that it causes is that stress can lead to worsening of symptoms of mental illness? Has that happened to anyone here—their symptoms get worse when they are under a lot of stress? Lots of people with mental illness tell us that when they are stressed out or dealing with a lot of stress, they often get more depressed, more delusional, or have more hallucinations. And as we have talked about in this group before, lots of times when symptoms get worse, people with mental illness will use drugs or alcohol as a way to cope with those symptoms. Does anyone remember the problem with using drugs or alcohol to cope with symptoms of mental illness? That's right, using doesn't help symptoms go away. In fact, symptoms tend to get worse when you are using*

Note to Therapist: You can recap dopamine information or information that clients discussed in the session on coping with symptoms.

So a second way that victimization and substance abuse are related is that being a victim of violence can lead to a worsening of your symptoms of mental illness, which can lead to relapse.

(c) Victimization leads to a person feeling numb and isolated and angry and depressed, which leads to drug and alcohol use to get rid of these feelings. *Another way that victimization and substance abuse are related is that victimization often makes people feel numb and isolated and angry. People who have been victimized or experienced violence will often turn to drugs or alcohol as a way to deal with these feelings of numbness and isolation and anger. These are very difficult feelings to deal with and oftentimes people find that using will take these feelings away for a brief period of time. What is the problem with using drugs and alcohol to deal with feelings of numbness or isolation? That's right—it doesn't last, it doesn't help in the long run.*

(d) Often a partner who is violent will provide drugs or alcohol to a user to keep that person dependent and in the violent relationship. *There is another way that victimization and substance abuse are related. Often people are victimized by partners who use drugs. Sometimes these partners don't want the person to get strong or healthy or to leave the relationship. So a partner will get drugs for a person in order to keep them dependent and in the relationship and keep them from getting strong enough to get out of the violent relationship. Has anyone here known anybody who has ever been in a situation like this—a relative or a friend or someone else they know? So being the victim of violence can involve a partner who is responsible for the violence getting drugs for the person in order to keep him or her in the relationship.*

What can you do?

(a) **Understand that violence, in any form, is wrong and it needs to be stopped.** *It is not your fault, even if you were using at the time.*

(b) **Do not keep it inside.** *Talking about what happened will help you cope with the feelings that victimization brings up. If you do not talk about it, you will have stress or symptoms or feel angry and isolated and this will put you at very high risk to use drugs and alcohol. Ways to talk about it:*

Call a hotline (**Note to Therapist:** Give out list of hotline numbers, reassure group members that hotlines are confidential).
Talk to a therapist or counselor.
Talk about it in group.
Talk to a trusted friend or family member.

(c) **End the relationship.**

Call the police, restraining orders, etc.
Find somewhere safe to go— (**Note to Therapist:** Distribute a list of shelters to group members); contact family members.
Talk to your counselor or therapist about things that you can do or places you can go.

(d) **If you can't leave, be safe in your house.** *Can you talk to your partner about this?*

Note to Therapist: Role-play client talking to his or her partner and expressing negative feelings about this. Use the following steps:

1. *Make eye contact.*
2. *Say exactly what the person did that upset you:*
   "It really made me feel—when you—."
3. *Say why it upset you:*
   "This upset me because—."
4. *Make a suggestion to keep this from happening in the future:*
   "In the future, could you please—."
5. *Go out if your partner is using or will be coming home high or drunk.*
6. *Find a place where you can be safe.*

   (e) Other, client-generated ideas. *Has anyone had to deal with this or known anybody who had to deal with this and what did he or she do that helped?*

As a reminder:

Refusal skills: Eye contact, state no, give reason, suggest alternative/leave.
Escape: Eye contact, state no, give reason, escape/leave immediately.
Avoidance: Eye contact, state no, give reason, suggest alternative/leave.

SKILL SHEET: DEALING WITH A PARTNER WHO USES DRUGS (OPTIONAL)

Goals

Group members will understand discuss why having a partner who uses drugs is a high-risk situation and will learn and practice strategies for coping with this situation.

Instructions to Therapists

1. **Conduct urinalysis before group and follow procedures in Urinalysis Contingency section.**
2. **Review goals and complete goal setting.**
3. **Brief review of last session:** Tailor this according to where in the schedule this session is completed.
4. **Today's session:** *Today we are going to talk about a high-risk situation that is probably relevant to a lot of people here, either now or at some time in the past, and that is how to cope with a partner who uses drugs and alcohol. Has anyone here ever been with a partner who used drugs and alcohol? What was that like? What would happen if you wanted to stop using for a while or go to treatment and try to stay clean? That's right—it's really hard to stay clean when you are involved with someone who is using drugs and alcohol. Why do you think it's so hard to stay clean if your partner is using? (Note: generate a list of reasons why a using partner makes it hard to stay clean.)*

So there are a lot of reasons why it's really hard to stop using or cut down on your use when you are with a partner who is continuing to use drugs and alcohol. This situation gets even more complicated because often you really care about the partner that you are with and you try to do what you want to do without hurting them or making them feel bad. But it's hard to stop using drugs when they are there with drugs all the time. Let's now think of some things that you could do in that situation so that you can work on staying clean even if you are faced with a partner who is using.

5. **Coping strategies.**

Note to Therapist: These are general guidelines. For each, develop a specific script for the client and have the client practice talking to the partner via role-plays.

(a) **Explain the situation.** *Tell the person that you are trying to stay clean or cut down your use and why.*

(b) **Stop seeing the person.** *If this person is unable to accept what you are doing and is unable to support your efforts to stay clean or cut down on your use, it might be time to think about whether it's best not to see that person any more. This is really hard because lots of times you care a lot about the person. But staying clean is also really important, and sometimes can be more important that staying with a partner who is using.*

(c) **Take a break from seeing that person.** *If you are unable to stop seeing your partner, talking about taking a break might be a good idea. Explain to your partner that you are trying to stay clean, you are involved in treatment, and you need a few weeks/months to get going with this, and so don't want to be around others who are using because it's too tempting.*

(d) **Limit your time with that person—only do things together that don't involve using drugs.** *See your partner for meals, for activities that don't involve drug use. This may mean limiting your time together to certain times of the day (i.e., if your partner uses at night then see him or her* *during the day), or limit your time together to certain activities (if your partner doesn't use in the mornings in order to get to work, see each other for breakfast; go to a meeting together).*

(e) **Other, client-generated ideas.** *Has anyone had to deal with this and what did you do that helped?*

Note to Therapist: *Incorporate skills that clients have learned in other sessions into these role-plays. For example, if a client is telling a partner that they are trying to stay clean and want to take a break from the relationship for a month, the client can follow these steps:*

1. *Make eye contact.*
2. *Tell partner that you are trying to stay clean from drugs.*
3. *Give a reason why you are trying to stay clean.*
4. *Suggest a relationship break and why.*
5. *Tell partner when you will contact him or her again, remind the partner not to contact you, and leave.*

As a reminder:

Refusal skills: *Eye contact, state no, give reason, suggest alternative/leave.*
Escape: *Eye contact, state no, give reason, escape/leave immediately.*
Avoidance: *Eye contact, state no, give reason, suggest alternative/leave.*

SKILL SHEET: CREATING A DRUG-FREE SOCIAL NETWORK (OPTIONAL)

Goals

Group members will discuss why meeting people who don't use drugs is an important part of their own not using and will learn and practice strategies for coping with this situation.

Instructions to Therapists

1. **Conduct urinalysis before group and follow procedures in Urinalysis Contingency section.**
2. **Review goals and complete goal setting.**
3. **Brief review of last session.** Tailor this according to where in the schedule this session is completed.
4. **Today's session.** *We have been told that it is very hard to stop using drugs when all your friends and everyone you see is using. Has anyone here experienced that? Why is it hard to stop when your friends and others around you are using?*

Note to Therapist: Get all clients to participate in this discussion). Today we want to talk about ways to find, meet, and get to know people who don't use drugs or alcohol. Being with people who don't use drugs is critical to staying clean. Why do you think being around people who don't use is so important to staying clean?

Sometimes figuring out how to change people, places, and things is really hard. Many people have been using drugs for so long, they forget the things that they used to like to do or other things that they could do instead of using, and they no longer know what to do with their time if they are not using. Let's talk about how to meet new people in order to create a group for yourself that doesn't use drugs.

5 **Coping strategies.**

Note to Therapists: these are general guidelines. For each strategy, develop a specific script for the client and practice having the client talk to the partner via role-plays.

(a) **Do things that support staying clean from drugs.** (**Note to Therapist:** generate a list with clients)

Go to AA/NA meetings
Go to other group treatment sessions
Go to a church group/meeting

(b) **Use social skills to meet new people.** *You might remember that at the very beginning of this group we talked about social skills—ways to get along with and talk to other people. You also might remember that the very first skill we learned was to start a conversation and make plans with someone. This is an important skill when you are working on staying off drugs—you need to know how to talk to people and make plans with people who don't do drugs. There are often times when you start a conversation with someone and you find out you have something in common. As a result you may want to become friends with that person. One way to start a friendship is to make plans to do something fun.*

Steps of the skill:

Step 1: *Make eye contact and say hello. Why is it important to make eye contact with someone when you are talking to them? This gets the person's attention. What if you were talking to someone but you were looking at their feet instead of their face? What do you think they would think of that? They wouldn't know that you were talking to them or they might not be able to hear you.*

Step 2: *Ask a general question. This starts the conversation and gives the person a chance to talk with you. Some examples of general questions are listed on your handout: How are you? What's up? What's new? How have you been? What do you think about this weather? These are all questions that get a conversation started.*

Step 3: *Invite the person to do something fun with you. What sorts of things would it be fun to do with someone you just met that you liked? Well, you could go to a movie, get something to eat or just have a cup or coffee, or just take a walk. On your handout are some ways to ask a person to do something fun with you. Can anyone think of any other fun activities that we could add?*

Step 4: *Confirm the invitation with the person, then give a reason and say good-bye. Why do you think it is important to confirm the invitation? That's right—just to make sure that the person knows what you are going to do and when you are going to do it. Why do you think it is important to give a reason why you have to go? That's right, it's a polite way to end the conversation. In your handouts there is a list of ways to confirm the plans and say goodbye.*

(c) Do other nonusing activities with someone.

Note to Therapist: Generate a list with clients; for example, have a meal together, go to a movie, go for a walk.

(d) Visit someone who doesn't use drugs. [C]*Chances are while you're using you heard from some friend or family member who was very concerned about you and wanted you to stop using. Now that you are not using, call that person, visit them, do things with them since you are now trying to stay clean.*

(e) Other, client-generated ideas. [C]*Has anyone had to deal with this and can you tell us what helped?*

Note to Therapist: Incorporate skills that clients have learned in other sessions into these role-plays. For example, if a client is sitting next to someone, use skills from sections on making small talk and making plans with a friend in the role-plays:

Making Small Talk	Making Plans with a Friend
1. Make eye contact and say "Hello"	1. Make eye contact and say "Hello"
2. Ask a general question	2. Ask a general question
3. Make small talk by asking questions about an appropriate topic	3. Invite the person to do something fun with you
4. Give a reason, and say good-bye	4. Confirm the invitation with the person, give a reason, say good-bye

As a reminder:

Refusal skills: *Eye contact, state no, give reason, suggest alternative/leave.*
Escape: *Eye contact, state no, give reason, escape/leave immediately.*
Avoidance: *Eye contact, state no, give reason, suggest alternative/leave*

SKILL SHEET: GENERAL ASSERTIVENESS TRAINING (OPTIONAL)

Goals

Group members will understand that being assertive will help them stay clean and they will learn and practice general assertiveness skills.

Instructions to Therapists:

1. **Conduct urinalysis before group and follow procedures in Urinalysis Contingency section.**
2. **Review goals and complete goal setting.**
3. **Brief review of last session. Tailor this according to where in the schedule this session is completed.**
4. **Today's session.** *There are many situations that require you to say how you are feeling about something, but lots of times this is a hard thing to do. Sometimes you want to tell someone that you don't want to do something, and other times you want to tell someone that you don't like what that person is doing to you. Saying what you want to say in a firm and clear manner is called being assertive. People tell us that it can be scary to be assertive, to tell someone how you feel about something and stick to it without backing down. Has anyone here ever had trouble being assertive and saying how you feel about something? Why was that difficult for you?*

The reason why saying how you feel is important is that if you don't say what's on your mind, everything just stays bottled up inside of you. Why is it a problem to let your feelings bottle up inside of you? That's right—if you don't say what's on your mind, eventually you won't be able to hold it in any more and you might wind up really angry or upset or exploding in a rage because you have been feeling so bad.

There are a few ways to be assertive: One is when you express negative feelings, stand up for your rights, and refuse unreasonable demands. Examples of appropriate negative assertion include: standing up to someone who is treating you unfairly or inappropriately; telling someone you don't want to do something that you think is unreasonable; and expressing justified anger or annoyance to someone.

Another way to be assertive is to express positive feelings: affection, approval, appreciation, and agreement. For example, thanking someone for doing you a favor; telling someone that he or she has done a really good job; and complimenting someone on his appearance or improvement.

Finally, you can be assertive by refusing to do things that you don't want to do. You might remember that we talked about this at the very beginning of group when we learned skills for refusing requests and offering an alternative. Telling people politely but firmly that you do not want to do something will help you feel less put upon by others.

People with mental illness tend to avoid or escape from situations in which they may be criticized or in which there may be conflict. The result is that people frequently take advantage of those with mental illnesses. Assertiveness is one of the most critical skills for people with mental illness to learn in order to avoid and reduce distress and avoid mistreatment. Positive assertion is similarly important in order to be able to develop and sustain friendships.

5. **Coping strategies.**

Note to Therapist: These are general guidelines. For each strategy, develop a specific script for the client and practice having the client talk to the partner via role-plays.

(a) Expressing negative feelings.

Note to Therapist: Review the importance of each negative feeling with group members.

    i. *Make eye contact.*
    ii. *Say exactly what the person did that upset you:*
       "It really made me feel—when you—."
    iii. *Say why it upset you:*
       "This upset me because—."
    iv. *Make a suggestion to keep this from happening in the future:*
       "In the future, could you please—."

(b) Expressing positive feelings.

Make eye contact.
Say what the person did that made you feel good:
    "It really made me feel—when you—."
Say why it made you feel good:
    "This made me feel—because—."
Say thank you and tell the person you appreciate it:
    "Thanks so much. I really appreciate it."

(c) Refusing a request and offering an alternative. (see BTSAS session on Refusing Requests for details and handouts)

    i. *Make eye contact and say "Hello."*
    ii *Tell the person that you cannot do what he (she) asked you to do.*
    iii. *Give a reason why you cannot do what was asked.*
    iv. *Offer an alternative.*

SKILL SHEET: ANGER MANAGEMENT (OPTIONAL)

Goals

Group members will discuss and practice anger management skills.

Instructions to Therapists

1. **Conduct urinalysis before group and follow procedures in Urinalysis Contingency section.**
2. **Review goals and complete goal setting.**
3. **Brief review of last session.** Tailor this according to where in the schedule this session is completed.
4. **Today's session.** *Today we are going to talk about what to do when you are angry. We all get angry. It's important to learn what to do when you are angry. Lots of times people handle anger badly—they get in fights or scream or yell or hurt themselves. Who here gets into fights or screams and yells when they get angry? Tell us a little bit about that. Why is getting in fights or screaming and yelling not a good thing to do when you are angry? Right—those things are bad both because they hurt you and others but also because they don't solve the problem and end whatever was making you angry in the first place. Often what happens when you are angry and you do something bad like get into a fight is that you get into even more trouble and wind up feeling angrier than ever. It's much better to do something that will not hurt anyone but that will also solve the problem so that you don't have to feel angry any more. We call this anger management—skills that you can learn so that when you get angry you will be able to feel better and solve the problem without getting into a fight or screaming and yelling and getting even more angry.*
5. **Steps for Anger Management.**

Step 1: Keep calm. *Why is it important to keep calm? That's right—if you can stay calm, you are better able to tell someone how you are feeling and solve the problem. If you don't keep calm, you might do something that can get you into trouble, like get in a fight. Why is fighting likely to get you into trouble? What are some ways to keep calm? Generate a list with group members: Take a deep breath, count to 10, leave the situation for a few minutes.*

Step 2: Say how you are feeling and why. *Why is it important to say how you are feeling and why? It lets the other person know what's going on with you and tells them why you are so upset. Lots of times people don't even know that they have done something that makes us angry. Other times they don't have any idea that we are angry with them. By telling them calmly and clearly, you are letting them know how you feel and what made you feel that way.*

"I am feeling—because you—."
Example: *"I am feeling angry because you did not show up to drive me to my appointment."*

Step 3: *Say why this made you angry. "This made me angry because—." Example: "This made me angry because I missed my appointment."*

Step 4: *Make a suggestion to keep this from happening in the future. "In the future, could you please—."*

Steps For Anger Management

Step 1:   Keep calm.

Step 2:   Say how you are feeling and why.

Step 3:   Say why this made you angry.

Step 4:   Make a suggestion so this doesn't happen again.

SKILL SHEET: EMPLOYMENT SKILLS (OPTIONAL)—
CONNECTING WITH JOB TRAINING, HOW TO PREPARE FOR A JOB INTERVIEW

Goals

Group members will discuss the skills that are needed to gain employment and will create a plan for trying out some of these skills.

Instructions to Therapists

1. **Conduct urinalysis before group and follow procedures in Urinalysis Contingency section.**
2. **Review goals and complete goal setting.**
3. **Brief review of last session.** Tailor this according to where in the schedule this session is completed.
4. **Today's session.** *Today we want to talk about things you need to know to get a job. Lots of times people who have long histories of using drugs have not worked in many years. Once they are clean they start to think about getting a job but are not sure where to start or what to do. Have any of you thought about getting a job at some point? You may not be thinking about it right now, but if you ever do start to think about getting a job, we hope you will know a few things about how to get the process started.*
5. **Coping strategies/things to do.**

Note to Therapist: These are general guidelines. For each, develop a specific script for the client and practice having the client talk to the partner via role-plays.)

(a) Talk to your counselor, social worker, or doctor. *The first thing to do is to talk with someone who knows something about the resources that might be available to you in terms of seeking employment. Your counselor, social worker, or doctor will be able to help you think through whether this is the right time to get a job, what sort of job might be good for you and fit into your schedule, how to deal with people on the job, how to find out about different jobs, and other things that you will need to know in order to find a job. Your counselor, social worker, or doctor can also be someone that you can talk to as you go through the process of looking for a job and someone who can give you advice along the way. They might also know about special programs that train people with mental illness for certain jobs, or programs that provide help to people trying to find a job after many years of not working.*

(b) Connect with job training. *This is something to ask your counselor, social worker, or doctor about. A job training program is the best way to get back into the swing of working when you haven't been working for a while. This type of program teaches people things that they need to know to do certain jobs and can tell you what is involved in lots of different jobs. Has anyone here ever been to a job training program before? What was it like for you?*

(c) Think about what sort of a job you might like, what sort of a job you could do. *Why do you think it's important to give some thought to what sort of job you might like? Also, you have to remember that what you might like might not always be a realistic choice. I might want to be a racecar driver but it's pretty unlikely that I'll be able to do that, right? You have to give some thought to what you might like to do and what might fit into your life. For example, you will still have to go to doctors' appointments and therapy appointments, so the type of job you consider has to be something that can work around these appointments that you already have. You also have to try for something that you think you can do and do pretty well. For example, you don't want to pick a job where you have to be around lots of people if you don't think* *that you would be able to be around lots of people and deal with it comfortably. Writing a list of things you might like to do is a good first step (see attached handout). Getting your thoughts about what you like to do, what you think you can do, and what other commitments you have is a good way to get things clear and organized as you starting thinking about getting a job.*

(d) Tips for preparing for a job interview. *Usually an employer will want to interview you before he or she decides whether or not you are right for the job. Doing a job interview is not all that hard, but some people find it a little bit nerve wracking or stressful. We have found that the more people think about the interview beforehand and prepare for it, the less stressful it is for them. How many people here have ever been to a job interview? Could you tell us a little bit about what happened at the interview?*

Tips

> *Think before the interview about why you would want to work at the job. What do you think you would like about it?*
>
> *Talk with your counselor, social worker, or doctor before the interview about what to expect. Suggest that they help you out by role-playing an interview so that you can get some practice answering questions.*
>
> *Arrange transportation to the interview ahead of time. Take a "trial run" a week before to make sure you know the way, whether you are driving or taking the bus. If someone is driving you, arrange for them to get you there at least 30 minutes early.*
>
> *Dress cleanly and simply.*
>
> *Be very polite.*
>
> *Answer all questions to the best of your ability. If you don't know something, tell the interviewer you don't know.*
>
> *Make eye contact when you are talking to an interviewer.*

(e) Practice general job interview steps. (Note to Therapists: *Discuss each interview step with group in terms of why each step is important):*

> **Step 1:** *Enter the room, shake hands, say hello.*
>
> **Step 2:** *When asked, say why you would like to have the job and why you think you would do it well.*
>
> **Step 3:** *Answer questions as best you can. Make good eye contact when answering questions.*
>
> **Step 4:** *At the end of the interview, ask when you might hear from the job, shake hands, say thank you, and say goodbye.*

(f) Other, client-generated ideas. *Has anyone had to deal with this and what did he or she do that helped?*

Note to Therapist: The therapist can complete the attached handout with group members as part of the group. After reviewing "Tips," engage group members in role-plays of mock interviews. Have clients watch for polite language and eye contact. Make role-plays fairly short and simple, and follow the steps outlined above.

As a reminder:

> **Refusal skills:** Eye contact, state no, give reason, suggest alternative/leave.
>
> **Escape:** Eye contact, state no, give reason, escape/leave immediately.
>
> **Avoidance:** Eye contact, state no, give reason, suggest alternative/leave

What Kind of Job Might Be Good For Me

1. What am I looking for in a job? (Circle Yes or No)

   Working with other people............... Yes   No

   Work that is interesting.................... Yes   No

   Work that is part-time..................... Yes   No

   Work that is near my home............... Yes   No

   Work that is low stress..................... Yes   No

2. What kind of job would I like? What do I like to do? What am I good at?

   _____

   _____

   _____

   _____

   _____

   _____

3. What appointments or meetings do I have to go to during the week:

   Appointment/meeting   Day of the week and time

   _____   _____

   _____   _____

   _____   _____

   _____   _____

   _____   _____

   _____   _____

SKILL SHEET: RELAXATION TRAINING

Goals

Group members will discuss the benefits of using relaxation training and will try it out in session.

Instructions to Therapists

1. **Conduct urinalysis before group and follow procedures in Urinalysis Contingency section.**
2. **Review goals and complete goal setting.**
3. **Brief review of last session.** Tailor this according to where in the schedule this session is completed.
4. **Today's session.** *As we have discussed before, the goal of the relapse prevention section of the group is to think about high-risk situations and plan ahead so if you get into a situation, you will know what to do to cope with that particular situation and not have a full-blown relapse. We have talked about lots of different high-risk situations including one that is important for a lot of people: coping with stress. All of us get stressed out, and lots of people use alcohol or drugs to cope with stress. Has anyone here used alcohol or drugs to cope with feeling stressed out? It's really important to learn how to handle stress without using alcohol or drugs. A while ago we talked about things that you can do to cope when you feel stressed, including doing pleasant activities, talking to someone, trying to solve the problem, or talking to your doctor about your medication. Today we are going to talk about another thing that you can do when you are stressed out —relaxation.*

Relaxation training is a skill that you can learn to help you feel calmer or less tense. There are lots of times when you might feel tense or stressed out and you don't know what to do to feel calm again. Or, you might get a craving and need something to do to help you wait it out without using. Sometimes it's hard to know what to do when you are stressed or having a craving. Relaxation can help—when you are tense, or stressed, or having a craving, or in a lot of other situations. It's also an easy way to cope with stress. After practicing these skills and getting good at them, you will see that they are easy to use and can help you relax even when you don't have a lot of time or when you are not at home.

Relaxation takes practice to get good at it. So in group we will do some relaxation and that will give you a chance to practice it and see how it works. You can then practice it at home or when you feel tense or stressed out or when you have a craving. Once you practice it for a while and get good at it, relaxation can help you feel less tense and more relaxed.

A reason that relaxation is helpful is because of the connection between our minds and our bodies. When you feel stressed out, your body gets tense and tight and it's hard to relax. You might even get a craving to use drugs or alcohol because you need to relax and feel less tense.

If you can relax your mind, then your body will feel relaxed too. Relaxation helps people get their minds and their bodies relaxed and calm, which as I said is very helpful when you are stressed out or tense or having a craving. You can't be tense and relaxed at the same time. So doing relaxation and getting yourself calm and relaxed is a good way to feel better and less tense and less stressed-out. In the past you may have turned to drugs or alcohol to help when you are stressed out or tense. Since our goal here is to help you reduce drug use or stop using drugs, we want to teach you another way of getting calm and relaxed, a way that does not involve drugs or alcohol.

The type of relaxation that we are going to do here in group is called "The Soles of the Feet Technique." This type of relaxation comes from the Far East and we know that it is helpful in dealing with urges to use, cravings, and negative feelings like being tense or stressed out. I want to do some relaxation with you all today, and when we are finished you can tell me what you thought of it. We will do this periodically in group so that you get practice using relaxation. This technique involves getting comfortable, doing some deep breathing, and clearing the tension out of your body.

5. **Relaxation Script.** *Sit back in your chair and close your eyes. Get real comfortable: lean back so that your back is supported in the chair, rest your head on the back of the chair, put your hands in your lap or let them hang down by the sides of the chair. Pull your feet up until your feet rest flat on the floor. That's good, nice and easy, get real comfortable and start to feel how your body is getting comfortable in the chair. Check yourself for comfort. Get real comfortable. Think about each part of your body and make sure it is comfortable. Your head is resting on the chair. Your back is supported by the chair and is resting comfortably. Your arms are loose and sitting in your lap or hang down. Your legs are resting comfortably on the floor and you can feel the floor underneath them.*

Now that you are comfortable, take several slow, deep breaths. Take a deep breath way down into your belly. Let your breathing slow down and start to feel relaxed. Each breath continues to relax you. Now take a deep breath in and hold it. Now slowly exhale, let the breath out, and let all the tension out with it. Feel calm and relaxed as you breathe slowly. Again take a deep breath and hold it. Now slowly exhale, let the breath out, and let all the tension out with it. Feel calm and relaxed as you breathe slowly. Each breath leaves you more and more relaxed. Focus your thoughts on your breathing, with each breath making you feel more and more relaxed. You are breathing quietly, peacefully. Feel the calm that spreads over your body with each breath. Now you feel relaxed over your whole body. Every part is feeling relaxed and calm and quiet. You are breathing slowly and peacefully and your body is feeling calm and relaxed. Each breath cleans your whole body and mind. Relax and feel the peace and calm that has spread throughout your body with each deep breath.

Now focus on your feet. Think about your feet inside your shoes and how your feet are filling up your shoes. Feel the bottoms of your feet touch the floor underneath them. Focus on the soles of your feet and how they are touching the floor. Your feet are on the floor and the soles of your feet are touching the floor. As you breathe deeply, in and out, in and out, focus on the soles of your feet. The soles of your feet are heavy, they are heavy against the floor. Now think about your breathing. Imagine with your next deep breath that the clean, pure air is spreading throughout your whole body, collecting all of the tension and stress. The air takes the stress and tension from your body. Imagine this air leaving through the soles of your feel. See the tension leaving your body with each breath. Imagine another breath entering your mouth and taking all the tension and stress with it as it leaves your body through the soles of your feet. As you exhale you feel your body clean and relaxed, deeply relaxed.

Now scan you body for any last bit of tension or stress. Let all the tension go down, through your legs, and out of your body through the soles of your feet. Your face is relaxed. Your forehead is smooth and your face is completely relaxed. Smooth and relaxed. You have let go of all the tension and worry, it goes down your body, through your legs, and out through the soles of your feet. Now your neck and shoulders are relaxed. Your shoulders droop and relax and your neck is free of tension. Free and relaxed. The tension in your shoulders moves down your body, through your legs, and out through the soles of your feet.

Now take a deep breath and as you exhale feel the relaxation spread throughout your body and your back. The tension in your body and your back is running through your legs and out the soles of feet. You feel free and relaxed. Your arms are heavy and relaxed. Heavier and heavier. More and more deeply relaxed. Heavy and relaxed. Letting go, letting go of all the tension. Letting it run out through the soles of your feel. Your legs are relaxed. They get heavier and heavier, more and more deeply relaxed. Letting go of the last bit of tension and stress. Letting any remaining tension run down your legs, out through the soles of your feet.

Now your whole body is feeling relaxed. Feel yourself being calm and relaxed. You are feeling peaceful and calm and relaxed. Now slowly start to open your eyes. Move around in your chair and when you are ready, open your eyes.

6. **Review and end group.**

Chapter **11**

GRADUATION AND TERMINATION

INTRODUCTION

Ending a treatment group can be an anxiety-producing situation for many clients who have done well in treatment. The message delivered throughout treatment is that clients are learning skills that they can take with them to maintain success in the future. However, it is not unusual for clients to feel that their success is tied to the urine testing and attendance at the group. Consequently, four BTSAS sessions deal with graduation, termination, and future plans.

Several topics are covered in these four sessions. First, progress made by the graduating client is reviewed, with an emphasis on positive reinforcement for whatever goals the person has achieved. Second, the most useful coping strategies for the graduating client are identified, and the client is prompted to use them whenever necessary. Third, short- and long-term goals are discussed and revised as needed, and an effort is made to anticipate potential near term problems in achieving goals. Finally, plans are made for the transition to aftercare and, where necessary, alternatives are identified for assistance/support that was provided by the group over the previous six months.

SPECIAL ISSUES IN GRADUATION AND TERMINATION

Well before graduation, the client should be informed that the end of his or her involvement in the BTSAS program is approaching.

Informing Clients of Their Progress

We recommend that the client receive periodic information on his or her progress in the program over the course of the 52 sessions (i.e., two sessions per week). We use attendance at BTSAS as a source of reinforcement for clients, such that a review of attendance is an opportunity to praise a client for continuing in the program and making a sustained effort to attend sessions. This is especially important for clients who are continuing to use drugs and are not reaching their substance use reduction goals. In such cases, clients can be praised for their efforts at attending sessions, illustrating their continued interest in working hard toward reducing their drug use. For clients who are meeting their goals with respect to drug use, reinforcing attendance is just an additional way to provide praise and encouragement.

Another benefit of this sort of periodic assessment of attendance is that clients are informed throughout the program of how much longer they have until graduation. This can serve as a motivator, as many clients with SPMI have little or no experience completing or graduating from any program, treatment related or otherwise. Importantly, it also means that most clients will not be surprised to hear that graduation is approaching, and will view their leaving BTSAS as a positive thing and a hard-earned accomplishment.

Open Enrollment and Termination

Remember that due to the open nature of BTSAS enrollment, clients graduate on different timetables. That is, this is not a closed group in which all participants started and will end together. Rather, clients leave the program on differing timetables and at different points in the curriculum. This is important to keep in mind, as issues related to termination from the group will need to be worked into other content when a client is nearing the end of his or her 52-session experience. The last four groups that a client attends should have some discussion of upcoming termination and include the issues described in detail below. Because other clients will not be graduating, this discussion of termination issues cannot take up the entire group. Rather, termination issues for a particular client should be introduced where appropriate and should take 5 to 10 minutes of group time.

Difficulty Leaving BTSAS

BTSAS has a different feel from other substance abuse treatment programs, and most SPMI clients we have worked with have noticed it. For this reason, a client might be nervous or anxious about leaving the BTSAS program. A successful client may attribute this success to the program rather than to his or her own efforts. If a client is convinced that a particular treatment component is essential for his continued success, the therapist should emphasize the importance of the client's own skills and achievements in making progress in the BTSAS program. In addition, if a client has shown good success in BTSAS, the therapist should attempt to find a referral that can continue some version of what the client requests (e.g., semiregular urine testing).

DROPOUT

Clients will have dropped out of BTSAS and not had four sessions to discuss termination issues. In our research, we have defined dropping out as missing eight sessions in a row without a reason (i.e., eight unexcused absences). Clinically speaking, the definition of dropping out might need to be tailored to different settings or circumstances. Whatever the definition of dropping out, in the event that a client does leave the BTSAS program early, several things must happen. First, the BTSAS therapist must inform the client's treatment team as soon as the client misses several sessions in a row and looks likely to be a dropout. Second, it is useful to attempt to find the client and determine the circumstances that led to the patient's dropping out. Often dropout is preceded by an increase in or return to drug use. Other times clients have other entanglements in their lives that lead to dropout, such as termination of housing, overlapping appointments, or medical problems. Finding out the circumstances is useful in the event that such precipitating problems can be solved with the help of the BTSAS therapist, or understanding the event can enable the BTSAS therapist to refer the client to another professional who can help. This might not keep the client in BTSAS, but may help to keep the client connected to mental health treatment, which is clearly better than losing the client to all treatment entirely. Third, when the client has missed several sessions and appears likely to drop out, it is useful to contact the client, let him know that he is in danger of being removed from the program, and if possible to engage in some problem solving that might help the client return. Importantly, the client should be reminded that he is welcome to participate in the BTSAS program even if he is not abstinent, and the therapist should talk to the client in a supportive tone ("We miss you in the group and hope you will return; you are a valuable group member") rather than an accusatory one ("You need to come back to group or you will be terminated").

TERMINATION SESSIONS

About four sessions before graduation, the therapist should announce to the group that a client is approaching graduation and generate some praise from the group that the client has made it to the end of the program (remember, with 52 sessions, this is no small accomplishment!).

Review of Progress

The therapist should then review the client's progress in the group, and solicit positive statements from the client regarding the accomplishments that have been made. It is important for the therapist to review the client's problem list at the start of the program and be sure to review progress in all of these areas. In our research protocols, this meant reviewing the problems that the client reported at his baseline ASI and comparing how these problems have improved (or not worsened) during six months of BTSAS. The therapist can also review the list of negative consequences that was generated during the first motivational interview, and use this list as a starting point for reviewing a client's progress. The following is a list of accomplishments that can be included in this review. As you can see, it is important to include accomplishments that are related to substance abuse treatment.

Reduced use of goal drug
Stopped use of goal drug
Periods of abstinence from goal drug
Reduced use of secondary drug
Stopped use of secondary drug
Periods of abstinence from secondary drug
Perfect/near perfect attendance at BTSAS sessions
Regular attendance at BTSAS sessions
Not dropping out of the BTSAS program
Taking psychiatric medications regularly
Attending most/all psychiatric/mental health clinic appointments
Maintained housing over the six months of the program
Any health improvements/health has not worsened
Eating better/looking better
Spending money on things other than drugs

For many clients this review will be relatively easy, since by the end of their involvement in the BTSAS program, they will have made significant reductions in drug use, stopped altogether, or had significant periods of abstinence during the preceding six months. For other clients, progress might be difficult to spot. Such clients may have attended sporadically over the six months of the program, made few if any changes in their drug use, and may not be experiencing any obvious benefits of their involvement in BTSAS. The following is a sample exchange between a therapist and a client who has not made much progress in reducing his drug use:

Therapist: As you know, we are coming up to your graduation in about two weeks. I want to take a few minutes now to review the progress you have made since you started in the program six months ago.

Client: I'm still using.

Therapist: It's true that you are still struggling with ways to stop using crack. Stopping drug use is an extremely difficult thing to do, and lots of people find it really hard to stop. I know that you are finding it hard to stop. Let me take a moment though to review some of the things I think you have accomplished in the last six months. The first thing is that you are even graduating from this program—that you made it for six months without dropping out. That is a tremendous accomplishment. Did you think you would graduate when you first started?

Client: No way. I haven't graduated from anything. I always leave.

Therapist: So one really great accomplishment is that you kept coming to group and here you are about to graduate. I have tallied all the groups you have come to, and you have made 33 groups so far—that's more than once per week! You have done a great job getting here, which we therapists really appreciate. Another thing I think you have done really well is be a really good and important group member. You talked a lot in group, shared your experiences, gave support to other group members, were always the first one to volunteer to do role-plays, answered questions—just made the most of your time here and really worked hard when you were here. That's not always easy and you have been terrific at working hard. That's also a big accomplishment.

Client: I didn't think of that as something good. But I guess it is. I don't talk much in my other groups, but I do talk here.

Therapist: So that's three things so far: graduating from the program, having really good attendance, and working hard when you are here. What's another thing you have accomplished in the last six months?

Client: I don't know.

Therapist: Think hard. You can come up with something.

Client: Well, I'm still in the clinic.

Therapist: That's right! Six months ago you were almost kicked out of the clinic for missing your appointments with your counselor and your psychiatrist. How have you been doing with those appointments?

Client: I've made all of my psychiatrist appointments. I have missed some of the others, but I have called to let Ms. Jones know I wouldn't be there. She likes that.

Therapist: Excellent! So you now make all of your psychiatrist appointments and most of your therapy appointments and you are still in the clinic and haven't been kicked out. Tremendous! What about your medication—how are you doing with that?

Client: I take it.

Therapist: How often?

Client: All the time now.

Therapist: And what were you doing six months ago when you first got here?

Client: I wasn't taking my medication all the time.

Therapist: That's right! You see where I'm going with this— another thing you have made excellent progress in is in taking your medication. And your symptoms are much better controlled as a result. So it seems there is a lot that you have done over the last six months that is really, really good.

The key here is to find some things, *any* things, the client has accomplished. These can be within-group behaviors (being a good group member), or within-clinic behaviors (attending clinic appointments), or improved management of SPMI (taking medications), etc.

Identification of Most Useful Coping Strategies

About three sessions before graduation, the therapist should have a discussion with the client about the coping strategies that she has found useful as she progressed through the program and achieved the accomplishments that were identified in the previous session. Remember that this should only take a few minutes of group time. It is important to have the client generate helpful strategies and review why they were helpful, rather than just telling the client what you think was helpful to her. That is, the therapist needs to get the client to talk about what has been helpful. If the client is not talking much, the therapist can offer input and solicit comments and ideas from other group members. This is another domain that will differ depending on the progress the client has made and the things she has achieved. The following is a sample exchange between a therapist and a client who has reduced her drug use significantly:

Therapist: So now that you are gearing up to graduate and you have really cut down your drug use, I want to ask you what things you think were helpful in you being able to change and to reduce your use.

Client: Lots of things. I just feel better. I take my meds and I see my doctor. Coming here has been good too because you are nice to me and you don't yell at me or tell me I'm bad when I mess up.

Therapist: Those are all important things that have been helpful. Sounds like once you graduate from this group, there are still lots of things you can keep doing—like taking your meds and seeing your doctor and going to your clinic appointments—so that you can keep making progress.

Client: Yeah, that's true.

Therapist: What else do you think has helped you?

Client: Spending my money when I get it. I got myself new clothes, got my hair done, got my nails done. I look good.

Therapist: Excellent! Spending your money on things other than drugs is good for two reasons—you get things that you need instead of drugs, and you look good when you have what you need. That's great!

Compare this with the following sample of an exchange between a therapist and a client who does not think many things have been helpful to him:

Therapist: Last group we reviewed some of the accomplishments you have made since you started here, like still being in the clinic and coming to so many of our groups that you are now graduating. What do you think has helped you be able to do these things?

Client: I'm still using. Just getting here isn't really great.

Therapist: I see it differently. When you first started here you were having a lot of trouble just getting here. The fact that now you get here and it's no trouble at all is, to me, really great. Ed, don't you agree?

Client 2: Yeah. When you first came here, you were mean and you didn't talk at all. Now you talk and you're nice and we talk in the waiting room.

Client: I guess.

Therapist: So what has helped you be able to get to your clinic appointments and get to our groups so regularly?

Client: I don't know.

Therapist: Any ideas? What's one thing that helps you get up and out of the house on group days or clinic days?

Client: I know I have to do it so I can get my medication.

Therapist: That's great! It sounds like you have come to see that your medication can really be helpful, and knowing that gets you here to the clinic. What about coming to our groups? What has helped you get here for the past six months?

Client: I want to stay in the clinic. I have to be here to stay. And these groups aren't so bad.

Therapist: I'll take that as a big compliment! These groups are OK, and it's important for you to get to them so you can stay in the clinic. Excellent!

The rule here, as it is throughout BTSAS, is not to argue with or attempt to convince the client of your view of things. That is, if a client is truly struggling to see improvement, your goal is not to demand that he or she see it. Rather, your job is to acknowledge the client's view, point out the things that you see as important, and tell him or her the reasons why you think they are important. The client may agree or disagree, but you have provided some information and been reinforcing and positive in the process.

List of Short- and Long-Term Goals

About three sessions before graduation, the therapist should have a brief discussion with the client about short- and long-term goals following graduation from the BTSAS program. "Short-term" should be viewed as for the foreseeable future, and short-term goals should focus on continuing the progress that has been made since starting in BTSAS. Long-term goals should be discussed briefly and should be very concrete and straightforward and realistic. At this point, the therapist should have an idea of some sort of goal that, if the client continues to do well, he or she could achieve. For the sample client above who made a lot of progress, short-term goals should be to keep up with her reductions in drug use and to keep taking her medications, which she considers to be one of the big reasons she was able to reduce her use. A long-term goal might be to try out something she suggested at some point during the six months of the BTSAS program, such as saving some money or seeing some relatives again. In this case, the therapist could also suggest that the client try to completely stop using drugs as a long-term goal:

Therapist: So in the short-term, you want to keep doing what you're doing, because you have been really successful. What are your thoughts on stopping drug use altogether?

Client: I have thought some about that. Right now I'm using once or twice per week. It's hard to stop completely.

Therapist: Yes it is, and I think it's great that you can say that outright and be honest about it. It is hard to stop completely. However, if you're doing this well right now, totally stopping would probably be a great thing. It's something to think about as you graduate and go forward.

Client: Yeah, I have been thinking about it. I'll probably try it soon.

Therapist: That's great! It's a good long-term goal. You have made lots of progress and when you are ready to stop the last two times per week that you use, I know you'll be able to do it.

Notice that the therapist did not keep going until the client said she would stop using drugs. Rather, it was a discussion about a suggestion, and the client was reinforced for thinking about it.

Treatment Referral

Treatment referral for graduating BTSAS clients involves several components. The first is to ensure that clients continue with any treatment they have been attending for their mental illness. Most clients will have been receiving simultaneous treatment for their SPMI, and they should be urged to continue with that care. The BTSAS therapist should notify the treatment team that the client is graduating from BTSAS, as well as discuss with the client the importance of continuing to attend his or her mental health treatment.

Graduation from BTSAS requires that the therapist and the client consider options for referral for further substance abuse treatment. Some clients will be in other substance abuse treatment groups or programs, and clients should be encouraged to continue with whatever additional treatment they have been attending (other substance abuse treatment providers should be informed of the client's upcoming BTSAS graduation).

For many clients, BTSAS will have been their sole form of substance abuse treatment over the previous six months. In such cases, the sort of referral to make, or whether to make one at all, requires thought and collaboration among the BTSAS therapist, the client, and members of the client's mental health treatment team. Some clients will clearly need a referral to another substance abuse treatment program, and the available options in the clinic should be explored and discussed. There are several different scenarios to consider. First, there may be clients who make it through BTSAS but clearly require more intensive substance abuse treatment than a bi-weekly outpatient program can provide. In such cases, options for inpatient care or detoxification should be considered, or referral to a program or clinic that specializes in substance abuse treatment. Many such treatment programs are not equipped to care for clients with SPMI, so any referral needs to be well-thought out and will require ongoing collaboration between the new program and the mental health treatment team.

Second, there will be clients who continue to need outpatient substance abuse treatment. Such clients should be referred to an appropriate program. Importantly, a simple referral is not sufficient for clients with SPMI. The BTSAS therapist should make contact with potential programs and gather the necessary information so that the client can make an informed decision. Then the BTSAS therapist should contact the clinician in the new program and actively coordinate an intake appointment. This might require some problem solving in the client's final BTSAS sessions during goal setting to make sure that the client knows that making this intake appointment is of high priority.

Third, there will be clients who have made significant progress and had a block of abstinence who may want to take a break from substance abuse treatment. Again, this is a decision that should be reached following collaboration with the client, the BTSAS therapist, and members of the client's mental health treatment team. There are cases in which a break from substance abuse treatment would be warranted. If a client has stopped using drugs, does not use any secondary drugs of abuse, is meeting all mental health treatment requirements, has a stable housing situation, and has some social support in his or her environment, then that client may be ready for a trial break from substance abuse treatment. We organize this in the following way: We first organize a meeting with all relevant parties (client, BTSAS therapist, counselor, psychiatrist, caregiver, or significant other). In that meeting, the BTSAS therapist, the counselor, or the psychiatrist tells the client that this is a trial period in which the client can take a break from substance abuse treatment. A plan should be generated and discussed, and the client is informed of the things that need to happen in order for this break to continue (take medication, attend all clinic appointments, attend appointments with psychiatrist), as well as the things that will trigger a return to substance abuse treatment (relapse, not keeping up with mental health treatment, etc). This is also a good time to suggested that the client attend some self-help meetings as an adjunct source of support for abstinence.

GRADUATION PARTY

The final session includes a graduation party, in which participants receive diplomas. A sample diploma is provided here. The graduation party can include snacks. Generally the graduation involves the therapist summarizing some of the termination discussions, including the progress the client has made and the short-term goals the client has identified. Sometimes the client wants to make a short speech thanking the group members; clients may speak but do not have to. Occasionally group members might want to speak to wish the graduating client well. We have also invited members of the client's mental health treatment team including counselors, psychiatrists, and case managers, or anyone else who has been integral to a client's attending BTSAS groups and supportive of his or her progress. In some cases, clients invite partners or other significant family members or friends to the graduation party.

SUMMARY

Graduation from the BTSAS program represents a significant accomplishment for clients with SPMI who often have a history of treatment failure. The therapist must direct the activities that surround graduation and termination such that clients feel positive about their BTSAS experience, recognize the progress they have made, and are connected to more substance abuse treatment if needed.

CERTIFICATE OF
ACHIEVEMENT

AWARDED TO

_____

For Successful Completion of

Behavioral Treatment of Substance Abuse in SPMI

At The Community Mental Health Center
This 29th day of January 2005

_____   _____

Sue Smith,
Therapist

Jim White,
Therapist

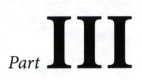

Part **III**

Chapter **12**

DEALING WITH COMMON PROBLEM SITUATIONS

A s with any clinical intervention, there are tricks to making the program more effective, and pitfalls that experienced clinicians learn to avoid over time. BTSAS is no different. Group members do not always behave as expected or desired, and BTSAS therapists need to have a repertoire of strategies to prevent or deal with problems that may arise. Many problems can be anticipated and prevented by carefully planning the group and tailoring the treatment to individual needs. However, even with optimal planning, some problems are likely to arise. Moreover, not every dual disordered person is a suitable candidate for BTSAS at every point in time. In some cases it might be better for the person and for the group if participation were delayed. This is especially true for people who are not really interested in reducing drug use, but have been pressured to come by clinicians, family members, or the court system.

The following sections provide some tips for structuring groups and for dealing with common problems. These ideas can be extrapolated for the idiosyncratic issues that the clinician will confront over time. Chapter 13 will also provide recommendations for how to deal with problems associated with specific BTSAS components (e.g., goal setting, urinalysis).

COMMON PROBLEMS IN CONDUCTING BTSAS GROUPS

It is crucial for group leaders to tailor the content and approach of *all* their groups based on the varying needs and abilities of the group members.

General Issues

Depending on the group members, the same basic social skills content areas can be presented with different levels of complexity and different expectations for the group members' performance. For example, in teaching drug refusal skills to very impaired persons, role-play rehearsals can be brief and uncomplicated, and the leaders can limit feedback to the basics, such as "Did the person say 'No?'" and "Did the person leave the situation?" In contrast, in teaching the same skill to a higher functioning group, the leaders might teach more sophisticated skills, including dealing with highly confrontational individuals (like drug dealers) or highly tempting situations (e.g., a girl friend who uses and offers sex after smoking crack). Similarly, feedback can address more subtle aspects of behavior, such as voice inflection, use of gestures, and offering alternatives to drug use. The range of content can also be adjusted depending on group members' cognitive abilities and what they will need to do in their particular social setting.

Following the Group Format

Prior to participating in BTSAS, most dual disordered persons will have experienced other group therapy approaches that were less structured, more insight-oriented, and where members were encouraged to "just let their feelings out." When first attending a BTSAS group, people might be surprised at its structure and at its teaching approach, and they may have difficulties initially in adapting to the group format.

The leaders should provide a clear description and explanation for the format of BTSAS groups in their initial interviews with prospective members, and again when they start. Early sessions should include a brief orientation/lesson plan so members know what to expect that day. In general, members should be provided with a curriculum so they are attuned to what will be coming in the future, as well as what will happen in a particular session.

When members drift from the format, the leaders can gently but firmly redirect them to the task at hand ("Right now I'd like you to hold your comments while you watch Steve do a role-play"). Praising group members who make progress in following the format is also beneficial. For example, to a person who previously interrupted role-plays and has now begun to observe them quietly, the leaders could say, "Miguel, I liked the way you waited until Steve finished his role-play before you gave feedback."

Usually people are able to follow the group format after several sessions. The open enrollment format is especially conducive to orienting new members as we do not ask much of them during the first week. New participants can observe other group members and learn appropriate behavior by modeling from their peers.

Care should be taken not to discredit or devalue the importance of any other type of treatment a patient has received or is participating in (especially double trouble or 12- step type programs). Acknowledge differences between approaches and suggest how they can be complementary, but emphasize that the most important thing is for the person to find strategies that work for them.

Reluctance to Role-play

Some new group members feel uncomfortable or awkward speaking in front of others. This may make them reluctant to role-play. However, several strategies are embedded in BTSAS to mitigate this problem. First, social modeling (observing peers) and positive reinforcement for effort is very effective in overcoming resistance. Second, therapists never force the person to do something they do not want to do. Rather, the leaders acknowledge the person's feelings and that his or her discomfort is understandable. It is helpful to let the person know that many people feel shy when they first try role-playing, but that they gradually get used to it and may even start to enjoy it. The person can be reminded that role-plays are very brief and that everyone in the group will be doing them. Some people are concerned that they will be criticized or teased. The leaders can point out that the emphasis of skills training is on providing positive feedback and suggestions for helping people be even more effective at using the skills. Negative comments and criticism are avoided in the group.

Third, reviewing the rationale for role-playing is important. The most common rationale is that "People need to practice the skills they are learning so that they can really know how to do them. It's like learning to play the piano or play basketball. You have to practice to get skillful." The leaders emphasize that by role-playing, people usually feel more comfortable when a situation comes up in real life where they need to use the skill. It may be helpful to encourage group members to identify examples of specific situations in their lives when the skill would be useful.

Fourth, BTSAS makes consistent use of the behavioral principle of shaping: developing new skills or overcoming resistance by gradually exposing the person to the task and gradually adding more and more difficult elements or gradually raising performance criteria. This is a form of teaching that minimizes failure and frustration, because the person is only asked to do what she can do or can almost do correctly. The following dialogue is representative of a supportive approach to encourage participation:

I can see that you are having a tough time today, and I appreciate you being here and making an effort. Remember that you are here because you've said that you don't want to continue using as you have been using in the past. Right now, you may not want to role-play/stop using. My job here is to help you get ready for the day when you are ready to make that commitment. The way I can best do that is to help you role-play/come up with a reason why you don't want to use at all. Let's see what we can help you to come up with.

If the member still doesn't want to role-play, the therapist may suggest only role-playing one or two of the steps of the day's skill, or suggest that the member role-play from his or her seat. In the same manner, the therapist or other group members can suggest alternative reasons that the member may find appropriate for the future when he or she *does* want to commit to abstinence.

Facilitators should be particularly aware of the members' *culture,* including gender, racial, ethnic, and socioeconomic factors and aspects of the *drug culture* that influence values, language, styles of interaction. Role-plays should be done in the most realistic manner possible. This means that facilitators should be familiar with vocabulary that would most often be used in the situations being role-played; types and brands of alcoholic drinks, various drug use practices (routes of administration, nicknames for drugs, etc.), and 12-step program vocabulary (sponsor, making amends, various slogans). Asking for specifics when eliciting role-play scenarios with group members is one way to gain this sort of information. While it may not always be an option, it is also important for both facilitators and group members portraying confederates to role-play one's own gender whenever possible.

Problems with Attention (Distractibility) and Memory

The cognitive impairments common to schizophrenia, such as distractibility, poor attention, impaired executive functioning, and memory problems, can interfere with some people's ability to benefit from groups. The repetition, overlearning, and behavioral rehearsal that are built into the social skills model can help compensate for some of these cognitive difficulties. Several other strategies may also be used to address cognitive impairments.

The treatment room should be minimally distracting and located in a quiet area of the treatment facility. The room should be arranged to facilitate eye contact with the leader, and visual cues such as posters, schedules, and signs may be used to assist individuals with memory impairments. Smaller groups and shorter training sessions are sometimes indicated for people who have significant cognitive impairments. We use cotherapists whenever possible because it is difficult for one person to coordinate the curriculum, role-playing, urinalysis, and also attend to each participant's individual needs. The clinician who is not serving as the primary leader should constantly be scanning the group and may unobtrusively signal individuals who appear distracted to gently remind them to focus on the leader. Questions may be directed to individuals who appear distracted to prevent them from drifting away from the work of the group. If people have trouble paying attention to role-plays, the leader should assign them the task of watching for specific target behaviors. For example, the group leader could ask, "I would like you to report on Tony's eye contact at the end of the role-play."

Group leaders should periodically remind people of the goals of the session in terms of what task they are working on. They should frequently ask people to repeat instructions and should ask questions designed to confirm comprehension of group materials. For example, the leader might ask, "What is Dan's role in the role-play? What is Yolanda's role? What are the goals of this skill?" If comprehension appears poor, the skills or skill components should be further simplified. As indicated previously, we also make extensive use of visual materials and handout both to serve as prompts for what is required, and to minimize demands on memory. For example, when we introduce role-plays we generally ask members to read the steps from their handouts. Similarly, when covering didactic material we may ask members to read brief segments of the material so they are not simply listening to a lecture. The more behaviorally engaged the members are the greater their ability to remain focused and the greater their interest in what is being taught.

Ambivalence about Committing to Treatment

At times, some group members may experience a desire to discontinue group participation or have difficulty committing to the treatment process. This is to be expected for anyone with a substance use problem and may be accentuated by the ambivalence that is often characteristic of schizophrenia.

This situation should be addressed without confrontation. The therapist should indicate that shifts in motivation are common, that they are not an indication of failure, and that it is important to continue learning skills so they are in the person's repertoire when he or she does decide to try and reduce substance use. The following is an example of the supportive, but directive approach to be employed:

> We like that you have been part of this group with us. You may not feel like talking about drugs and alcohol today, but you are an important part of this group. The other members learn from what you have to say and the things you contribute by being here. You don't have to role-play today if you don't feel up to it. We can take it session by session for a while and work with you on staying in the group. People sometimes have a hard time with group meetings about drugs and alcohol and we'll work hard to help you.
>
> I understand that this is not a good time for you to get off crack, but you were motivated to use less when you started treatment, and you will probably become motivated again down the line. This is still a good time to learn strategies that will be helpful when you do want to quit or cut back, so we can increase your chance of being successful.

Poor Attendance

One of the most fundamental problems leaders encounter when they conduct BTSAS groups is getting members to attend on a regular basis. The scientific literature on treatments for substance abuse consistently indicates that better outcomes are associated with better attendance at treatment programs. This problem is not unique to substance abuse treatment; most professionals working with people who have SPMI report that it is an ongoing struggle for them to attend programs of any kind. Several strategies are helpful in boosting attendance.

From the very first contact, it is helpful for the leaders to express warmth and a positive expectation about participation in treatment. The leaders need to convey the expectation that the group will help people to achieve personal goals and that they will enjoy attending. For people who express extreme reluctance, have short attention spans, or have a poor attendance record with other programs, it is desirable to set small goals for initial attendance. For example, for the first group, the leaders might ask the person to give it a try for 10 minutes and make very few demands during those 10 minutes. People who observe the process of the group are usually reassured by what they see and become more receptive to attending the group. As the person becomes more comfortable during short periods in the group, the leaders can gradually increase their expectations for how long the person will attend.

Other reinforcers, such as money, food, increased privileges (in the case of an inpatient facility), recreational opportunities, or time with a favorite staff member also help provide motivation for increasing attendance. Some community residences develop a reward system where goals for attendance and participation are set each month, and people who achieve their monthly goals are invited to a party.

Progress toward these attendance goals is recorded on a chart in the room where the social skills group is held. The party includes pizza and interactive games.

At times the leaders might feel discouraged when a particular person does not attend the group. However, it is important not to give up. With encouragement, even people who do not attend any other treatment programs may attend BTSAS groups. We have found several strategies to be helpful. Members are given appointment cards after each session. We call members the evening before (or the morning of) sessions for members who have particular difficulty attending regularly. Whenever possible we enlist the aid of a *concerned significant other* who can help prompt the person to come. This could be a housemate, family member, case worker, minister, or anyone else the person trusts and has given us permission to contact. Finally, members should never be criticized for an absence when they do come back, even if it is several weeks later. The reminders and requests for attendance should always be upbeat and friendly and convey both an expectation of attendance and of appreciation for coming. Notably, members need to learn that they should come even when they have used drugs: that they will not be censured or made to feel guilty.

Some participants are really not participants at all: they come very inconsistently, using treatment groups almost as a drop-in program. While we just indicated that the general approach is to encourage and reinforce attendance, people who come so erratically may be doing themselves an injustice by feeling/acting as if they are in treatment when they are not. They also may be setting a bad example for other members. In an effort to deal with this problem in our research program we decided that a subject who missed eight consecutive group sessions was considered a "dropout" from the group. If the subject expressed a desire to rejoin the group after that period, there was a mandatory "time-out" or waiting period of approximately one month before the subject could reenter the group. Additionally, before reentering, the therapist met with the person one-on-one to determine if it was appropriate for the person to come back, and if so, to complete another motivational interview to reflect any changes in the patient's motivation to reduce substance use. The eight-session limit is somewhat arbitrary, and each clinical program may wish to set a different criterion. Regardless, it is important to establish an objective standard in order to avoid arguments or preferential treatment. Different rules may be warranted for members who miss sessions due to illness, incarceration, or inpatient psychiatric or drug treatment.

MEMBERS WHO CONTINUE TO USE SUBSTANCES

BTSAS clients may continue to use their goal drug throughout their time in the program, or they may use or abuse other substances while they are trying to reduce or stop their goal drug. There are several important issues to consider when planning for how to respond to continued drug use.

Harm Reduction Approach Applied To Goal Drug

Clients do not have to be abstinent or committed to abstinence. We employ a harm reduction approach and view decreased use as a positive step that will reduce persons' overall level of harm. There are several reasons why we believe that this is a useful approach with this population. First, as we have previously discussed, behavior change is particularly difficult for people with SPMI. Overall change is best conceptualized as a long-term process with many components, some of which have little to do with drug use per se. For example, for many participants a substantial amount of time is needed for them to feel comfortable simply attending sessions and remaining in a room with a group of people for over an hour twice per week. Because this is a long-term process, any reductions in use made at any point are significant in and of themselves, and may bring the client closer to eventually attempting abstinence. Second, dual disordered persons often abuse or are dependent on multiple substances, making it highly unlikely that total abstinence from all substances could be achieved at the start of treatment. Members select a goal drug at the start of treatment and they focus on reducing or stopping their use of this goal drug. Participants are encouraged to select abstinence as their treatment goal, but reducing use is praised, especially when a participant is unwilling to attempt abstinence. Once abstinence is achieved with the goal drug, we encourage members to turn their attention to other, secondary drugs of abuse. Third, a requirement of total abstinence could very well turn some members off to the group entirely, especially those members who are not considering change. Thus although therapists are directive and determine the content of group sessions, they are not confrontational or critical of members and their substance use, and the tone of BTSAS sessions is empathic and reinforcing. This emphasis on harm reduction means that we get a mix of participants at different levels of use and motivation. Some are using daily and have not thought about cutting down. Others have started decreasing their substance use, and others may have a few days or weeks of clean time.

Stages of Change

We employ Prochaska and DiClementi's Transtheoretical Model (TTM; 1982) of change to conceptualize motivation throughout treatment. Consistent with a harm avoidance perspective, we attempt to help patients move to higher stages of change (i.e., greater motivation to quit) by consistently setting goals for reduced use and teaching members techniques to decrease use when they choose to do so. The therapists should determine (either clinically or by examination of structured assessment instruments administered during research assessments) what stage of change each group member has reached in addressing their substance use problem: precontemplation, contemplation, preparation, action, or maintenance. For those persons in precontemplation (e.g., no clear desire to reduce use), the focus should remain on basic skills and steps for conversation/refusal sessions. Persons who appear to be focusing with more certainty on some sort of recovery (reduction of use or abstinence) can be focused on substance reduction and how it relates to the conversation and refusal skills they learn from early on in group.

Strategies for Clients with Poly-Substance Abuse

Clients participating in a BTSAS program often will use and perhaps abuse or be dependent on multiple substances. While they must select heroin, cocaine, or marijuana as their goal drug as a part of their BTSAS participation, clients will often come to the program using some combination of these drugs, or drinking and abusing other drugs, both illicit and prescribed. BTSAS includes one session during the *relapse prevention* section on "Other Drugs of Abuse" as a high-risk situation leading to relapse. However, we have learned that secondary substance use or poly-substance abuse/dependence is often an important issue for BTSAS clients, which impacts their engagement in the program, the quality of their experience in the program, and their ability to complete the program. In this section we review some of the most common poly-drug use combinations and issues, and describe some of the ways in which the BTSAS program and its therapists need to address this issue.

There are three general types of other drug use in BTSAS clients: (1) comorbid alcohol use/abuse/dependence; (2) poly-substance dependence; and (3) secondary drug use.

Comorbid Alcohol Use/Abuse/Dependence

Alcohol use and associated disorders are particularly prevalent in dually diagnosed SMI clients. Alcohol is the most widespread substance of abuse among schizophrenia patients (Mueser, Yarnold, & Bellack, 1992; Mueser, Bennett, & Kushner, 1995), and people with major mental illnesses, including bipolar disorder and schizophrenia, show the greatest risk of developing comorbid alcohol use disorders of any patient population (Reiger et al., 1990). The ECA Study (Reiger et al., 1990) found that 33.7% of individuals with schizophrenia spectrum disorders and 46.2% of those with bipolar I disorder met criteria for an alcohol use disorder. Others estimate that between 12 and 50% of people with schizophrenia suffer from alcohol use disorders at some point in their lives (Mueser, Bellack, & Blanchard, 1992). Grant and Hartford (1995) found that among respondents with major depression, 32.5% met criteria for alcohol dependence during their lifetime, as compared to 11.2% of those without major depression. The combination of SMI and alcohol disorders exerts a profound impact on the course and severity of both disorders, including more severe symptoms of mental illness, more frequent hospitalizations, higher rates of violence and suicide, increased risk for HIV and AIDS, greater rates of homelessness, poor self-care, unstable living environments, and problems in social functioning (see Drake et al., 1990 for a review). Clearly drinking and the problems it generates are important issues to address in dually diagnosed SMI clients.

Alcohol has several unique qualities that make it particularly attractive to SMI clients. First, drinking is widespread and engaged in nonproblematically by most people. The perception is that drinking is a normal, acceptable way to celebrate occasions or improve mood when done in moderation, and is done by the vast majority of people. SMI clients, many of whom want to do things that make them appear and feel "normal," will drink as a way to do something mainstream and socially accepted. Importantly, there is a fine line between acceptable drinking and alcohol abuse, and perceptions of where this line begins and ends may not be shared by client and therapist. For example, a client may see nothing wrong with drinking a few beers over the weekend, while the therapist may believe that any drinking by an SMI client with drug dependence is ill-advised. Or a client with a pattern of some problems associated with use may not view these problems as particularly significant in comparison to those he has experienced because of drug use. Second, alcohol is easy to obtain and inexpensive. The fact that buying alcohol is legal and easy is a plus for SMI clients in that it does not require any great demands on cognitive functioning or entail any social risks. Alcohol is also cheap, which puts it within range for even the most financially strapped clients—most are able to easily come up with a few dollars a day to purchase alcohol if they want to (in contrast with the time, effort, and risk it can take to raise enough money for drugs). Third, alcohol can be and often is used alone by SMI clients. It does not require much interaction with others to obtain or use alcohol, which stands in contrast to the more social nature of illicit drug use. This is a benefit for SMI clients who often show deficits in social skills and find it difficult to interact successfully with other people.

Drinking in addition to drug use has implications for engaging and maintaining clients in the BTSAS program. First, the content of a BTSAS group may not map on directly to drinking. For example, refusal skills may not be as important in this population, since clients often obtain and use alcohol alone and offers to drink are not as frequent as offers to use drugs. Another example is the emphasis in BTSAS on teaching clients to identify and avoid drug-related triggers and high-risk situations, which might be different from those for drinking. In addition, it is difficult to avoid many alcohol-related triggers (seeing alcohol in restaurants, and on advertisements and billboards) and high-risk situations (gatherings with family and friends, passing liquor stores and bars) that are legal and prevalent in mainstream society and not as secret or underground as many drug-related triggers might be. Second, there are implications for clinicians in treating drug abuse while a client continues to drink. For example, some clients may wind up increasing their drinking in order to "make up" for reduced drug use. Other issues include clients attending BTSAS groups following drinking or coming to groups intoxicated. We have, over the years, struggled with the idea that focusing on drugs in BTSAS may send a message to alcohol-abusing clients that drinking is OK. Clients who drink can be more unpredictable and have more chaotic lives, which can impact their engagement, attendance, and participation in BTSAS.

Poly-Substance Dependence

Many SMI clients will have true poly substance dependence—while they have selected one drug as their goal drug, they will have one or more other drugs that they use with the same intensity and level of problems as their self-selected goal drug. The most frequent combination of poly-substance dependence that we have encountered is the combination of cocaine and heroin, which when used together is referred to by our clients as a "speedball."

Poly-substance dependence has many important implications for the BTSAS program. Most importantly, clients with poly-substance dependence are simply more difficult to work with than are clients with a single substance use disorder. They generally have more, and more severe problems, both with substances and with other life issues. Our experience has been that BTSAS therapists working with these clients often feel as if there is so much going on with this one person that it is difficult to keep BTSAS focused and on track. This is often a process going on within the client has well—with two or more equally problematic substances, a client may feel that there is just too much to try to tackle at one time. If not addressed, these feelings can lead to hopelessness in both the therapist and the client, and can do much to decrease motivation for change. In addition, poly-substance dependence can make the selection of a goal drug more difficult. Generally, the goal drug is the substance that causes the most harm, whether or not it is the substance used most frequently (see chapter 7 for a more extensive discussion of the range of factors that are involved in selecting the goal drug). When two or more drugs are viewed by the client as equally problematic, it becomes unclear how to select the goal drug and where the focus of the intervention should be. Finally, a practical consideration for clients with poly-substance dependence is that because use of multiple drugs is so problematic, reducing use of one drug may not make a noticeable amount of difference in the client's life. That is, while BTSAS is built on the foundation of small steps and positive reinforcement of even the slightest change, clients with multiple substance dependence may change use of one drug but not experience a reduction in substance-related problems. Clearly this could be demoralizing.

Secondary Drug Use

We define secondary drug use as use or abuse of drugs that is not as intense and does not generate the same degree of negative consequences as the goal drug, but is still either time consuming for the client or generates some additional problems in the client's life. For example, many SMI clients will come to BTSAS due to cocaine dependence, but also use marijuana fairly regularly or meet criteria for marijuana abuse. Some of the most frequently used secondary drugs among the clients we have worked with are marijuana, as well as prescription drugs used to get high that include Clonazepam (Klonopin) or methadone.

Use or abuse of secondary drugs brings with it several issues that impact BTSAS. Probably the most significant issue, especially in cases of drug use that do not rise to the level of abuse or dependence is that clients may not want to change their use of the secondary drug. Rather, clients often see continued use of a secondary drug as unrelated to use of their goal drug and report that they intend to continue this use both during and after the BTSAS program. For example, clients who smoke marijuana periodically or regularly may view their use as nonproblematic, and view it as a way to reduce feelings of tension or stress. This is particularly relevant when the secondary drug is a legal substance and one that is prescribed by the psychiatrist for relief of some psychiatric symptom. For example, Klonopin is an anticonvulsant that is often prescribed to SMI clients to treat symptoms of anxiety. We have found that SMI clients who use Klonopin as a secondary drug (i.e., use it more often than it is prescribed, in order to get high rather than to control anxiety symptoms) generally do not view this use as problematic because it is "medicine" rather than a drug. A related issue is that while some nonproblematic substance use may be the end point for a particular client, there is a danger of other clients in the group adopting the same notion for themselves when it is much less relevant. For example, a client who has stopped all use of his goal drug but continues periodic and nonproblematic use of marijuana might be considered a treatment success. For another client who has not fully stopped her cocaine use and smokes marijuana on a more regular basis, the secondary drug use may be a more significant treatment issue. Importantly, there will be cases in which the client does not even bring up his or her use of a secondary drug, but the therapist finds out in some other way. For example, a client may come to a session smelling of alcohol, or may consistently come up positive for a secondary drug such as marijuana on the urinalysis test. In other cases another treatment provider may report secondary drug use in referring the client to the BTSAS program. In such cases, figuring out how to address secondary drug use is complicated by the fact that the client has not directly told the therapist about the use in the first place.

How to Address Poly-Substance Abuse or Secondary Substance Use in BTSAS

There are several guidelines and strategies for addressing other substance use and abuse in the context of BTSAS.

Don't Panic

There will be clients who initially do not want to address use of other or secondary substances, or perhaps do not want to change this use at any point in the program. This is OK. Remember that BTSAS takes a harm reduction approach that views any reductions in use of any substance made at any point as a significant treatment goal on its own, and one that improves health and reduces risk on its own. This means that we accept that other drug use is a part of the overall picture for some clients, and we reinforce any steps that take the client closer to abstinence. We will not get there for all clients. However, we believe that we are likely to be more helpful to clients and more effective in treating substance abuse if we keep the clients attending treatment, and clients are more likely to attend if we do not require them to be abstinent from all drugs at the start of the program or push total abstinence as the only goal of the BTSAS program.

A special case in this context is the client who is dependent on two substances and uses both equally, as in the case of combined cocaine and heroin use (speedballs). In this situation the therapist can address both drugs together in the context of the group. Goal setting can revolve around reduced use of both cocaine and heroin, and role-plays can involve the client refusing use of both drugs. However, it is typically best to have the client select one drug for the urinalysis contingency, in the hope that maybe sometimes the client will be clean of at least one of these drugs and so can receive the financial reward for a negative test.

Don't Ignore It

If other substance use is an issue for a client, then it should not be ignored. In keeping with the philosophy of BTSAS as accepting and reinforcing, use of other substances should be treated in an open and nonjudgmental way, as fact rather than as something to be avoided. Clients will take the lead on this from the therapist. If the therapist does not bring something up and avoids talking about it, the client will too. If the therapist talks about something in a calm and reasonable way, the client is likely to do the same. Acknowledging use of drugs other than the goal drug will promote honesty—therapists are better off knowing about all drug use, primary or secondary. There are many places within the BTSAS program to ask about and briefly discuss secondary drugs of abuse: the motivational interview, goal setting, skills training sessions, education sessions, and relapse prevention sessions may all be places where secondary drug use can be brought into the discussion.

In cases where the client has not reported any secondary use, the therapist can ask about it, either directly or indirectly via a group discussion of a related topic. For example, suppose a client who has been working on cocaine as a goal drug consistently tests positive in the urinalysis for marijuana but has not brought up his marijuana use in group. The therapist has several options. First, if the therapist has some idea of the marijuana use prior to the client beginning the BTSAS program (i.e., from the referral source), then the first motivational interview (MI) is a great place to bring this up. As we reviewed in chapter 6, the MI starts with some introductory conversation, and as part of this, the therapist can ask the client not only about his goal drug but also about other substances the client has used in the past and now. Getting this information out in the open at the start of the program is useful in that it promotes honesty from the start and ensures that both client and therapist know all there is to know about the client's current use. In addition, the marijuana use can be brought up separately from the goal drug in each of the sections of the MI, providing the therapist with information on consequences and motivation for change that will be useful throughout the client's time in the program.

Second, the therapist could ask the client to stay after group and could ask the client about his marijuana use in a supportive and nonjudgmental way ("I have noticed that your urinalysis has been positive for marijuana for the past few weeks. You have never talked about using marijuana and I wanted to check in with you about this. Would you mind telling me a bit about your use?"). Third, the therapist could make the marijuana use part of the discussion during the urinalysis feedback and goal-setting components of the session ("Bob, your test was clean for your goal drug cocaine which is terrific! That makes it two weeks that you have come in here clean from cocaine! That is terrific! I did notice that today your test is positive for marijuana. Tell me what your marijuana use was like this week."). Fourth, the topic of the group session can be directed toward a discussion that might prompt the client to discuss his marijuana use. Certain sessions, such as "Other Drugs of Abuse" (relapse prevention) and "Coping with Stress/Negative Affect" (relapse prevention), will lend themselves particularly well to this approach. The therapist must decide which of these options to use based on his or her knowledge of the client and how the client will react to this sort of discussion, as well as the topic of the session and whether a discussion of secondary drugs can be logically fit in.

Start Where the Client Is

As we reviewed above (as well as in chapter 2), our ideas about motivation for change are based on the Stages of Change Model, which acknowledges that people come to treatment at different stages of motivation, with many being opposed to or ambivalent about change. Importantly, a client may be in one stage for one drug (action for the goal drug) and another stage for other drugs (for example, precontemplation for alcohol use). A therapist may need to do different things for the same client who is in different stages of readiness to change for different substances. For example, suppose a client has selected cocaine as his goal drug (i.e., action stage) but also drinks regularly and with some problems and expresses no desire to reduce his drinking (i.e., precontemplation stage). The therapist is addressing the cocaine via the majority of skills and information provided by the BTSAS group. However, the therapist can also encourage the client to discuss his drinking during goal setting in the following way:

> Your goal is to stay clean from cocaine between now and the next session. That's great! You have talked in the past about your drinking and been honest that you are not at this point considering cutting down how much or how often you drink. It is really great that you have talked about this honestly. I think it might be time for you to reconsider that, given what you have told us about how you have been drinking a bit more recently and you have had a few problems related to your drinking such as hangovers and fights when you were drunk. While I am not telling you what to do and I think that you are the best person to figure out what is going on with you, I am wondering if some part of your goal this week can be related to your drinking.

The therapist can also provide information on the harmful effects of drinking as part of an education session, or privately ask the client to consider a referral for his drinking. Alternatively, a client who is interested in improving his health as a reason to reduce/stop drug use could be encouraged to get a physical examination as a way to see what specific health issues the client needs to address and as a way to examine objectively whether and how alcohol is impacting health. The important issue here is that clients need different kinds of help, depending on their motivation to change for different substances. Remember that the client is attending BTSAS—this attendance and willingness to work on changing one drug should be viewed as the starting point from which the therapist may eventually be able to lead the client in a new direction on other drugs.

Use Assessment as a Way to Ask Questions

In chapter 5 we reviewed the uses and types of assessment that fit in with the BTSAS program. Using assessment to gather information on secondary substance use and abuse is an excellent way to get the client talking about this in an objective way. Assessment should cover both the nature of the use (quantity, frequency, years of regular use, problems associated with use) as well as the level of motivation to change associated with secondary substance use.

Be Reinforcing

It is important to reinforce any discussions of secondary drug use, especially those that focus on its harmful consequence or the client's need to decrease his or her secondary substance use. This means being vigilant for any mention of secondary use, supportive when the client discusses this, and tailoring your response to the client's level of readiness to change. For example, consider the following two ways of responding to a client's report of drinking at the start of a session:

Scenario 1

Client: It was tough for me to get here today. I was drinking last night and I had too much and I feel really sick today.

Therapist: Your drinking is a real problem. We talk a lot about your goal drug, but you need to stop drinking too.

Client: It was a one-time thing. I had too much last night but I don't usually do that. My drinking is fine.

Scenario 2

Client: It was tough for me to get here today. I was drinking last night and I had too much and I feel really sick today.

Therapist: I'm glad you were able to make it here today. Thank you for the effort—you add a lot to the group and I appreciate you getting here even when you're not feeling so good. It sounds like your drinking left you feeling pretty bad today. Tell me about that.

Client: I woke up with a sick feeling in my stomach and a really bad headache. I still have a headache actually and I feel wiped out. I have a lot to do today and all I want to do is go home and go to sleep.

Therapist: Wow, that sounds pretty bad. And on the one hand you have things to get done today and one of your goals has been keeping up with things like getting to all your appointments and not missing things. On the other hand you feel sick and this might get in the way of you keeping your appointments. What are you going to do?

Client: Well, I'm going to make sure that when I have a lot to do, I don't drink the night before.

Therapist: That's an excellent idea! If you plan ahead, you can plan to not drink the night before you have important things to do. Good thinking! How about if we work that into your goal setting today? Your main goal can be to continue to stay clean from cocaine—a goal you have been doing a great job with. How about a smaller goal of not drinking the night before those days when you have a lot to do. Which days between now and the next session do you have a lot to do?

In scenario 2, by being empathic and reinforcing, the therapist evoked a suggestion for reduced use from the client rather than suggesting it to him. This then provided something for the therapist to strongly reinforce and work into the framework of the BTSAS session.

Be Gently Persistent Where Appropriate

Within the reinforcing and positive tone that is the hallmark of BTSAS, the therapist can make it clear that he or she is going to be persistent and continue to bring up the client's secondary substance use. This can be done by gently checking in about the client's secondary use during goal setting or during another section of the session ("You were clean for your goal drug today! That's great! You are up to $3.50 now—congratulations! What was your marijuana use like since our last group?"). Timing is everything here: for a client who is new to the program and having enough difficulty focusing on her goal drug, talk of a secondary drug can wait. In contrast, a client who has been in the program for a while and seen improvement with use of his goal drug is a better candidate for brief and gentle reminders of the need to pay some attention to his other drugs of abuse. The therapist should communicate that the reason for this persistence is genuine concern about the client rather than any need for the client to be abstinent to remain in treatment or to avoid punishment. For example:

Therapist: OK Sue, let's set up your role-play. You said that you need to practice saying no to your boyfriend, and that he brings drugs to your apartment and wants to use with you in your apartment.

Client 1: Yeah, he brings the drugs and we use them together. Since I'm trying to have clean urines for crack, now when he comes over he smokes the crack and I smoke some weed.

Therapist: So you have been able to tell him that you don't want to use crack. That's great! You have really made some changes in your crack use and you have had clean urines for crack for a few weeks now. Great work! The thing that concerns me though is that he is there with the crack and that if you smoke weed, you might be less good at using your drug refusal skills and wind up smoking crack. Has that ever happened to anyone here—you used some other drug and using that drug led you to use your goal drug?

Client 2: That happens to me. When I drink I wind up using crack. If I want to stop using crack, I can't drink because when I drink I go out and look for the crack and if I find it I use it.

Therapist: What do you think about that Sue?

Client 1: I don't know.

Therapist: My concern is that you are doing such a great job with using your drug refusal skills, and I don't want anything to get in the way of you refusing to use crack with your boyfriend because you are working really hard to achieve your goal of stopping your use of crack. So let's do a role-play and practice you telling your boyfriend that you don't want to use anything today. Since he has the drugs on him and wants to use in your apartment, how would you feel about telling him to come back when he doesn't have drugs? Would he do that?

Client 1: It would be OK I guess. If I told him I didn't want him to do crack in my apartment, he would try to get me to let him in.

Therapist: What could you tell him that would make him understand that you don't want to use?

Client 1: I could say that I need to have a clean urine.

Therapist: Excellent idea! So first you make eye contact and then you tell him that you don't want to use any drugs. Then you could tell him that you are trying to have a clean urine. That's a great reason!

Other Strategies

A few other strategies should be kept in mind. There is a session in the *relapse prevention* section of the BTSAS program on "Other Drugs of Abuse." This session can be done at a different time in the program if it is particularly relevant to a group of clients, or could be repeated if needed during the optional sessions at the end of the program. In addition, if a client's secondary use turns into abuse or dependence, or poly-substance dependence becomes too problematic to be handled in the context of an outpatient group treatment program, the BTSAS therapist should work with the mental health treatment team to refer the client to a more intensive program. This is especially true in cases in which the poly-substance use or any attempt to stop use is life-threatening or puts the client at extremely high risk for harm (frequent IV heroin use, attempts to stop drinking in the context of high risk for severe withdrawal symptoms).

CRISIS SITUATIONS AND BTSAS

BTSAS is designed to provide substance abuse treatment to dually diagnosed SPMI clients as one component of a multifaceted mental health service that includes psychiatric medication and follow-up, counseling, and general case management or social work services as needed. As such, it is important for BTSAS therapists to link with the rest of a client's treatment team and to work with the other professionals on that team in order to provide complete service to a client. This collaboration of substance abuse and mental health service providers is necessary due to the many severe and overlapping problems that these clients tend to bring to the treatment setting. In no situation is this need for partnership more clear than when a SPMI client experiences some sort of crisis. By crisis, we are referring to a relatively sudden and intense situation that is able and likely to have an extremely negative outcome, such as psychiatric decompensation or relapse, becoming homeless, or becoming lost to treatment. Dually diagnosed SPMI clients may experience crises for a range of reasons. The more frequent crises we have encountered in our work with this population include: loss of housing due to continued drug use, termination from mental health treatment due to continued drug use, and drug withdrawal and the need for more intensive drug treatment services.

Loss of Housing Due to Continued Drug Use

In our dually diagnosed SPMI population living in inner-city Baltimore, loss of housing due to continued drug use is a frequent problem. In BTSAS, we have a firm commitment to harm reduction, and we encourage clients to attend groups even if they are actively using drugs. However, many supervised housing programs, community residences, and government-funded therapeutic living situations often require clients to be abstinent and will immediately force clients to leave who are found using drugs. In addition, most temporary housing options, such as short-term shelters and other programs that will provide housing for up to several weeks, also require clients to commit to not using drugs, and will refuse to take clients who are known or recently drug users. For example, many temporary housing programs require 28 to 30 days with no drug use or a clean urinalysis for entry. These sorts of requirements can be impossible for many active users with SPMI. We have had many clients relapse, lose housing, and become homeless within days, initiating a downward spiral of treatment dropout, failure to take medication, and decompensation of symptoms that leads to dropping out of the BTSAS program and other mental health treatment.

Several strategies can help a BTSAS therapist assist a client who is experiencing a housing crisis. First, know the housing options in your area and establish contact with them when you set up your BTSAS program. This contact should involve the BTSAS therapist visiting the housing program, meeting the staff, and presenting the BTSAS model, goals, and philosophy to the program. Establishing this contact will help in the event a BTSAS client faces an acute need for housing—knowing a program and the program professionals knowing you and your program can only help a referral move more quickly and efficiently. Second, make sure the client understands that you are available to help him or her in the event of a housing crisis. Let the client know that you are connected with several housing programs, and if he or she needs help with housing you will be there to provide it. Third, when a client is referred to the BTSAS program, talk with his or her treatment team about housing and options for the client in the event of a housing crisis. If the team has thought about this as a potential issue and devised a plan of action, it can only help in terms of solving a problem during the heat of a crisis.

Termination from Mental Health Treatment Due to Continued Drug Use

Like housing programs, many treatment centers that serve SPMI clients require abstinence and will terminate clients from psychiatric treatment if they miss sessions due to drug use or are using and so are failing to comply with treatment recommendations. Clinics have reasons for upholding this policy, including that to continue a client in treatment when he or she is actively using sends the wrong message and makes it seem as though the clinic is condoning the drug use. In BTSAS, we take all eligible clients who want to participate, even those who are actively using. There will be times when a client's use is too severe to treat on a bi-weekly outpatient basis, and then the BTSAS therapist must explore other treatment options. Otherwise, most clients who are actively using are still encouraged to and reinforced for treatment attendance. We have reviewed our reasons for this approach previously in our discussion of harm reduction. The fact that BTSAS encourages active drug users to attend treatment while most other clinics will terminate users from treatment means that the BTSAS therapist needs to have a plan for this sort of situation. In our work with clients in BTSAS, we have had numerous times when clients were either threatened with termination from mental health treatment, or were in fact kicked out of treatment due to use. This situation is, in our experience, uniformly bad for SPMI clients, resulting in dropout from BTSAS, any other treatment, and often a return to heavy drug use. Here again, the BTSAS therapist can plan ahead in several ways to be prepared for this situations. First, the BTSAS therapist should talk with others on the treatment team and in the clinic prior to implementing the BTSAS program and discuss options for clients who are not complying with mental health treatment. If all members of the treatment team and the larger clinic staff understand the BTSAS philosophy, it is likely that some guidelines can be implemented that can deter termination from mental health treatment. For example, guidelines for recognizing clients who are at risk for missing too many clinic appointments could be developed such that the BTSAS therapist and the rest of the treatment team starts to problem solve with the client long before the situation becomes critical. In addition, there could be an agreed-upon number of appointments that a client would have to miss before being terminated from the mental health clinic, so that standards would not differ across clinicians. It is also important to establish with the mental health treatment program what is the minimum amount of treatment a client can attend without being terminated from the program. Oftentimes a client is scheduled for two or three appointments in a week (such as individual sessions and groups), but attendance at only one would be sufficient to keep the client's case active. This information can be used to help a client succeed at attending one session, with the number of sessions increasing over time.

Second, there are many tools with the BTSAS program that can be utilized to improve a client's attendance at mental health services. For example, the BTSAS therapist can use BTSAS participation as leverage to help clients get to other clinic appointments by scheduling these appointments immediately after a BTSAS group and escorting the client to the appointment once the BTSAS session ends. In addition, attendance at clinic appointments can be the focus of goal setting within BTSAS sessions, which allows the client and BTSAS therapist to do in-depth problem solving around attendance and potential solutions. This is useful in that the client will often tell the BTSAS therapist the reasons for his or her nonattendance at clinic appointments, and many times the reasons are fairly practical or reasonable and can be easily solved. We have had clients who were unable to make clinic appointments early in the morning but kept having their appointments scheduled for early in the morning. By focusing on this issue in goal setting, the client and therapist developed a role-play around talking to the counselor about changing the time of the appointment, and the client then practiced this role-play in preparation for having the actual conversation with his or her mental health service provider. The BTSAS therapist can also provide outreach in the form of phone calls reminding clients of their clinic appointments and helping clients to problem solve barriers to attendance during these phone calls.

Third, the BTSAS therapist must make sure the client knows that BTSAS participation does not have to end if the client relapses or is at risk for termination from his or her mental health treatment. This is a good point to make at the start of treatment, as well as during treatment if a client is struggling with use and attendance at mental health treatment. Many SPMI clients, having been terminated from treatment before for their use, will not realize that BTSAS attendance is not dependent on abstinence.

Drug Withdrawal or Need for More Intensive Drug Treatment

There will be times when clients experience symptoms of drug withdrawal, or when a client's substance use is simply too severe to be effectively treated within a twice per week outpatient program. Some clients require inpatient care for their substance use disorders. As with the other crises we have reviewed, it is always better to be informed ahead of time and to have a plan to cope with withdrawal or the need for more intensive treatment. First, it is critical that the BTSAS therapist know and be able to recognize common withdrawal symptoms for different drugs of abuse so that he or she will immediately know when drug withdrawal is becoming a problem. Clients should be informed that drug withdrawal can be dangerous, and that any large scale decreases or termination in use should be discussed in the group and with members of his or her mental health treatment team. This discussion should be done in a positive and reinforcing way, given that at its core it is about a client wanting to make a positive change in drug use. In addition, knowing when a client needs more treatment than BTSAS can provide is also critical. Cues such as a client attending BTSAS sessions high or intoxicated and persistent daily or heavy use, despite BTSAS participation, suggest that a client is unable to refrain from use for even a brief period of time. If he or she is unable to attend some sessions without using, it is unlikely that BTSAS can have any real impact, and suggests that the client needs a greater level of care. Second, the BTSAS therapist must know the procedures in the clinic for referring a client for detoxification, as well as how and where to admit clients to inpatient or intensive outpatient substance abuse treatment. This information can be a bit tricky and depends on a client's health insurance or lack thereof, and it is important that the BTSAS therapist know in advance of a client's participation in the process for making a referral, and the eligible programs to refer to if this is necessary. Finally, the clients should know at the start that referral to another program may be an option under certain circumstances. BTSAS is done with a collaborative spirit; informing clients up front of what they can expect can only make it easier to talk about referrals and to implement them if they are needed.

SUMMARY

The structure of BTSAS and its reinforcing qualities make it easier than many other treatments to implement successfully. However, problems still occur and some individuals are not appropriate group participants at certain times. This is especially true when they are pressured to come by clinicians, family members, or the court system. This chapter addressed several common problems, including helping members adapt to the structure and strategies of BTSAS, as well as ways of dealing with members who continue to use drugs. We also reviewed crisis situations that can arise, such as loss of housing, removal from other clinical services, and drug withdrawal symptoms.

Chapter **13**

IMPLEMENTING BTSAS IN CLINIC SETTINGS: STRATEGIES AND POTENTIAL MODIFICATIONS

Since the mid-1980s, researchers have discussed the importance of transporting empirically supported treatments from the research supported university setting into community settings. For a variety of reasons, the rate of transfer of innovative evidenced based treatments has been very slow (Addis, 2002). The U.S. Surgeon General (2000) found that the majority of clients with severe mental illness do not receive evidence-based treatments. Other research suggests that treatment interventions with an abundance of research support are not practiced widely in community settings (Goisman, Warshaw, & Keller, 1999). One reason cited for this slow dissemination is the insistence by treatment developers on complete adherence to a manual or treatment protocol (Wiltsey Stirman, Crits-Christoph, & DeRubeis, 2004). Typically manuals offer no suggestions for how to modify or adapt treatments to better fit into the realities of community settings. This chapter outlines potential adaptations and modifications of the BTSAS treatment as well as strategies for implementing this empirically supported treatment.

POSSIBLE ADAPTATIONS AND MODIFICATIONS

Innovative mental health interventions often target a specific problem or particular psychiatric diagnosis. From a community mental health perspective, however, implementing an intervention that targets only one segment of their treatment population may be considered irrelevant or inefficient given the variability of diagnostic profiles found in these settings.

Diagnostically Homogenous vs. Heterogenous Groups

Though our treatment was developed for people with schizophrenia, the treatment philosophy and teaching techniques and strategies would clearly benefit people with other serious and persistent mental illnesses and co-occurring substance use disorders. Consequently, in our randomized clinical trial, we chose to expand our group to include people with other types of serious and persistent mental illnesses in order to evaluate the broader applicability of the treatment. The outcome data from this trial indicate that the treatment is quite effective at impacting substance behavior in a broader population of consumers. Given this, providing the group treatment to people with a variety of serious and persistent mental illnesses is a legitimate modification. We do, however, have certain guidelines and recommendations regarding the selection of group participants.

First, we recommend that BTSAS groups include only consumers with DSM-IV Axis I psychiatric diagnoses, such as schizophrenia, schizoaffective disorder, bipolar disorder, and recurrent major depression(American Psychiatric Association, 2000). The treatment was not designed to treat people with substance use disorders who have severe Axis II psychiatric disorders, such as borderline personality disorder. Furthermore, the serious and persistent component of the mental illness is critical in that it indicates a predetermined level of disability resulting from mental illness. For example, to be eligible for the group it might be required that in addition to an Axis I psychiatric diagnosis that all participants also be receiving Social Security benefits for psychiatric disability and have been unemployed for more than one year as a result of their mental illness. The number of previous psychiatric hospitalizations is also frequently used to determine the severity and persistence of a mental illness.

A second recommendation is to have group members be compatible on important behavioral dimensions in order to enable the group to run smoothly and help individuals feel comfortable. For example, it would not be advisable to place a person with major depression in a group of four to five people with chronic schizophrenia who have primarily negative symptoms and poor hygiene. If you are putting together a group with a mixture of Axis I psychiatric diagnoses, it is important to consider level of functioning, verbal ability, and ability to focus. Obviously, given the nature of serious and persistent mental illness, symptoms and level of functioning will vary over time. The overall goal, however, is to have the group members be as compatible as possible on important behavioral measures.

Group Size

The optimal group size is four to six patients. This relatively small size maximizes the possibility that each participant has the opportunity to repeatedly practice the social skill targeted during the group session as well as enabling the cotherapists to repeatedly check in with participants to ensure they understand what is being discussed. It may not be practical, however, from a management point of view to have two therapists occupied twice per week for 90 minutes to work with only four to six patients. To help address this, the group size could be expanded to six to eight patients. More than eight members, however, would make it very difficult to involve group members in the series of role-plays required for effective social skills treatment.

Managed Care Limitations on Number of Sessions Per Week

A second major obstacle for clinics in implementing evidenced-based practices is the limits that managed care places on the number of visits per week. Often managed care companies limit the number of therapy sessions (nonmedication visits) to 24 per year. With sound clinical argument, a therapist might be able to increase the number of authorized visits to one per week for a year. Our treatment, however, was designed to occur twice weekly for 90 minutes for six months. This level of structure and consistency allows for sufficient repetition of necessary skills and information to impact substance use behavior in this population. If managed care refuses authorization for 48 sessions in six months, the BTSAS treatment can be modified in the following manner. First, the treatment could be offered one time per week for 12 months as opposed to two times per week for six months. This is not an optimal form of the treatment, but it may be the only option in certain community settings. Down sides to offering group once a week are the reduced opportunity to closely monitor drug use (e.g., urine analysis would only occur once per week) and problem solve regarding strategies for managing triggers, cravings, and urges to use. Obviously, the greater the exposure to positive support the better the chances are that group members will be able to modify their drug use behaviors. To compensate for this, group members could be asked to come in for brief check-ins to both provide a urine analysis as well as to enable the therapist to provide support and strategies for reducing or maintaining drug free behavior.

A second way to modify treatment is to maintain the six-month duration of the treatment, but reduce the content or material covered. Although the social skills training section needs to remain intact, the Education and Coping Skills section as well as the Problem Solving Relapse Prevention section could be modified. For example, in the Education and Coping Skills section, the sessions on HIV and hepatitis C could be removed. If the majority of group members do not have schizophrenia, the educational session covering the interaction between drugs/alcohol and schizophrenia could be eliminated. To adjust for this change in curriculum, therapists could provide handouts to group members that simply and clearly discuss the interaction between illicit substances and prescribed medication and the impact of illicit substances on psychiatric symptomatology. Individual therapists or case managers could be asked to review this information with their patients during their individual sessions.

Other adaptations might include a reduction in the number of topics covered in the PS/RP section. We have proposed and outlined nine topics for this segment of the BTSAS treatment. Therapists could identify or select one or two of these topics that are particularly relevant to their clinic population as opposed to covering all nine of the proposed topics.

One Therapist as Opposed to Two

It is preferable that social skills groups be conducted by two leaders because it is challenging for one person to teach the skills, set the pace, and maintain control of the group on a continuing basis. In addition, the use of coleaders can greatly facilitate the demonstration and modeling of new skills, as well as aid in the coaching of clients during role-plays. However, a practical reality is that clinics will not be able to provide two therapists to run the treatment. It may be too costly for underresourced clinics to have two therapists occupied with one group. For meeting this challenge we offer the following suggestions.

If clinics are affiliated with a teaching institution or have access to students, one possibility is to recruit a student or trainee as a cotherapist. Possibilities include nursing students, psychiatry residents, psychology and social work interns, psychology graduate students looking for more clinical experience prior to internship application. It would also be worth considering master's level students who are interested in applying for their doctorate in clinical psychology and would like to have more clinical experience to bolster their applications. The trainees would not be financially compensated for their time, but would receive training in the application of an evidence-based treatment as well as have exposure to a clinical population.

Alternatively, a relatively high functioning consumer with significant clean time could be recruited as an assistant. This person could help with the practical issues of running the group such as collecting the urines, helping with the flipchart, modeling the skill for the group, and participating in the role-plays as the confederate. Benefits of using a consumer as an assistant are the exposure of group members to a consumer role-model and the empowerment of a consumer with skills and responsibility for helping others—which will positively contribute to his or her sense of self and recovery.

Consumer assistants, however, need to be carefully selected. Particular attention needs to be given to the relationship the consumer has or may have over time with group members. For example, do group members attend or have the potential to attend other groups with this consumer? Is there overlap or the potential for overlap in housing situations? Optimally, this person needs to be relatively unknown to group members in order to help prevent relational difficulties or dual roles developing both outside and inside of group.

If there is no other alternative but to have one therapist running the group, she will have to very deliberately select individuals for group who are not likely to present with disruptive behaviors, are psychiatrically stable, and easy to manage. To help facilitate the demonstration of role-plays, she will have to demonstrate the target skill, provide coaching of clients during the role-play, and set the pace of the group, in addition to the practical issues of collecting urines and assigning homework. This will be demanding but not impossible. To ease the burden, the group size could be limited to four members as opposed to six.

STRATEGIES FOR IMPLEMENTING THE BTSAS INTO COMMUNITY CLINICS

A common approach to implementing new treatments into clinical settings is to present staff with the positive outcomes associated with the treatment (Torrey, Drake, Dixon, Burns, Flynn, & Rush, 2001). This approach has worked effectively for pharmaceutical companies, but has been less successful with the dissemination of psychosocial or behavioral treatments. A better strategy is the "knowledge utilization method," in which treatments are promoted more actively and transported by identifying and addressing organizational barriers to adoption and detailed discussion with various stakeholders (Wiltsey Stirman et al., 2004).

Integration into Clinic Services

All models of dissemination emphasize the necessity of careful planning because of the challenges associated with introducing change into existing organizational structures and cultures. The planning phase itself involves assessment of the community setting or target system and securing collaboration with administrators and therapists. The attitude of members of the target system, resources available to support the new treatment, and the needs of the community mental health setting are all important factors to consider. For example, both clinicians and administrators need to feel that the treatment would benefit a large number of their consumers. Given the pervasiveness of substance abuse among seriously and persistently mentally ill individuals this is rarely a problem. Several researchers advise conducting a readiness analysis to help identify any obstacles that may interfere with the adoption of the new treatment (Backer, 1995, 2000; Lehman, Greener, & Simpson, 2002). A readiness analysis typically involves the assessment of the motivation to change among staff and administrators, adequacy of resources to support the treatment (e.g., staff time), and the organizational climate (e.g., the extent to which employees view the work environment as positive and beneficial), all of which will impact the delivery of a new intervention (Lehman et al., 2002). Paper and pencil assessments are available to facilitate this analysis (Backer, 1995; Lehman et al., 2002).

The successful implementation of a new treatment such as BTSAS is often influenced by how the decision is made to adopt the intervention. There is evidence to suggest that mandates, or "top-down" decisions to adopt made solely by administrators, lead to faster, but less successfully sustained dissemination (Backer, Liberman, & Kuehnel, 1986; Henggeler, Schoenwald, Liao, Letourneau, & Edwards, 2002). In part, the tendency toward "mandate drift" may be due to the perception of staff that the administrators are indifferent to their needs and day-to-day realities. Clinicians may resent having treatment strategies imposed upon them by administrators who may be seen as lacking clinical expertise. Collective decisions are less susceptible to this type of resistance, but the decision process will generally require more time, as individuals within the agency will need to be consulted in the decision process (Rogers, 1995; Wiltsey Stirman et al., 2004).

As mentioned previously, what is advised in the dissemination theories is the use of a task force, advisory board, or planning committee that involves all stakeholders, including, if possible, consumers, mental health practitioners, and agency heads. Torrey and colleagues (2002) found that the involvement of such stakeholders was critical to the successful implementation of integrated dual diagnosis treatment (IDDT; Drake et al., 2001) and significantly helps overcome therapist reluctance.

Working with Mental Health Professionals

It is critical to build the treatment into the clinical service structure. BTSAS was designed to be an integral part of community mental health service systems, not simply as an add on therapy such as a wellness group or a medication management group. As such, the point of referral for consumers ideally should come at intake and it is essential to establish a collaborative relationship with professionals and agencies involved in the day-to-day treatment of clients participating in a social skills group.

Establishing relationships with other professionals is a rewarding but not always easy task. It requires patience, flexibility, and commitment on the part of the leaders. In many cases, the integration of social skills training into a hospital setting, day treatment program, or supervised living situation requires a formal orientation of the staff to the program. As with the introduction of any new therapeutic intervention, it is not unusual for there to be some resistance or suspicion on the part of the staff. The leaders must address directly any discomforts or concerns that may arise among the staff members and work toward building enthusiasm among them for the skills training approach.

The leaders should explain how social skills training and the techniques involved can be useful not only in addressing clients' skill deficits, but also in helping staff members respond to clients' problematic behaviors. It is also helpful for group leaders to have an idea of what problems the staff members are currently experiencing in working with the clients and then be able to explain how skills training can be used to specifically address those problems. In addition to substance use, some common problems facing staff at community residences include frequent arguments among the clients and refusal to do chores or to take prescribed medication. These problems, although common, make the staff's job more stressful and any resistance in managing them is usually well received.

There are many ways that group leaders can orient staff members to the philosophy and principles of social skills training. A copy of chapter 3 in this book, which covers our treatment philosophy, would provide detailed information. Workshops outlining the principles of behavioral training and social skills techniques offer an interactive and efficient way to provide information to the staff.

Group leaders should also remain in contact with the staff through regularly scheduled meetings. Attending weekly treatment team meetings is ideal. The group leaders can use this meeting as a way to monitor what is happening outside of group as well as provide staff members with information as to what topics or skills are being covered in the weekly group sessions. It gives group therapists the opportunity to hear about medication changes and to discuss any observed changes in symptom levels or patterns during group. Treatment team members can be helpful to BTSAS therapists by giving them information regarding the emergence of any stressful life events in the consumer's world. For instance, if a client has recently moved into a new housing situation and has a roommate who listens to very loud music, having the client actually practice in group asking the roommate to turn down the music would be quite helpful and reinforce skill acquisition and generalization. The more relevant the skills you teach are to the person's immediate life, the more likely the skills will be utilized and practiced outside of group.

A common question typically asked by other mental health professionals is how BTSAS integrates with other substance abuse treatment groups such as AA, NA, or double trouble groups. It is important to explain to staff members that BTSAS is not meant to replace self-help groups such as these, but should be viewed as an additional treatment intervention. A pitfall to be aware of is when different substance abuse treatment philosophies exist between BTSAS therapists, staff members, or agencies. For example, staff members may not accept a harm reduction model. Housing or treatment programs may have a policy to discharge individuals who relapse at any given time (e.g., one strike and you are out). If this is the case, we suggest that group therapists request that while individuals are engaged in the BTSAS group that they be contacted in advance of individuals being discharged so that proactive planning may occur around securing alternative care or housing. In situations such as this, it is critical to develop a close and collaborative relationship with individuals' case managers. Providing staff members with articles or information supporting the use of a harm reduction model might help move them along the continuum of change toward greater acceptance of this model.

Covering Costs

Clinical trials and treatment development are well supported by federal research dollars, which makes it easier to cover costs for urine analysis contingencies, snacks and graduation party supplies, therapist training, ongoing supervision by experts in the field, and even therapist time. To help overcome this potential obstacle, we offer several strategies.

Vouchers or coupons for donated merchandise from local retailers can be used in place of money as a reward for urine analysis contingencies. Often times when local retailers, food or restaurant chains (e.g., Wal-Mart, Target, Subway, grocery stores, or smaller clothing stores) are approached by clinic staff or management for donated merchandise coupons to support an innovative project aimed at helping people in their community be drug free, they are more than happy to contribute. To increase the intrinsic value of the coupons, clinics might want to informally survey the patients to determine which retailers are more appealing and practical in terms of location. For example, staff might assume that coupons from Wal-Mart would be appealing, but consumers may have difficulty getting there by bus or feel overwhelmed by the size, and thus prefer a different and perhaps smaller, more manageable retailer.

Potential merchandise donors can be approached in person or by letter. If the decision is to approach them in person, bring a brief description of the project with you for them to keep. Make sure to have your contact information on this letter. In-person contact can be effective in that you can answer any questions the retailer may have regarding the project and its participants. On the other hand, mailing out letters is more efficient and enables one to solicit donations from many retailers simultaneously. Letters should be on clinic stationary and again, a description of the project and how the donated vouchers will be used should be included.

A possible strategy for securing funding for larger ticket items such as staff training, the purchase of manuals, and ongoing supervision is to respond to requests for applications offered by private foundation funding sources. Both national and local private foundations are often interested in contributing to community programs aimed at helping people get off drugs and alcohol—particularly those that target at risk populations. These applications are often only two to three pages in length and can provide anywhere from $1,000 to $50,000 in support. The downside to securing funds externally is that the money is only provided for one or two years. However, such funds might help pay for staff training, cost for manuals, and ongoing supervision for a year. These types of costs occur in the first couple of years of implementation. A good resource for identifying requests for applications is http://www. fdncenter.org/pnd/rfp/.

Another strategy to cover costs is to work on a community, state, or nationwide level by becoming involved in initiatives to provide evidenced-based treatments to mental health consumers. For example, several states, including Hawaii (Chorpita et al., 2002), Ohio (Biegel et al., 2003), Oregon (Chamberlain, 2003), New Hampshire and Maryland (Goldman et al., 2001), have begun such initiatives. In fact, agencies such as NIMH, the U.S. Substance Abuse and Mental Health Services Administrations (SAMHSA), and private foundations currently provide funding to states that are willing to adopt evidenced-base practices. Hence, partnering with state departments of mental health to promote and study the adoption of evidenced-based practices can ensure the availability of the funding to provide the infrastructure and training necessary for sustained adoption (Goldman, et al., 2001). Obviously, this is a time-consuming strategy;however, if it is successful it provides the most comprehensive and long term support for treatment implementation.

SUMMARY

This summary identifies for treatment providers and community mental health managers potential adaptations and modifications of the BTSAS treatment that might facilitate the transportation of this treatment into outpatient community settings. Possible strategies for implementing and adopting BTSAS into treatment services systems were described as well. Specifically, ideas for working with staff and covering costs were offered. Implementing innovative and manual based interventions into overworked and underresourced community settings can be an enormous challenge. Our goal was to offer individuals useful ideas for implementing our treatment.

REFERENCES

Addington, J., & el-Guebaly, N. (1998). Group treatment for substance abuse in schizophrenia. *Canadian Journal of Psychiatry, 43*(8), 843–845.

Addis, M. E. (2002). Methods for disseminating research products and increasing evidence-based practice: promises, obstacles, and future directions. *Clinical Psychology: Science and Practice, 9*(4), 367–368.

Albanese, M. J., Bartel, R. L., Bruno, R. F., Morgenbesser, M. W., & Schatzberg, A. F. (1994). Comparison of measures used to determine substance abuse in an inpatient psychiatric sample. *American Journal of Psychiatry, 151*(7), 1077–1078.

American Psychiatric Association. (1994). *Diagnostic and statistical manual of mental disorders* (4th Ed., DSM-IV). Washington, DC: Author.

American Psychiatric Association. (2000). *Diagnostic and statistical manual of mental disorders* (4th Ed., Text Rev., DSM-IV). Washington, DC: Author.

Annis, H. M., & Davis, C. S. (1989). Relapse prevention. In R. K. Hester & W. R. Miller (Eds.), *Handbook of alcoholism treatment approaches* (pp. 170–182). New York: Pergamon.

Appleby, L., Dyson, V., Altman, E., & Luchins, D. J. (1997). Assessing substance use in multiproblem patients: Reliability and validity of the Addiction Severity Index in a mental hospital population. *Journal of Nervous and Mental Disease, 185*(3), 159–165.

Appleby, L., Dyson, V., Altman, E., McGovern, M. P., & Luchins, D. J. (1996). Utility of the Chemical Use, Abuse, and Dependence scale in screening patients with severe mental illness. *Psychiatric Services, 47*(6), 647–649.

Backer, T. (1995). Assessing and enhancing readiness for change: Implications for technological transfer. In T. Backer, S. David, & D. Soucy (Eds.), *Reviewing the behavioral science knowledge base on technology transfer* (pp. 21–41). (NIDA Research Monograph 155, NIDA publication No. 95-4035). Rockville, MD: National Institute on Drug Abuse.

Backer, T. (2000). The failure of success: Challenges of disseminating effective substance abuse prevention programs. *Journal of Community Psychology, 28,* 363–373.

Backer, T., Liberman, R. P., & Kuehnel, T. G. (1986). Dissemination and adoption of innovative psychosocial interventions. *Journal of Consulting and Clinical Psychology, 54,* 111–118.

Baker, A., Boggs, T. G., & Lewin, T. J. (2001). Randomized controlled trial of brief cognitive-behavioural interventions among regular users of amphetamine. *Addiction, 96,* 1279–1287.

Bandura, A. (1969). *Principles of behavior modification*. New York: Holt, Rinehart, & Winston.

Barrowclough, C., Haddock, G., Tarrier, N., Lewis, S., Moring, J., O'Brien, R., et al (2001). Randomized controlled trial of motivational interviewing, cognitive behavior therapy, and family intervention for patients with comorbid schizophrenia and substance use disorders. *American Journal of Psychiatry, 158,* 1706–1713.

Bellack, A. S. (2004). Skills training for people with severe mental illness. *Psychiatric Rehabilitation Journal, 27,* 375–391.

Bellack, A. S., Bennett, M. E., Gearon, J. S., Brown, C. H., & Yang, Y. (2006). A randomized clinical trial of a new behavioral treatment for drug abuse in people with severe and persistent mental illness. *Archives of General Psychiatry, 63,* 426–532.

Bellack, A. S., & Blanchard, J. J. (1993). Schizophrenia: Psychopathology. In A. S. Bellack & M. Hersen (Eds.), *Psychopathology in adulthood: An advanced tex* (pp. 216–233). Needham, MA: Allyn & Bacon.

Bellack, A. S., & DiClemente, C. C. (1999). Treating substance abuse among patients with schizophrenia. *Psychiatric Services. 50,* 75–80.

Bellack, A. S., & Gearon J. S. (1998). Substance abuse treatment for people with schizophrenia. *Addictive Behaviors, 6,* 749–766.

Bellack, A. S., Gold, J. M., & Buchanan, R. W. (1999). Cognitive rehabilitation for schizophrenia: problems, prospects, and strategies. *Schizophrenia Bulletin, 25*(2), 257–274.

Bellack, A. S., Mueser, K. T., Gingerich, S., & Agresta, J. (1997). (Eds.). *Social skills training for schizophrenia: A step-by-step guide*. New York: Guilford.

Bellack, A. S., Mueser, K. T., Gingerich, S., & Agresta, J. (2004). *Social skills training for schizophrenia: A step-by-step guide* (2nd ed.). New York: Guilford.

Bennett, M. E., & Barnett, B. (2003). Dual-diagnosis. In M. Hersen & S. M. Turner (Eds.), *Adult psychopathology and diagnosis* (4th ed., pp. 36–71). New York: Wiley.

Bergman, H. C., & Harris, M. (1985). Substance abuse among young adult chronic patients. *Psychological Rehabilitation Journal, 9,* 49–54.

Biegel, D., Kola, L., Ronis, R., Boyle, P., Delos Reyes, C., & Wieder, B. (2003). The Ohio substance abuse and mental illness coordinating center of excellence: Implementation support for evidenced based practice. *Research on Social Work Practice, 13,* 531–545.

Bien, T. H., Miller, W. R., & Tonigan, J. S. (1993). Brief interventions for alcohol problems: A review. *Addiction, 88,* 315–336.

Breakey, W. R., Calabrese, L., Rosenblatt, A., & Crum, R. M. (1998). Detecting alcohol use disorders in the severely mentally ill. *Community Mental Health Journal, 34*(2), 165–174.

Carbonari, J. P., DiClemente, C. C., & Zweben, A. (1994). *A readiness to change scale: Its development, validation and usefulness.* Presented at the annual meeting of the AABT, San Diego, CA.

Carey, K. B., Carey, M. P., Maisto, S. A., & Purnine, D. M. (2002). The feasibility of enhancing psychiatric outpatients' readiness to change their substance use. *Psychiatric Services, 53,* 602–608.

Carey, K. B., Cocco, K. M., & Correia, C. J. (1997). Reliability and validity of the Addiction Severity Index among outpatients with severe mental illness. *Psychological Assessment, 9*(4), 422–428.

Carey, K. B., & Correia, C. J. (1998). Severe mental illness and addictions: Assessment considerations. *Addictive Behaviors, 23*(6), 735–748.

Carey, M. P., Carey, K. B., & Kalichman, S. C. (1997). Risk for human immunodeficiency virus (HIV) infection among persons with severe mental illnesses. *Clinical Psychology Review, 17,* 271–291.

Carroll, K. M., Power, M. E. D., Bryant, K., & Rounsaville, B. J. (1993). One-year follow-up status of treatment-seeking cocaine abusers: Psychopathology and dependence severity as predictors of outcome. *Journal of Nervous and Mental Disease, 181,* 71–79.

Carroll, K. M., Rounsaville, B. J., & Gawin, F. H. (1991). A comparative trial of psychotherapies for ambulatory cocaine abusers: Relapse prevention and interpersonal psychotherapy. *American Journal of Drug and Alcohol Abuse, 17,* 229–247.

Chamberlain P. (2003). *Treating chronic juvenile offenders: Advances made through the Oregon multidimensional treatment foster case model. Law and public policy.* Washington, DC: American Psychological Association.

Chiauzzi, E. J. (1991). *Preventing relapse in the addictions: A biopsychosocial approach.* New York: Pergamon.

Chorpita, B. F., Yim, L. M., Donkervoet, J. C., Arensdorf, A., Amundsen, M. J., & McGee, C. (2002). Toward large scaled implementation of empirically supported treatment for children: A review and observations by the Hawaii Empirical Basis to Services Task Force. *Clinical Psychology: Science and Practice, 9,* 165–190.

Cocco, K. M., & Carey, K. B. (1998). Psychometric properties of the Drug Abuse Screening Test in psychiatric outpatients. *Psychological Assessment, 10*(4), 408–414.

Corse, S. J., Herschinger, N. B., & Zanis, D. A. (1995). The use of the ASI with persons with severe mental illness: Face validity. *Psychosocial Rehabilitation Journal, 19*(1), 9-18.

Daley, D. C., Salloum, I. M., Zuckoff, A., Kirisci, L., & Thase, M. E. (1998). Increasing treatment adherence among outpatients with depression and cocaine dependence: Results of a pilot study. *American Journal of Psychiatry, 155,* 1611–1613.

Daley, D. C., & Zuckoff, A. (1998). Improving compliance with the initial outpatient session among discharged inpatient dual diagnosis clients. *Social Work, 43,* 470–473.

Dawe, S., Seinen, A., & Kavanagh, D. (2000). An examination of the utility of the AUDIT in people with schizophrenia. *Journal of Studies on Alcohol, 61*(5), 744–750.

DiClemente, C. C., Carbonari, J. P., Montgomery, R. P. G., & Hughes, S. O. (1994). The Alcohol Abstinence Self-Efficacy scale. *Journal of Studies on Alcohol, 55,* 141–148.

DiClemente, C. C., Fairhurst, S. K., & Piotrowski, N. A. (1995). Self-efficacy and addictive behaviors. In J. Maddux (Ed.), *Self-efficacy, adaptation and adjustment: Theory, Research and Application.* New York: Plenum.

DiClemente, C. C., & Hughes, S. O. (1990). Stages of change profiles in outpatient alcoholism treatment. *Journal of Substance Abuse, 2,* 217–235.

Dixon, L. (1999). Dual diagnosis of substance abuse in schizophrenia: Prevalence and impact on outcomes. *Schizophrenia Research, 35,* S93–S100.

Dixon, L., Haas, G., Weiden, P., Sweeney, J., & Frances, A. (1990). Acute effects of drug abuse in schizophrenic patients: Clinical observations and patients' self-reports. *Schizophrenia Bulletin, 16*(1), 69–79.

Drake, R. E., & Bellack, A. S. (2005). Psychiatric rehabilitation. In B. J. Sadock & V. A. Sadock (Eds.), *Kaplan and Sadock's comprehensive textbook of psychiatry* (pp. 1476–1486). Philadelphia: Lippincott, Williams & Wilkins.

Drake, R. E., Essock, S. M., Shaner, A., Carey, K. B., Minkoff, K., Kola, L., Lynde, D., Osher, F. C., Clark, R. E., & Rickards, L. (2001). Implementing dual diagnosis services for clients with severe mental illness. *Psychiatric Services, 52,* 469–476.

Drake, R. E., McHugo, G. J., & Noordsy, D. L. (1993). Treatment of alcoholism among schizophrenic outpatients: 4-year outcomes. *American Journal of Psychiatry, 150,* 328–329.

Drake, R. E., Mueser, K. T., Brunette, M. F., & McHugo, G. J. (2004). A review of treatments for people with severe mental illnesses and co-occurring substance use disorders. *Psychiatric Rehabilitation Journal, 27,* 360–374.

Drake, R. E., Mercer-McFadden, C., Mueser, K. T., McHugo, G.J., & Bond, G.R. (1998). Review of integrated mental health and substance abuse treatment for patients with dual disorders. *Schizophrenia Bulletin, 24,* 589–608.

Drake, R. E., Osher, F. C., Noordsy, D. L., Hurlburt, S. C., Teague, G. B., & Beaudett, M. S. (1990). Diagnosis of alcohol use disorders in schizophrenia. *Schizophrenia Bulletin, 169*(1), 57–67.

Dumaine, M. L. (2003). Meta-analysis of interventions with co-occurring disorders of severe mental illness and substance abuse: Implications for social work practice. *Research on Social Work Practice, 13,* 142–165.

First, M. B., Spitzer, R. L., Gibbon, M., & Williams, J. B. W. (1994). *Structured clinical interview for DSM-IV Axis I disorders.* New York: Biometrics Research Department, New State Psychiatric Institute.

Gearon, J. S., Bellack, A. S., Rachbeisel, J., & Dixon, L. (2001). Drug-use behavior and correlates in people with schizophrenia. *Addictive Behaviors, 26*(1), 51–61.

Gearon, J. S., Kaltman, S. I., Brown, C., & Bellack, A. S. (2003). Traumatic life events and PTSD in substance disordered women with schizophrenia. *Psychiatric Services, 54*, 523–528.

Goisman, R, Warshaw, M., & Keller, M. (1999). Psychosocial treatment prescriptions for generalized anxiety, panic disorder and social phobia, 1991–1996. *American Journal of Psychiatry, 156*, 1819–1821.

Goldman, H., Drake, R., Gorman, P., Hogan, M., Hyde, P., & Morgan, O. (2001). Policy Implications for implementing evidenced-based practices. *Psychiatric Services, 52*, 591–1597.

Grant, B. F., & Harford, T. C. (1995). Comorbidity between DSM-IV alcohol use disorders and major depression: Results of a national survey. *Drug and Alcohol Dependence, 39*, 197–206.

Grella, C. E. (1996). Background and overview of mental health and substance abuse treatment systems: Meeting the needs of women who are pregnant or parenting. *Journal of Psychoactive Drugs, 28*(4), 319–343.

Haddock, G., Barrowclough, C., Tarrier, N., Moring, J., O'Brien, R., Schofield, N. et al. (2003). Cognitive-behavioural therapy and motivational intervention for schizophrenia and substance misuse. 18-month outcomes of a randomized controlled trial. *British Journal of Psychiatry, 183*, 418–426.

Hall, S. M., Wasserman, D. A., & Havassy, B. E. (1991). Relapse prevention. In R.W. Pickens, C. G. Leukefeld, & C. R. Schuster (Eds.), *Improving drug abuse treatment* (pp. 279–292). Rockville, MD: National Institute on Drug Abuse. NIDA Research Monograph No. 106.

Heather, N. (1989). Brief intervention strategies. In R. K. Hester & W. R. Miller (Eds.), *Handbook of alcoholism treatment approaches* (pp. 93–116). New York: Pergamon.

Henggeler, S. W., Schoenwald, S., Liao, J., Letourneau, E., & Edwards, D. (2002). Transporting efficacious treatments to field settings: The link between supervisory practices and therapist fidelity in MST programs. *Journal of Clinical Child and Adolescent Psychology, 31*, 155–167.

Hesse, M. (2006). The Readiness Ruler as a measure of readiness to change poly-drug use in drug abusers. *Harm Reduction Journal, 3*, 1–5.

Higgins, S. T., Alessi, S. M., & Dantona, R .L. (2002) Voucher-based incentives. A substance abuse treatment innovation. *Addictive Behaviors, 27*(6), 887–910.

Jerrell, J. M., & Ridgely, M. R. (1995). Comparative effectiveness of three approaches to serving people with severe mental illness and substance abuse disorders. *Journal of Nervous and Mental Disease, 183*, 566–576.

Kemp, R., Hayward, P., Applewhaite, G., et al. (1996). Compliance therapy in psychotic patients: Randomised controlled trial. *British Medical Journal, 312*, 345–349.

Kemp, R., Kirov, G., Everitt, B., Hayward, P., & David, A. (1998). Randomised controlled trial of compliance therapy: 18-month follow-up. *British Journal of Psychiatry, 172*, 413–419.

LaForge, R. G., Maddock, J. E., & Rossi, J. S. (1999). Replication of the temptations and decisional balance instruments for heavy, episodic drinking on an adult sample [Abstract]. *Annals of Behavioral Medicine, 21*, S67.

Lehman, A. F. (1988). A quality of life interview for the chronically mentally ill. *Evaluation and Program Planning, 11*, 51–62.

Lehman, A. F., Dixon, L.B., Kernan, E., DeForge, B.R., & Postrado, L.T.(1997). A randomized trial of assertive community treatment for homeless persons with severe mental illness. *Archives of General Psychiatry, 54*, 1038–1043.

Lehman, A. F., Kreyenbuhl, J., Buchanan, R.W., Dickerson, F. A., Dixon, L. B., Goldberg, R., et al. (2004). The schizophrenia patient outcomes research team (PORT): Updated treatment recommendations 2003. *Schizophrenia Bulletin, 30*, 193–217.

Lehman, A. F., Myers, C. P., Dixon, L. B., & Johnson, J. L. (1994). Defining subgroups of dual diagnosis patients for service planning. *Hospital and Community Psychiatry, 45*, 556–561.

Lehman, A. F., Myers, C.P., Dixon, L. B., & Johnson, J. L. (1996). Detection of substance use disorders among psychiatric inpatients. *Journal of Nervous and Mental Disease, 184*(4), 228–233.

Lehman, W., Greener, J., & Simpson, D. (2002). Assessing organizational readiness for change. *Journal of Substance Abuse Treatment, 22*, 197–209.

Ley, A., Jeffery, D. P., McLaren, S., & Siegfried, N. (2003). Psychosocial treatment programmes for people with both severe mental illness and substance misuse. *The Cochrane Library, 3*, 1–37.

Lieberman, J. A., Kane, J. M., & Alvir, J. (1987). Provocative tests with psychostimulant drugs in schizophrenia. *Psychopharmacology, 91*, 415–433.

Marlatt, G. A., & Gordon, G. R. (1985). *Relapse prevention: Maintenance strategies in the treatment of addictive behaviors.* New York: Guilford.

Martino, S., Carroll, K. M., O'Malley, S. S., & Rounsaville, B. J. (2000). Motivational interviewing with psychiatrically ill substance abusing patients. *American Journal on Addictions, 9*, 88–91.

McCrady, B. S. (1993). Alcoholism. In D. H. Barlow (Ed.), *Clinical handbook of psychological disorders* (2nd ed., pp. 362–395). New York: Guilford.

McLellan, A. T., Kushner, H., Metzger, D., Peters, R., Smith, I., Grissom, G., et al. (1992). Addiction Severity Index (5th ed.). *Journal of Substance Abuse Treatment, 9*, 199–213.

McLellan, A. T., Luborsky, L., Woody, G. E., & O'Brien, C. P. (1980). An improved diagnostic evaluation instrument for substance abuse patients: The Addiction Severity Index. *Journal of Nervous and Mental Disease, 168*, 26–33.

McLellan, A. T., Luborsky, L., Woody, G. E., O'Brien, C. P., & Druley, K. A. (1983). Predicting response to alcohol and drug abuse treatments. Role of psychiatric severity. *Archives of General Psychiatry, 40*, 620–625.

Meir, V. J., & Hope, D. A. (1998). Assessment of social skills. In A. S. Bellack & M. Hersen (Eds.), *Behavioral assessment* (4th ed., pp. 232–255). Needham Heights, MA: Allyn & Bacon.

Miller, W. R. (1992). The effectiveness of treatment for substance abuse: Reasons for optimism. *Journal of Substance Abuse Treatment, 9*, 93–102.

Miller, W. R. (1995). Increasing motivation for change. In R. K. Hester & W. R. Miller (Eds.), *Handbook of alcoholism treatment approaches: Effective alternatives* (2nd ed., pp. 89–104). Needham Heights, MA: Allyn & Bacon.

Miller, W. R. (2000). Rediscovering fire: Small interventions, large effects. *Psychology of Addictive Behaviors, 14*(1), 6–18.

Miller, W. R, Andrews, N. R., Wilbourne, P., & Bennett, M. E. (1998). A wealth of alternatives: Effective treatments for alcohol problems. In W. R. Miller & N. Heather (Eds.), *Treating addictive behaviors* (2nd ed., pp. 203–216). New York: Plenum Press.

Miller, W. R., Benefield, R. G., & Tonigan, J. S. (1993). Enhancing motivation for change in problem drinking: A controlled comparison of two therapist styles. *Journal of Consulting and Clinical Psychology, 61*(3), 455–461.

Miller, W. R, Brown, J. M., Simpson, T. L., Handmaker, N. S., Bien, T. H., Luckie, L. F., Montgomery, H. A., Hester, R. K., & Tonigan, J. S. (1995). What works? A methodological analysis of the alcohol treatment outcome literature. In R. K. Hester & W. R. Miller (Eds.), *Handbook of alcoholism treatment approaches: Effective alternatives* (2nd ed., pp. 12–44) Needham Heights, MA: Allyn & Bacon.

Miller, W. R., & Heather, N. (1998). (Eds.). *Treating addictive behaviors* (2nd ed.). New York: Plenum Press.

Miller, W. R., & Rollnick, S. (1991). *Motivational interviewing: Preparing people to change addictive behaviors.* New York: Guilford.

Moggi, F., Ouimette, P .C., Finney, J. W., & Moos, R. H. (1999). Effectiveness of treatment for substance abuse and dependence for dual diagnosis patients: A model of treatment factors associated with one-year outcomes. *Journal of Studies on Alcohol, 60*(6), 856–866.

Monti, P. M., Abrams, D. B., Kadden, R. M., & Cooney, N. L. (1989). *Treating alcohol dependence: A coping skills training guide.* New York: Guilford.

Mueser, K. T., & Bellack, A. S. (1998). Social skills and social functioning. In K. T. Mueser & N. Tarrier (Eds.), *Handbook of social functioning in schizophrenia* (pp. 79–96) . Needham Heights, MA: Allyn & Bacon.

Mueser, K. T., Bellack, A. S., & Blanchard, J. J. (1992). Comorbidity of schizophrenia and substance abuse: Implications for treatment. *Journal of Consulting and Clinical Psychology, 60*(6), 845–856.

Mueser, K. T., Bennett, M., & Kushner, M. G. (1995). Epidemiology of substance use disorders among persons with chronic mental illnesses. In A. F. Lehman & L. B. Dixon (Eds.), *Double jeopardy: Chronic mental illness and substance use disorders* (Vol. 3, pp. 9–25). Longhorne, PA: Harwood Academic.

Mueser, K. T., Drake, R. E., & Wallach, M. A. (1998). Dual diagnosis: A review of etiological theories. *Addictive Behaviors, 23*, 717–734.

Mueser, K. T., Noordsy, D. L., Drake, R. E., & Fox, L. (2003). *Integrated treatment for dual disorders: A guide to effective practice.* New York: Guilford.

Mueser, K. T., Yarnold, P. R., & Bellack, A. S.(1992). Diagnostic and demographic correlates of substance abuse in schizophrenia and major affective disorder. *Acta Psychiatrica Scandinavica, 85*, 48–55.

Mueser, K. T., Yarnold, P. R., Levinson, D. F., Singh, H., Bellack, A. S., Kee, K., Morrison, R. L., & Yadalam, K. G. (1990). Prevalence of substance abuse in schizophrenia: Demographic and clinical correlates. *Schizophrenia Bulletin, 16*, 31–56.

Newman, F. (1999). *The whole lesbian sex book.* San Francisco: Cleis Press.

Peniston, E. G. (1988). Evaluation of long-term therapeutic efficacy of behavior modification program with chronic male psychiatric inpatients. *Journal of Behavior Therapy and Experimental Psychiatry, 19*, 95–101.

Petry, N. M. (2000). A comprehensive guide to the application of contingency management procedures in clinical settings. *Drug and Alcohol Dependence, 58*, 9–25.

Polcin, D. L. (1992). Issues in the treatment of dual diagnosis clients who have chronic mental illness. *Professional Psychology: Research and Practice. 23*(1), 30–37.

Prochaska, J. O., & Diclemente, C. C. (1982). Transtheoretical therapy: Toward a more integrative model of change. *Psychotherapy: Theory, Research, and Practice, 19*, 276–288.

Prochaska, J. O., Velicer, W. F., Rossi, J. S., Goldstein, M. G., Marcus, B. H., Rakowski, W., et al. (1994). Stages of change and decisional balance for 12 problem behaviors. *Health Psychology, 13*(1), 39–46.

Project MATCH Research Group. (1997). Matching alcoholism treatments to client heterogeneity: Project MATCH post treatment drinking outcomes. *Journal of Studies on Alcohol, 58*(1), 7–29.

Regier, D. A., Farmer, M. E., Rae, D. S., Locke, B. Z., Keith, S. J., Judd, L. L., et al. (1990). Comorbidity of mental disorders with alcohol and other drug abuse. *Journal of the American Medical Association, 264*, 2511–2518.

Ridgely, M. S., Goldman, H. H., & Willenbring, M. (1990). Barriers to the care of persons with dual diagnoses: Organizational and financing issues. *Schizophrenia Bulletin, 16*(1), 123–132.

Ridgely, M. S., Lambert, D., Goodman, A., Chichester, C. S., & Ralph, R. (1998). Interagency collaboration in services for people with co-occurring mental illness and substance use disorder. *Psychiatric Services, 49*, 236–238.

Rogers, E. (1995). Diffusion of preventive innovations. *Addictive Behaviors, 27*, 989–993.

Roll, J. M., Chermack, S. T., & Chudzynski, J. E. (2004). Investigating the use of contingency management in the treatment of cocaine abuse among individuals with schizophrenia: A feasibility study. *Psychiatry Research, 125*, 61–64.

Rosenberg, S. D., Drake, R. E., Wolford, G. L., Mueser, K. T., Oxman, T. E., Vidaver, R. M., et al. (1998). Dartmouth Assessment of Lifestyle Instrument (DALI): A substance use disorder screen for people with severe mental illness. *American Journal of Psychiatry, 155*(2), 232–238.

Saunders, J. B., Aasland, O. G., Babor, T. F., De La Fuente, J. R., & Grant, M. (1993). Development of the Alcohol Use Disorders Identification Test (AUDIT): WHO collaborative project on early detection of persons with harmful alcohol consumption: II. *Addiction, 88*, 791–804.

Saunders, B., Wilkinson, C., & Phillips, M. (1995). The impact of a brief motivational intervention with opiate users attending a methadone programme. *Addiction, 90*, 415–424.

Schuckit, M. A. (1983). Alcoholism and other psychiatric disorders. *Hospital and Community Psychiatry, 34*(11), 1022–1027.

Searles, J. S., Alterman, A. I., & Purtill, J. J. (1990). The detection of alcoholism in hospitalized schizophrenics: A comparison of the MAST and the MAC. *Alcoholism: Clinical and Experimental Research, 14*(4), 557–560.

Selzer, M. (1971). The Michigan Alcoholism Screening Test: The quest for a new diagnostic instrument. *American Journal of Psychiatry, 127*, 1653–1658.

Shaner, A., Robert, L. J., Eckman, T. A., Tucker, D. E., Tsuang, J. W., Wilkins, J. N., & Mintz, J. (1997). Monetary reinforcement of abstinence from cocaine among mentally ill patients with cocaine dependence. *Psychiatric Services, 48*, 807–810.

Sigmon, S. C., Steingard, S., Badger, G. J., Anthony, S. L., & Higgins, S. T. (2000). Contingency reinforcement of marijuana abstinence among individuals with serious mental illness: A feasibility study. *Experimental and Clinical Psychopharmacology, 8*, 509–517.

Skinner, H. (1982). The Drug Abuse Screening Test. *Addictive Behaviors, 7*, 363–371.

Sobell, L. C., & Sobell, M. B. (1992). Timeline follow-back: A technique for assessing self-reported alcohol consumption. In R. Z. Litten & J. P. Allen (Eds.), *Measuring alcohol consumption: Psychosocial and biochemical methods* (pp. 41–72). Totowa, NJ: Humana Press.

Stephens, R. S., Roffman, R. A., & Curtin, L. (2000). Comparison of extended versus brief treatments for marijuana use. *Journal of Consulting and Clinical Psychology, 68*, 898–908.

Stotts, A. M., Schmitz, J. M., Rhoades, H. M., & Grabowski, J. (2001). Motivational interviewing with cocaine-dependent patients: A pilot study. *Journal of Consulting and Clinical Psychology, 69*, 858–862.

Swanson, A. J., Pantalon, M. V., & Cohen, K. R. (1999). Motivational interviewing and treatment adherence among psychiatric and dually diagnosed patients. *Journal of Nervous and Mental Disease, 187*, 630–635.

Timko, C., & Moos, R. H. (2002). Symptom severity, amount of treatment, and 1 year outcomes among dual diagnosis patients. *Administrative and Policy in Mental Health, 30*, 35–54.

Toland A. M., Moss, H. B. (1989). Identification of the alcoholic schizophrenic: Use of clinical laboratory tests and the MAST. *Journal of Studies on Alcohol, 50*(1), 49–53.

Torrey, W., Drake, R., Dixon, L., Burns, B., Flynn, L., & Rush, A. J. (2001). Implementing evidenced-based practices for persons with server mental illnesses. *Psychiatric Services, 5*, 45–50.

Tracy, J. I., Josiassen, R. C., & Bellack, A. S. (1995). The neuropsychology of dual diagnosis: Understanding the combined effects of schizophrenia and substance use disorders. *Clinical Psychology Review, 15*, 67–97.

U.S. Department of Health and Human Services. (1999). *Mental Health: A report of the Surgeon General*. Rockville, MD: U.S. Department of Health and Human Services. National Institute of Health, National Institute of Mental Health.

Velicer, W. F., DiClemente, C. C., Prochaska, J. O., & Brandenberg, N. (1985). Decisional balance measure for assessing and predicting smoking status. *Journal of Personality and Social Psychology, 48*, 1279–1289.

Wilkins, J. N., Shaner, A. L., Patterson, C. M., Setoda, D., & Gorelick, D. (1991). Discrepancies between patient report, clinical assessment, and urine analysis in psychiatric patients during inpatient admission. *Psychopharmacology Bulletin, 27*(2), 149–154.

Wiltsey Stirman, S, Crits-Christoph, P., & DeRubeis, R. J. (2004). Achieving successful dissemination of empirically supported psychotherapies: A synthesis of dissemination theory. *Clinical Psychology: Science and Practice, 11*(4), 343–359.

Zanis, D. A., McLellan, A. T., & Corse, S. (1997). Is the Addiction Severity Index a reliable and valid instrument among clients with severe and persistent mental illness and substance abuse disorders? *Community Mental Health Journal, 33*(3), 213–227.

INDEX

DATE DUE